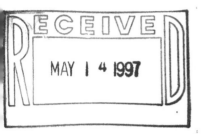

1997
YEAR BOOK OF
NUCLEAR MEDICINE®

Statement of Purpose

The YEAR BOOK Service

The YEAR BOOK series was devised in 1901 by practicing health professionals who observed that the literature of medicine and related disciplines had become so voluminous that no one individual could read and place in perspective every potential advance in a major specialty. In the final decade of the 20th century, this recognition is more acutely true than it was in 1901.

More than merely a series of books, YEAR BOOK volumes are the tangible results of a unique service designed to accomplish the following:

- to *survey* a wide range of journals of proven value
- to *select* from those journals papers representing significant advances and statements of important clinical principles
- to provide *abstracts* of those articles that are readable, convenient summaries of their key points
- to provide *commentary* about those articles to place them in perspective

These publications grow out of a unique process that calls on the talents of outstanding authorities in clinical and fundamental disciplines, trained literature specialists, and professional writers, all supported by the resources of Mosby, the world's preeminent publisher for the health professions.

The Literature Base

Mosby and its Editors survey more than 1,000 journals published worldwide, covering the full range of the health professions. On an annual basis, the publisher examines usage patterns and polls its expert authorities to add new journals to the literature base and to delete journals that are no longer useful as potential YEAR BOOK sources.

The Literature Survey

The publisher's team of literature specialists, all of whom are trained and experienced health professionals, examines every original, peer-reviewed article in each journal issue. More than 250,000 articles per year are scanned systematically, including title, text, illustrations, tables, and references. Each scan is compared, article by article, to the search strategies that the publisher has developed in consultation with the 270 outside experts who form the pool of YEAR BOOK editors. A given article may be reviewed by any number of editors, from one to a dozen or more, regardless of the discipline for which the paper was originally published. In turn, each editor who receives the article reviews it to determine whether or not the article should be included in the YEAR BOOK. This decision is based on the article's inherent quality, its probable usefulness to readers of that YEAR BOOK, and the editor's goal to represent a balanced picture of a given field in each volume of the YEAR BOOK. In addition, the editor indicates when to include figures and tables from the article to help the YEAR BOOK reader better understand the information.

Of the quarter million articles scanned each year, only 5% are selected for detailed analysis within the YEAR BOOK series, thereby assuring readers of the high value of every selection.

The Abstract

The publisher's abstracting staff is headed by a seasoned medical professional and includes individuals with training in the life sciences, medicine, and other areas, plus extensive experience in writing for the health professions and related industries. Each selected article is assigned to a specific writer on this abstracting staff. The abstracter, guided in many cases by notations supplied by the expert editor, writes a structured, condensed summary designed so that the reader can rapidly acquire the essential information contained in the article.

The Commentary

The YEAR BOOK editorial boards, sometimes assisted by guest commentators, write comments that place each article in perspective for the reader. This provides the reader with the equivalent of a personal consultation with a leading international authority—an opportunity to better understand the value of the article and to benefit from the authority's thought processes in assessing the article.

Additional Editorial Features

The editorial boards of each YEAR BOOK organize the abstracts and comments to provide a logical and satisfying sequence of information. To enhance the organization, editors also provide introductions to sections or individual chapters, comments linking a number of abstracts, citations to additional literature, and other features.

The published YEAR BOOK contains enhanced bibliographic citations for each selected article, including extended listings of multiple authors and identification of author affiliations. Each YEAR BOOK contains a Table of Contents specific to that year's volume. From year to year, the Table of Contents for a given YEAR BOOK will vary depending on developments within the field.

Every YEAR BOOK contains a list of the journals from which papers have been selected. This list represents a subset of the more than 1,000 journals surveyed by the publisher and occasionally reflects a particularly pertinent article from a journal that is not surveyed on a routine basis.

Finally, each volume contains a comprehensive subject index and an index to authors of each selected paper.

The 1997 Year Book Series

Year Book of Allergy, Asthma, and Clinical Immunology: Drs. Rosenwasser, Borish, Gelfand, Leung, Nelson, and Szefler

Year Book of Anesthesiology and Pain Management®: Drs. Tinker, Abram, Chestnut, Roizen, Rothenberg, and Wood

Year Book of Cardiology®: Drs. Schlant, Collins, Gersh, Graham, Kaplan, and Waldo

Year Book of Chiropractic®: Dr. Lawrence

Year Book of Critical Care Medicine®: Drs. Parrillo, Balk, Calvin, Franklin, and Shapiro

Year Book of Dentistry®: Drs. Meskin, Berry, Kennedy, Leinfelder, Roser, Summitt, and Zakariasen

Year Book of Dermatologic Surgery®: Drs. Greenway, Papadopoulos, and Whitaker

Year Book of Dermatology®: Drs. Sober and Fitzpatrick

Year Book of Diagnostic Radiology®: Drs. Federle, Clark, Gross, Dalinka, Maynard, Rebner, Smirniotopolous, and Young

Year Book of Digestive Diseases®: Drs. Greenberger and Moody

Year Book of Drug Therapy®: Drs. Lasagna and Weintraub

Year Book of Emergency Medicine®: Drs. Wagner, Dronen, Davidson, King, Niemann, and Roberts

Year Book of Endocrinology®: Drs. Bagdade, Braverman, Haas, Horton, Kannan, Landsberg, Molitch, Morley, Nathan, Odell, Poehlman, Rogol, and Ryan

Year Book of Family Practice®: Drs. Berg, Bowman, Davidson, Dexter, and Scherger

Year Book of Geriatrics and Gerontology®: Drs. Beck, Burton, Ostwald, Rabins, Reuben, Roth, Shapiro, and Whitehouse

Year Book of Hand Surgery®: Drs. Amadio and Hentz

Year Book of Hematology®: Drs. Spivak, Bell, Ness, Quesenberry, Wiernik, and Blume

Year Book of Infectious Diseases®: Drs. Keusch, Barza, Bennish, Poutsiaka, Skolnik, and Snydman

Year Book of Medicine®: Drs. Klahr, Cline, Petty, Frishman, Greenberger, Malawista, Mandell, and O'Rourke

Year Book of Neonatal and Perinatal Medicine®: Drs. Fanaroff and Klaus

Year Book of Nephrology, Hypertension, and Mineral Metabolism: Drs. Schwab, Bennett, Emmett, Hostetter, Kumar, and Toto

Year Book of Neurology and Neurosurgery®: Drs. Bradley and Wilkins

Year Book of Nuclear Medicine®: Drs. Gottschalk, Blaufox, Neumann, Strauss, and Zubal

Year Book of Obstetrics, Gynecology, and Women's Health: Drs. Mishell, Herbst, and Kirschbaum

Year Book of Occupational and Environmental Medicine®: Drs. Emmett, Frank, Gochfeld, and Hessl

Year Book of Oncology®: Drs. Ozols, Cohen, Glatstein, Loehrer, Tallman, and Wiersma

Year Book of Ophthalmology®: Drs. Wilson, Augsburger, Cohen, Eagle, Flanagan, Grossman, Laibson, Maguire, Nelson, Penne, Rapuano, Sergott, Spaeth, Tipperman, and Ms. Salmon

Year Book of Orthopedics®: Drs. Sledge, Poss, Cofield, Dobyns, Griffin, Springfield, Swiontkowski, Wiesel, and Wilson

Year Book of Otolaryngology–Head and Neck Surgery®: Drs. Paparella and Holt

Year Book of Pain®: Drs. Gebhart, Haddox, Jacox, Janjan, Marcus, Rudy, and Shapiro

Year Book of Pathology and Laboratory Medicine: Drs. Mills, Bruns, Gaffey, and Stoler

Year Book of Pediatrics®: Dr. Stockman

Year Book of Plastic, Reconstructive, and Aesthetic Surgery®: Drs. Miller, Cohen, McKinney, Robson, Ruberg, Smith, and Whitaker

Year Book of Podiatric Medicine and Surgery®: Dr. Kominsky

Year Book of Psychiatry and Applied Mental Health®: Drs. Talbott, Ballenger, Breier, Frances, Meltzer, Schowalter, and Tasman

Year Book of Pulmonary Disease®: Dr. Petty

Year Book of Rheumatology®: Drs. Sergent, LeRoy, Meenan, Panush, and Reichlin

Year Book of Sports Medicine®: Drs. Shephard, Drinkwater, Eichner, Torg, Anderson, and Mr. George

Year Book of Surgery®: Drs. Copeland, Bland, Deitch, Eberlein, Howard, Luce, Seeger, Souba, and Sugarbaker

Year Book of Thoracic and Cardiovascular Surgery®: Drs. Ginsberg, Wechsler, and Williams

Year Book of Urology®: Drs. Andriole and Coplin

Year Book of Vascular Surgery®: Dr. Porter

1997

The Year Book of NUCLEAR MEDICINE®

Editor-in-Chief
Alexander Gottschalk, M.D.

Associate Editors
M. Donald Blaufox, M.D., Ph.D.
Ronald Neumann, M.D.
H. William Strauss, M.D.
I. George Zubal, Ph.D.

Editor Emeritus
Paul B. Hoffer, M.D.

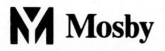 **Mosby**

St. Louis Baltimore Boston Carlsbad Chicago Naples New York Philadelphia Portland
London Madrid Mexico City Singapore Sydney Tokyo Toronto Wiesbaden

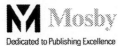

Mosby
Dedicated to Publishing Excellence

A Times Mirror
Company

Vice President and Publisher, Continuity Publishing: Kenneth H. Killion
Director, Editorial Development: Gretchen C. Murphy
Developmental Editor: Kris Horeis
Acquisitions Editor: Li Wen Huang
Illustrations and Permissions Coordinator: Lois M. Ruebensam
Director, Continuity–EDP: Maria Nevinger
Project Supervisor, Editing: Rebecca Nordbrock
Senior Project Manager, Production: Max F. Perez
Freelance Staff Supervisor: Barbara M. Kelly
Director, Editorial Services: Edith M. Podrazik, B.S.N, R.N.
Information Specialist: Kathleen Moss, R.N.
Information Specialist: Terri Santo, R.N.
Circulation Manager: Lynn D. Stevenson

1997 EDITION
Copyright © March 1997 by Mosby–Year Book, Inc.

Printed in the United States of America
Composition by Reed Technology and Information Services, Inc.
Printing/binding by Maple-Vail

Mosby–Year Book, Inc.
11830 Westline Industrial Drive
St. Louis, MO 63146

Editorial Office:
Mosby–Year Book, Inc.
161 North Clark Street
Chicago, IL 60601

International Standard Serial Number: 0084–3903
International Standard Book Number: 0–8151–3820–2

Table of Contents

Journals Represented

Mosby and its Editors survey more than 1,000 journals for its abstract and commentary publications. From these journals, the Editors select the articles to be abstracted. Journals represented in this YEAR BOOK are listed below.

Acta Neurologica Scandinavica
Acta Radiologica
American Heart Journal
American Journal of Cardiology
American Journal of Kidney Diseases
American Journal of Neuroradiology
American Journal of Orthopedics
American Journal of Roentgenology
American Journal of Sports Medicine
Annals of Neurology
Archives of Disease in Childhood
Brain
British Journal of Radiology
Cancer
Cephalalgia
Chest
Circulation
Clinical Cancer Research
Clinical Endocrinology (Oxford)
Clinical Infectious Diseases
Clinical Nuclear Medicine
Clinical Radiology
Digestive Diseases and Sciences
European Heart Journal
European Journal of Cancer
European Journal of Nuclear Medicine
Gut
Health Physics
IEEE Transactions on Medical Imaging
International Journal of Radiation, Oncology, Biology, and Physics
Investigative Radiology
Journal of Bone and Joint Surgery (American Volume)
Journal of Clinical Epidemiology
Journal of Clinical Oncology
Journal of Computer Assisted Tomography
Journal of Magnetic Resonance Imaging (JMRI)
Journal of Neurology, Neurosurgery and Psychiatry
Journal of Neuropsychiatry and Clinical Neurosciences
Journal of Nuclear Cardiology
Journal of Nuclear Medicine
Journal of Pediatric Surgery
Journal of Pharmacology and Experimental Therapeutics
Journal of Rheumatology
Journal of Urology
Journal of the American College of Cardiology
Magnetic Resonance in Medicine
Medical Physics

Neurology
Neuroradiology
Pediatric Radiology
Pediatrics
Quarterly Journal of Medicine
Radiology
Skeletal Radiology
Stroke
World Journal of Surgery

STANDARD ABBREVIATIONS

The following terms are abbreviated in this edition: acquired immunodeficiency syndrome (AIDS), cardiopulmonary resuscitation (CPR), central nervous system (CNS), cerebrospinal fluid (CSF), computed tomography (CT), deoxyribonucleic acid (DNA), electrocardiography (ECG), [fluorine-18]-fluorodeoxyglucose (FDG), gadolinium-diethylenetriamine-pentaacetic acid (Gd-DTPA), health maintenance organization (HMO), human immunodeficiency virus (HIV), intensive care unit (ICU), intramuscular (IM), intravenous (IV), magnetic resonance (MR) imaging (MRI), nuclear magnetic resonance (NMR), positron emission tomography (PET), ribonucleic acid (RNA), and single-photon emission CT (SPECT).

NOTE

The YEAR BOOK OF NUCLEAR MEDICINE® is a literature survey service providing abstracts of articles published in the professional literature. Every effort is made to assure the accuracy of the information presented in these pages. Neither the editors nor the publisher of the YEAR BOOK OF NUCLEAR MEDICINE® can be responsible for errors in the original materials. The editors' comments are their own opinions. Mention of specific products within this publication does not constitute endorsement.

To facilitate the use of the YEAR BOOK OF NUCLEAR MEDICINE® as a reference tool, all illustrations and tables included in this publication are now identified as they appear in the original article. This change is meant to help the reader recognize that any illustration or table appearing in the YEAR BOOK OF NUCLEAR MEDICINE® may be only one of many in the original article. For this reason, figure and table numbers will often appear to be out of sequence within the YEAR BOOK OF NUCLEAR MEDICINE®.

Publisher's Preface

Publication of the 1997 YEAR BOOK OF NUCLEAR MEDICINE marks the end of a brief yet exceptional period of editorship by John G. McAfee, M.D., and Frans J. Th. Wackers, M.D. Both of these talented editors provided the readers of the YEAR BOOK with discerning and informative literature and editorial commentary of the highest caliber. We extend our sincere thanks to Drs. McAfee and Wackers for their ever-present commitment to the YEAR BOOK OF NUCLEAR MEDICINE.

With this 1997 edition, we wish to welcome Ronald Neumann, M.D., from the nuclear medicine division of the National Institutes of Health Clinical Center, and H. William Strauss, M.D., from the division of nuclear medicine at the Stanford University School of Medicine. We look forward to working with these distinguished experts.

Introduction

The editors of the YEAR BOOK OF NUCLEAR MEDICINE have approached their work in a new way this year. In the past, we have selected articles for publication year round but have usually waited for them to be abstracted before writing our editorial comments. To improve the quality of our publication, this year we not only selected the articles at regular intervals, we also wrote our editorial comments at the time we selected the articles. With this system, work is being completed throughout the year rather than all at once at the end, improving the publication process. The time saved in production is being applied to our literature survey schedule, allowing us to provide our readers with more current literature reviews than this book has contained in the past.

We have worked with this new system of article selection for the past year. From the editor's point of view, the new system requires more rev up and rev down time because of the multiple increments required to select and comment on these papers. However, as it provides more current material, and therefore a higher-quality publication for the reader, the additional effort will be worth it. All in all, it looks like an interesting process, and we hope it will add to the value of the YEAR BOOK OF NUCLEAR MEDICINE for our readers.

Unfortunately, this change has a sad spinoff, as well. The new system requirements (of effort and availability throughout the entire year) simply do not fit into the schedules of Drs. John G. McAfee and Frans J. Th. Wackers. Regretfully, they have informed me that they can no longer continue as editors for the YEAR BOOK OF NUCLEAR MEDICINE. I am sorry to lose them both, as they did a terrific job for all of us. At the same time, I am delighted to welcome Drs. Ronald Neumann and H. William Strauss as new members of the Editorial Board. They bring proven talent and interests to the YEAR BOOK, and I look forward to reading their insights, and I am sure you do as well.

Alexander Gottschalk, M.D.

1 Pulmonary

Introduction

It will come as no surprise to learn that the bulk of this year's selections are articles about pulmonary embolism. These begin with the application of the revised Prospective Investigation of Pulmonary Embolism Diagnosis (PIOPED) criteria. A controversial paper from Pennsylvania about embolism diagnosis in different patient populations follows shortly (Abstract 1–4). This chapter continues with our new effort to evaluate low-probability criteria and finishes with a pulmonary embolism mimic and a discussion of reversed mismatch. Oncologic imaging was popular this year, and lung cancer staging and detection of recurrence have become active areas for PET. This chapter goes on to consider some interesting technical applications or case presentations and finishes with a new approach to develop a "hot spot" clot imaging technique to detect pulmonary embolism.

Alexander Gottschalk, M.D.

Modified PIOPED Criteria Used in Clinical Practice
Freitas JE, Sarosi MG, Nagle CC, et al (St Joseph Mercy Hosp, Ann Arbor, Mich; Univ of Washington, Seattle; William Beaumont Hosp, Royal Oak, Mich)
J Nucl Med 36:1573–1578, 1995
        1–1

Introduction.—In the evaluation of patients with suspected pulmonary embolism, radionuclide ventilation-perfusion (V/Q) scintigraphy has played a major role by depicting the sequelae of pulmonary embolism as V/Q mismatch. To improve the sensitivity and specificity of V/Q scintigraphy in the detection of pulmonary embolism, various interpretive schemes or algorithms have been advanced. Based on the results of a retrospective analysis, the original criteria in the Prospective Investigation of Pulmonary Embolism Diagnosis (PIOPED) for V/Q scan interpretation should be modified by categorizing a single moderate perfusion defect as intermediate rather than low probability. Extensive matched V/Q with a clear chest radiograph should be modified as low probability rather than as indeterminate probability. The validity of the "stripe sign" was confirmed as an indication that a segmental perfusion defect showing the sign probably was not caused by pulmonary embolism. A prospective study was conducted to determine whether the new knowledge gleaned from the retrospective analysis of the PIOPED study would improve the clinical usefulness of V/Q scintigraphy.

Methods.—Six-view V/Q imaging using 74 MBq (2 mCi) of technetium-99m macroaggregated albumin was performed on 1,000 patients (593 women and 407 men). If the perfusion was abnormal, a ventilation study was performed using ^{99m}Tc-pentetate (DTPA) aerosol, contrast pulmonary selective angiography, and Doppler sonography with leg compression as needed. The V/Q studies had 4 categories: normal, low, intermediate, or high (Table 1). Ventilation was not performed in 402 patients because perfusion was normal. Angiography was performed in 133 patients considered to be group A. The remaining 867 patients comprised group B. To detect subsequent thromboembolic events, patients were followed for a mean of 13.9 months.

Results.—The V/Q assigned pulmonary embolism probabilities were distributed as follows: high probability 5.7%, intermediate probability 17.4%, low probability 41.4%, and normal 35.5%. In group A patients,

---

TABLE 1.—Assignment of Ventilation-Perfusion Probability of Pulmonary Embolism

Begin with Perfusion Scan Probability = Normal.
1. Are there any Q defects?
     No → PROB = NORMAL. **STOP.**
     Yes → PROB = LOW. *Continue to question 2.*
2. Are there any Q defects > 25% of a segment?
     No → PROB = LOW. **STOP.**
     Yes → *Continue to question 3?*
3. Are there any chest radiograph abnormalities overlapping Q defects (>25% of segment)?
     No → PROB = LOW. *Continue to question 5.*
     Yes → *Continue to question 4.*
4. Are all Q defects >25% of a segment matched by much larger chest radiograph defects?
     No → PROB = INTERMEDIATE. *Continue to question 5.*
     Yes → PROB = LOW. **STOP.**
5. Are there any Q defects > 25% of a segment *not* matched by chest radiograph abnormality?
     No → **STOP.**
     Yes → *Continue to question 6.*
Perform Ventilation Scan
6. Are ALL >25% of a segment Q defects matched by V defects despite normal chest radiograph?
     No → *Continue to question 7.*
     Yes → PROB ≥ LOW. *Continue to question 9?*
7. Are there ≥2 large Q defects "much larger than" corresponding V or chest radiograph defects? Answer **no** if V and chest radiograph are normal in defect regions or only one large defect is present.
     No → PROB = INTERMEDIATE. *Continue to question 8.*
     Yes → PROB = HIGH. **STOP.**
8. Are there >2 segmental equivalent Q defects with normal V and normal chest radiograph?
     No → PROB = INTERMEDIATE. **STOP.**
     Yes → PROB = HIGH. **STOP.**
9. Do matched V and Q defects cover >50% of the combined lung fields?
     No → PROB = LOW. **STOP.**
     Yes → PROB = INTERMEDIATE. **STOP.**

(Reprinted by permission of the Society of Nuclear Medicine, from Freitas JE, Sarosi MG, Nagle CC, et al: Modified PIOPED criteria used in clinical practice. *J Nucl Med* 36:1573–1578, 1995.)

there was a determination of a 27.1% prevalence of pulmonary embolism. In the group B patients, who did not have angiograms, there was a determination of a 7.5% prevalence of pulmonary embolism. Pulmonary embolism was diagnosed in 101 patients, 36 by angiography (5 of 6 in the high probability category (Fig 1) and 65 by a combination of sonography,

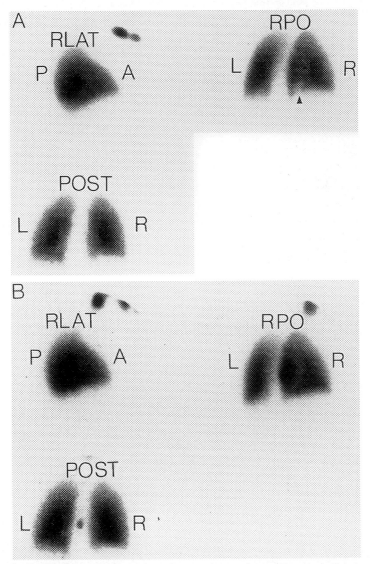

FIGURE 1.—A, selected perfusion images demonstrate a moderate right posterior basal perfusion defect (*arrows*). **B,** selected ventilation images demonstrate mismatched ventilation to this segment. (Reprinted by permission of the Society of Nuclear Medicine, from Freitas JE, Sarosi MG, Nagle CC, et al: Modified PIOPED criteria used in clinical practice. *J Nucl Med* 36:1573–1578, 1995.)

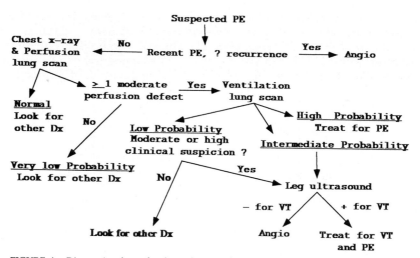

FIGURE 4.—Diagnostic scheme for the evaluation of patients with suspected pulmonary embolism. (Reprinted by permission of the Society of Nuclear Medicine, from Freitas JE, Sarosi MG, Nagle CC, et al: Modified PIOPED criteria used in clinical practice. *J Nucl Med* 36:1573–1578, 1995.)

lung scan, and clinical assessment. The positive predictive value of a high-probability V/Q study for pulmonary embolism was 98.2%. The positive predictive value of an intermediate-probability V/Q study for pulmonary embolism was 24.1%, whereas the low probability for pulmonary embolism was 0.5%

Conclusion.—There is better discrimination between the intermediate- and low-probability scan categories using a perfusion test followed by a ventilation V/Q study using the modified PIOPED interpretation criteria than the original criteria of the PIOPED study. The authors provide the diagnostic algorithm shown in Figure 4.

▶ As a modifier of the PIOPED criteria and a co-creator of the "stripe sign," you can easily imagine that I am delighted to see these results. If you look at these data, you will note that the authors did extremely well diagnosing their low-probability group compared to the original PIOPED study. And I would love to tell you it's because they did such a good job using the revised rather than the original low-probability PIOPED criteria. However, this cannot be the only reason, because these authors also did much better with their high-probability readings than PIOPED did, and they used the same high-probability criteria as the original PIOPED readers.

It seems to me that several variables may be working here. In the first place, we have had almost a decade of experience since the PIOPED readings were made, which I hope counts for something. Second, these authors used a different technique than PIOPED, the postperfusion aerosol. However, I know of no comparison data to prove that this is better than the original PIOPED technique using preperfusion xenon-133, and I can think of reasons to argue this both ways. Third, the patient population studied here is clearly different than the PIOPED population. To my knowledge, all of the tertiary care centers in the PIOPED study had an incidence of intermediate-probability scans in the 30% to 40% range, and normal scans were usually well under 10%; PIOPED also had about twice as many high-probability readings. In short, I think the PIOPED patients were sicker, and PIOPED had a larger group of difficult intermediate studies.

Of all the variables listed above, I think the last is most important. However, I also think that the population seen at the community hospital from which these authors report data is more likely to fit the patient population of many of the readers of the YEAR BOOK OF NUCLEAR MEDICINE. Therefore, I believe you should consider these data to be extremely encouraging. I certainly do.

A. Gottschalk, M.D.

Ventilation/Perfusion Lung Scan Probability Category Distributions in University and Community Hospitals
Lowe VJ, Bullard AG, Coleman RE (St Louis Univ; Central Carolina Heart, Lung, and Allergy Clinic, Sanford, NC; Duke Univ, Durham, NC)
Clin Nucl Med 20:1079–1083, 1995   1–2

Introduction.—The Prospective Investigation of Pulmonary Embolism Diagnosis (PIOPED) is a prospective, randomized trial of diagnostic ventilation-perfusion (V/Q) scintigraphy in patients with suspected PE. The interpretive criteria for V/Q scintigraphy used in the PIOPED study, from which the probability of pulmonary embolism is determined, have come into widespread use. However, these criteria were based on patients seen at tertiary care centers, who may differ from those seen at other types of centers. Possible differences in patient population were examined by comparing the distribution of V/Q scan results at a university hospital and a community hospital.

Methods.—The retrospective study included 54 V/Q scans performed at a university medical center and 49 scans performed at a community hospital during a 1-year period. Each scan was interpreted using the PIOPED criteria, and the distribution of probability categories was compared for the 2 groups.

Results.—Seventeen percent of scans performed at the university hospital were normal or very low probability, compared with 27% for scans performed at the community hospital. Thirty-one and 59 percent of scans, respectively, were considered low probability. Probability was intermediate in 39% of scans performed at the university hospital vs. 10% for those performed at the community hospital, and high for 13% and 4% of scans, respectively.

Conclusions.—The patient populations seen at university and community hospitals may differ in their prevalence of PE. The posttest probability of this diagnosis depends on its prevalence and on the sensitivity and specificity of V/Q scanning. Thus, the posttest probability data from the PIOPED study should only be applied by institutions with similar patient populations. The clinical management approach sugested by the PIOPED study does not necessarily apply to patients undergoing V/Q scanning at a community hospital.

▶ I rest my case.

A. Gottschalk, M.D.

Comprehensive Analysis of the Results of the PIOPED Study
Worsley DF, Alavi A (Vancouver Hosp and Health Sciences Ctr, Canada; Univ of Pennsylvania, Philadelphia)
J Nucl Med 36:2380–2387, 1995   1–3

Background.—There are effective treatments for pulmonary embolism (PE), but their use requires accurate diagnosis. The multicenter Prospective Investigation of Pulmonary Embolism Diagnosis (PIOPED) study, sponsored by the National Heart, Lung, and Blood Institute, evaluated several conventional diagnostic methods for PE, with an emphasis on ventilation-perfusion (V/Q) lung scanning. The findings of the PIOPED study were reviewed, including new data from the study population and comprehensive criteria for interpreting V/Q scans.

Methods.—The analysis included PIOPED data from the years 1990–1994. The study included a total of 1,487 adult patients with suspected acute PE who had a completed V/Q lung scan. The patients were randomized to undergo angiography according to the study protocol, i.e., if their V/Q lung scan was abnormal, or at the discretion of the attending physician. Pulmonary angiography was performed in 81% and 60% of these groups, respectively.

Results.—The results suggested that clinically significant PE could be ruled out in a patient whose V/Q lung scan was normal. The information provided by the V/Q scan was most useful when it suggested a very low, low, or high probability of PE in a patient whose clinical findings were consistent with these results. Further studies to determine the presence or absence of acute venous thromboembolism were likely to be required in patients whose V/Q scan suggested an intermediate probability of PE or those with conflicting PE and clinical findings. Although mismatched vascular defects helped to identify patients with PE, their absence did not exclude it. Of 399 study patients with PE, only 10 died of PE and only 1 of the patients died untreated.

Conclusions.—Ventilation-perfusion lung scanning is a useful test in the evaluation of patients with suspected PE. The PIOPED results have been used to modify the criteria for interpretation of V/Q lung scans, which should reinforce its central role in patients with suspected PE (Fig 3). Still, many patients will need peripheral venous imaging or pulmonary angiography to confirm or exclude the diagnosis.

High Probability
- ≥ 2 large (> 75% of a segment) segmental perfusion defects without corresponding ventilation or CXR abnormalities.
- 1 large segmental perfusion defect and ≥ 2 moderate (25-75% of a segment) segmental perfusion defects without corresponding ventilation or CXR abnormalities.
- ≥ 4 moderate segmental perfusion defects without corresponding ventilation or CXR abnormalities.

Intermediate Probability
- 1 moderate to < 2 large segmental perfusion defects without corresponding ventilation or CXR abnormalities.
- Corresponding V/Q defects and CXR parenchymal opacity in lower lung zone.
- Single moderate matched V/Q defects with normal CXR findings.
- Corresponding V/Q defects and small pleural effusion.
- Difficult to categorize as normal, low or high probability.

Low Probability
- Multiple matched V/Q defects, regardless of size, with normal CXR findings.
- Corresponding V/Q defects and CXR parenchymal opacity in upper or middle lung zone.
- Corresponding V/Q defects and large pleural effusion.
- Any perfusion defects with substantially larger CXR abnormality.
- Defects surrounded by normally perfused lung (stripe sign).
- >3 small (< 25% of a segment) segmental perfusion defects with a normal CXR.
- Nonsegmental perfusion defects (cardiomegaly, aortic impression, enlarged hila).

Very Low
- ≤3 small (< 25% of a segment) segmental perfusion defects with a normal CXR.

Normal
- No perfusion defects and perfusion outlines the shape of the lung seen on CXR.

V/Q = Ventilation-perfusion
CXR = Chest radiograph

FIGURE 3.—Amended Prospective Investigation of Pulmonary Embolism Diagnosis ventilation-perfusion lung scan interpretation data. (Reprinted by permission of the Society of Nuclear Medicine, from Worsley DF, Alavi A: Comprehensive analysis of the results of the PIOPED study. *J Nucl Med* 36:2380–2387, 1995.)

▶ As far as it goes, this is a good review article. These authors do not agree with the concept of stratifying patients into categories including those with and without cardiopulmonary disease. This in turn means that they continue to lump all the high-probability criteria together. Dr. Paul Stein and I have shown that you can use different high-probability criteria for these 2 groups of patients and that, for those of you who have trouble sizing segmental perfusion defects, the use of "vascular lesions" will make the job much easier.[1, 2] If you do these things, you can take a lot of patients with mismatched defects between a single subsegmental (moderate) mismatched defect and 2 segmental (large segmental) mismatched defects and move them from the intermediate- to the high-probability category. Nevertheless, the chart above is a useful diagnostic compilation of much of the current literature describing data from the PIOPED study.

A. Gottschalk, M.D.

References

1. Stein PD, Gottschalk A, Henry JW, et al: Stratification of patients according to prior cardiopulmonary disease and probability assessment based on the number of mismatched segmental equivalent perfusion defects: Approaches to strengthen the diagnostic value of ventilation/perfusion lung scans in acute pulmonary embolism. *Chest* 104:1461–1467, 1993.
2. Stein PD, Henry JW, Gottschalk A: Mismatched vascular defects: An easy alternative to mismatched segmental equivalent defects for the interpretation of ventilation/perfusion lung scans in pulmonary embolism. *Chest* 104:1468–1471, 1993.

Comparison of Diagnostic Performance With Ventilation-Perfusion Lung Imaging in Different Patient Populations

Worsley DF, Alavi A, Palevsky HI, et al (Univ of Pennsylvania, Philadelphia)
Radiology 199:481–483, 1996   1–4

Introduction.—Previous studies have shown the value of ventilation-perfusion (V-P) lung imaging in the diagnostic evaluation of patients with suspected pulmonary embolism (PE). The diagnostic performance of V-P imaging in the identification of acute PE was investigated in different patient populations. In particular, the effects of age, chest radiographic abnormalities, or a history of cardiopulmonary disease or venous thromboembolism were investigated.

Methods.—A total of 1,493 adult patients with acute onset of signs or symptoms suggesting PE were evaluated. Pulmonary embolism was definitively diagnosed with pulmonary angiography and was excluded with pulmonary angiography and 1-year clinical follow-up. Ventilation-perfusion lung images were obtained and were interpreted by 2 independent readers. The diagnostic performance of V-P imaging was evaluated with receiver operating characteristic (ROC) analysis to examine the dependence of V-P imaging diagnostic accuracy on patient age, the presence or absence of cardiopulmonary disease, normal or abnormal findings on chest radiographs, and the presence or absence of a history of venous thromboembolism.

Results.—The majority of patients had abnormalities on the chest radiograph. A history of cardiopulmonary disease was present in 50%, and 19% had a history of venous thromboembolism. There were no significant differences in the diagnostic performance of V-P imaging among patients of varying ages, in patients with or without abnormalities on the chest radiograph, or in patients with or without a history of cardiopulmonary disease or venous thromboembolism.

Conclusions.—The diagnostic performance of V-P lung imaging for the identification of acute PE was reliable in varying patient populations. Specifically, the diagnostic performance was not dependent on patient age, abnormalities on chest radiography, or a history of cardiopulmonary disease or venous thromboembolism. Ventilation-perfusion imaging is therefore recommended as the initial test in the evaluation of suspected acute PE.

▶ I think these authors have thrown the "high-probability" baby out with the "overall" bath water. For example, these authors agree that "chronic thromboembolism is a well-documented cause of a false positive high-probability V-P imaging interpretation." They go on to point out, however, that in their data, "overall" V-P diagnostic performance looking at the entire population of patients with previous thromboembolism is the same as those with no history of thromboembolism. In short, they are masking the usefulness of knowing whether someone has had a prior PE when trying to make a high-probability diagnosis by combining this with the lack of usefulness for the intermediate- or low-probability interpretation. We think they have done the same thing for cardiopulmonary disease. If we take these data literally, there would be no reason to stratify patients. However, these authors agree that "patients with no history of cardiopulmonary disease require fewer mismatched V-P segments for a given positive predictive value." In short, the high-probability utility of stratification—the only utility that we have ever proposed[1, 2] is blunted by looking at the entire population of patients with previous cardiopulmonary disease, i.e., those with very low, low-, intermediate-, and high-probability studies when using the ROC technique. In short, I believe the shape of the ROC curves used in these studies is in large part determined by the low and intermediate probability diagnoses, and changes in the high-probability portion of the curve make too little change in the area under the ROC curve to show up.

These data troubled us enough to relook at the question with an entirely different set of Prospective Investigation of Pulmonary Embolism Diagnosis data, which we believe further verify our concept that stratification is a very useful idea to better define the high-probability diagnostic group. Please read on for this argument.

A. Gottschalk, M.D.

References

1. Stein PD, Gottschalk A, Henry JW, et al: Stratification of patients according to cardiopulmonary disease assessment based on the number of mismatched segmental equivalent perfusion defects: Approaches to strengthen the diagnostic value of ventilation/perfusion lung scans in acute pulmonary embolism. *Chest* 104:1461–1467, 1993.
2. Stein PD, Henry JW, Gottschalk A: Mismatched vascular defects: An easy alternative to mismatched segmental equivalent defects for the interpretation of ventilation/perfusion lung scans in pulmonary embolism. *Chest* 104:1468–1471, 1993.

Patient Stratification by Cardiopulmonary Status in the Diagnosis of Pulmonary Embolism

Gottschalk A, Stein PD, Henry JW (Michigan State Univ, East Lansing; Henry Ford Heart and Vascular Inst, Detroit)
J Nucl Med 37:570–572, 1996   1–5

Objective.—The findings of the Prospective Investigation of Pulmonary Embolism Diagnosis (PIOPED) suggested that less stringent criteria for the ventilation-perfusion (V/Q) scan diagnosis of pulmonary embolism (PE) should be used for patients without a history of cardiopulmonary disease than for those with such a history. This practice makes V/Q scanning more sensitive in diagnosing PE without reducing its specificity or positive predictive value. In response to questions about this concept, a new analysis for interpreting V/Q scans according to the presence or absence of previous cardiopulmonary disease was presented.

TABLE 1.—Consensus Estimates of Probability of Pulmonary Embolism on V/Q Lung
Scans in Patients Stratified According to Prior CPD

Consensus probability	CPD (n = 430)		No CPD (n = 292)	
	PE/total	(%)	PE/total	(%)
0%–10%	9/105	(9)	10/85	(12)
11%–20%	19/108	(18)	18/80	(23)
21%–30%	17/68	(25)	12/36	(33)
31%–40%	19/49	(39)	7/12	(58)
41%–50%	8/24	(33)	4/8	(50)
51%–60%	2/7	(29)	7/9	(78)
61%–70%	6/7	(86)	6/6	(100)
71%–80%	8/10	(80)	8/9	(89)
81%–90%	16/21	(76)	19/21	(90)
91%–100%	29/31	(94)	24/26	(92)
Totals	132/430	(31)	115/292	(39)

Abbreviations: V/Q, ventilation perfusion; *CPD*, cardiopulmonary disease; *consensus probability*, the subjective estimate of PE agreed on by the 2 PIOPED nuclear physicians interpreting the V/Q scan; *PE/TOTAL*, angiographically proven PE divided by the total number of patients examined by pulmonary angiography for each 10% probability estimate.
(Reprinted by permission of the Society of Nuclear Medicine, from Gottschalk A, Stein PD, Henry JW: Patient stratification by cardiopulmonary status in the diagnosis of pulmonary embolism. *J Nucl Med* 37:570–572, 1996.)

Methods.—Using data from the PIOPED database, the subjective consensus probability estimates made by the nuclear medicine specialists who served as readers in the original study were analyzed. No formal criteria were used in making these intuitive estimates. Separate evaluations of the estimates of probability of PE were made for patients with and without a history of cardiopulmonary disease.

Results.—Probability estimates made in patients with previous cardiopulmonary disease were generally correct. In contrast, the likelihood of acute PE was consistently underestimated in patients with no history of cardiopulmonary disease (Table 1). Logistic regression analysis suggested that the odds ratio for PE in patients with no history of cardiopulmonary disease vs. those with such a history was 1.62 (95% confidence interval, 1.10–2.38).

Conclusions.—Nuclear medicine specialists use their experience in correctly estimating the likelihood of acute PE in the V/Q scans of patients with previous cardiopulmonary disease. However, in patients with no previous cardiopulmonary disease, the subjective criteria used in making these estimates seem inadequate. For patients with no history of cardiopulmonary disease, fewer mismatched perfusion deficits are needed to make a high-probability estimate of PE.

▶ We were spurred on to write this paper because the group from Pennsylvania, using receiver operating characteristic using analysis of the entire database, found no basis for patient stratification. Our argument for stratifying patients as those with and those without cardiopulmonary disease has been described in detail previously,[1, 2] and these data further indicate that you can improve your diagnostic abilities in V/Q scan interpretation for acute pulmonary embolism by stratifying the patients. It is simple to do—try it, you will like it.

A. Gottschalk, M.D.

References

1. Stein PD, Gottschalk A, Henry JW, et al: Stratification of patients according to prior cardiopulmonary disease and probability assessment based upon the number of mismatched segmental equivalent perfusion defects: Approaches to strengthen the diagnostic value of ventilation perfusion lung scans in acute pulmonary embolism. *Chest* 104:1461–1467, 1993.
2. Stein PD, Henry JW, Gottschalk A: Mismatched vascular defects: An easy alternative to mismatched segmental equivalent defects for the interpretation of ventilation perfusion lung scans in pulmonary embolism. *Chest* 104:1468–1472, 1993.

Evaluation of Individual Criteria for Low Probability Interpretation of Ventilation-Perfusion Lung Scans

Stein PD, Relyea B, Gottschalk A (Henry Ford Heart and Vascular Inst, Detroit; Michigan State Univ, East Lansing)
J Nucl Med 37:577–581, 1996   1–6

Background.—The Prospective Investigation of Pulmonary Embolism Diagnosis (PIOPED) identified ventilation-perfusion (V/Q) lung scan findings that indicate a low probability for the presence of pulmonary embolus (PE), but the criteria still have a positive predictive value of up to 20%. The PIOPED data were reevaluated to determine very low probability criteria, for which the positive predictive value for PE is less than 10%.

Methods.—For patients in both arms of the PIOPED study who had undergone pulmonary angiography for suspected acute PE, the scan results were reexamined to determine the frequency of PE, compared with the frequency of various V/Q scan abnormalities, either singly or in combination.

Results.—Nonsegmental perfusion abnormalities, such as those associated with mediastinal or hilar enlargement, and perfusion defects smaller than associated radiographic abnormalities, each taken alone, had a positive predictive value for PE of less than less than 10%. In combination, these 2 findings still had a positive predictive value of less than 10%.

Conclusion.—It is possible to identify V/Q scan criteria for which the positive predictive value for PE is less than 10%.

▶ Our effort here was to develop a group of "very low probability" criteria (a positive predictive value of less than 10%) for PE that the pulmonologists would accept as a useful diagnostic group. As you know, pulmonologists like Russell Hull have categorized all low-probability studies as "nondiagnostic." Our hope here is to begin to pull out criteria that can be combined into a very low probability scan category to form a subgroup of low probability that would take patients out of the nondiagnostic category. We have other such criteria, not listed in this paper, that will be published shortly, and we hope to bring them to you next year.

In the meantime, there is hope that Dr. Hull and others will accept this. In the most recent algorithmic approach to pulmonary embolism, Drs. Stein, Hull, and Pineo recognize that the "near-normal" V/Q scan in PIOPED, together with an appropriate clinical probability, represent a group that did not need treatment.[1] Unfortunately, the near-normal group in PIOPED was a constellation of low, very low, and normal readings by the PIOPED readers and was not based on specific criteria. Therefore, we are hoping to extract criteria that could be used to identify this group of patients. In addition, the discussion of the low-probability diagnosis with a very difficult diagnostic case illustration has been presented by investigators from Stanford[2] for those of you interested in this problem.

A. Gottschalk, M.D.

References

1. Stein PD, Hull RD, Pineo GF: Strategy that includes serial non-invasive leg tests for diagnosis of thromboembolic disease in patients with suspected acute pulmonary embolism based on data from PIOPED. *Arch Intern Med* 155:2101–2104, 1995.
2. Kwok CG, Skibo LK, Segall GM: Low probability lung scan in a patient at high risk for pulmonary embolism. *J Nucl Med* 37:165–170, 1996.

Scintigraphic Lung Scans and Clinical Assessment in Critically Ill Patients With Suspected Acute Pulmonary Embolism
Henry JW, Stein PD, Gottschalk A, et al (Henry Ford Heart and Vascular Inst, Detroit; Michigan State Univ, East Lansing; Univ of Tennessee, Memphis)
Chest 109:462–466, 1996   1–7

Background.—It is difficult to make a clinical diagnosis of pulmonary embolism (PE) in a critically ill patient. The value of ventilation-perfusion (V/Q) lung scanning in patients in the ICU is unclear; it may be difficult to obtain a technically adequate scan of a patient who is receiving ventilatory support. Lung scanning and clinical assessment were evaluated for their diagnostic accuracy in critically ill patients with suspected acute PE.

Methods.—The analysis used data from the Prospective Investigation of Pulmonary Embolism Diagnosis (PIOPED). Four groups of critically ill patients were included: 89 patients with hypoxemia on room air who were not receiving ventilatory support, 46 patients who were receiving ventilatory support, 85 ICU patients who were not receiving ventilatory support, and 3 patients who were hypotensive but not hypoxemic and were not receiving ventilatory support. To determine the accuracy of lung scans and clinical assessment in diagnosing acute PE, comparisons were made between these patients and 627 noncritically ill patients who did not meet any of these criteria.

Results.—For all 4 groups of critically ill patients, the sensitivity, specificity, and positive predictive value of a high-probability lung scan were not significantly different from those in the noncritically ill patients. When the physicians judged an 80% to 100% likelihood of PE in a critically ill patient, they were correct 75% to 88% of the time. By comparison, the positive predictive value in noncritically ill patients was 77%. Clinical assessment also had a similar positive predictive value for critically ill and noncritically ill patients. Positive predictive value was generally improved when the results of clinical assessment agreed with those of lung scanning.

Conclusions.—Scintigraphic lung scanning and clinical assessment are no less accurate in diagnosing PE in critically ill patients than in noncritically ill patients. The combination of the 2 tests generally improves the positive predictive value for PE. Perfusion scanning without ventilation scanning may be done in some patients receiving ventilatory support, although this may increase the percentage of indeterminate scans.

▶ If your ICU folks try to tell you that the V/Q scan will not work for them because their patients are "too sick," these data should be helpful. As noted, the PIOPED data indicate that lung scans together with clinical assessment work well in this group of patients.

A. Gottschalk, M.D.

A "Changing Stripe Sign" in Serial Pulmonary Perfusion Imaging
Watanabe N, Oriuchi N, Suzuki H, et al (Gunma Univ, Maebashi, Japan)
Clin Nucl Med 21:111–114, 1996   1–8

Objective.—On pulmonary perfusion scintigraphy, the finding of a well-maintained rim of activity between a perfusion defect and the pleural surface is known as the stripe sign. The stripe sign's cause is unclear, but it may reflect morphological changes and ventilation abnormalities in the lung. It has been suggested to predict the absence of pulmonary embolism, and it does not generally change on serial perfusion imaging studies. A case in which the stripe sign resolved on serial pulmonary perfusion imaging was reported.

> *Case Report.*—Woman, 76, with diabetes mellitus had sudden chest pain with dyspnea after percutaneous transluminal coronary angioplasty for right coronary artery stenosis. Pulmonary perfusion scanning showed a stripe sign in the right lower lobe with subsegmental defects in the left lower lobe (Fig 1). Although pulmonary angiography was recommended, the patient was given anticoagulant therapy because of her worsening clinical condition. Combined pulmonary ventilation-perfusion scanning, performed the next day, showed partial reperfusion in the right lower lobe but no change in the subsegmental perfusion defects in the left lower lobe. When combined pulmonary ventilation-perfusion scintigraphy was

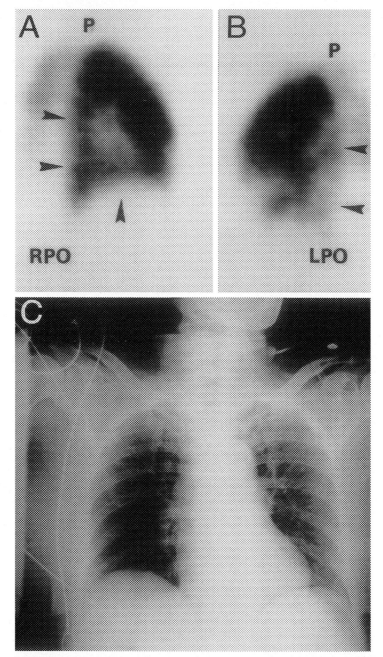

FIGURE 1.—Pulmonary perfusion (*P*) imaging. Right posterior oblique (*RPO*) image (**A**) showed a stripe sign in the right lower lobe (*arrowheads*). Left posterior oblique (*LPO*) projection image (**B**) showed subsegmental defect in the left lower lobe (*arrowheads*). Chest radiography showed no abnormalities. (Courtesy of Watanabe N, Oriuchi N, Suzuki H, et al: A "changing stripe sign" in serial pulmonary perfusion imaging. *Clin Nucl Med* 21:111–114, 1996.)

repeated 2 weeks later, the stripe sign was gone from the right lower lobe, with normal perfusion. The perfusion defects in the left lower lobe were still present, however. None of the scans showed any ventilation abnormality.

Discussion.—A patient with a "changing stripe sign" associated with acute pulmonary embolism was reported. When a patient without emphysema or a ventilation abnormality is found to have a changing stripe sign, the possibility of resolving pulmonary embolism should be considered. The persistent perfusion defects noted in this case were indistinguishable from diabetes-related vasculitis.

▶ Dr. Sostman and I never said it was perfect. We said that when there was a stripe sign present, the defect involved was not pulmonary embolism 93% of the time.[1] Even considering the right lung stripe sign, the authors also illustrate a left posterior oblique view indicating, to my eye, that the patient clearly had pulmonary embolism. There is a segmental lesion in the lingula and probably also a vascular lesion in the adjacent anterior basilar lower lobe segment. There is also a segmental defect in the apical segment of the lower lobe and either a lateral or posterior segment out in the lower lobe or both. Note that these are all segmental (vascular) defects even though they do not all have absent perfusion. I stress again that the *area,* not the degree of perfusion, is the critical thing when analyzing segmental (or vascular) lesions. Therefore, in this case, I believe that even though you may have disregarded the perfusion defect in the right lung because of the stripe sign, a diagnosis of high probability for pulmonary embolism seems secure. We also made this point in our paper (i.e., that the stripe sign usually allows the reader to move a case from intermediate to low probability without affecting the high-probability determination).

A. Gottschalk, M.D.

Reference

1. Sostman HD, Gottschalk A: Prospective validation of the stripe sign in ventilation-perfusion scintigraphy. *Radiology* 184:455–459, 1992.

Ventilation/Perfusion Reverse Mismatch in Septic Pulmonary Emboli

Spencer RP (Univ of Connecticut, Farmington)
Clin Nucl Med 21:328–329, 1996   1–9

Case Report.—Man, 33, with a history of IV substance abuse was hospitalized with fever, shortness of breath, tachycardia, and tachypnea. His breathing was labored and uneven. *Staphylococcus* species grew in a blood culture. On echocardiography, the patient was found to have vegetations on the tricuspid cardiac valve. On a chest radiograph, he had lesions evolving into consolidation with

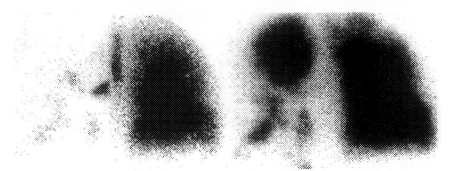

FIGURE 1.—A pulmonary ventilation study (**left**) was carried out after the patient had inhaled 2 mCi of technetium-99m–DTPA aerosol. The posterior image revealed nearly absent ventilation of the left lung, with minor entry into the lower segments. A perfusion study (**right**) with administration of 4.7 mCi of IV 99mTc-macroaggregated albumin demonstrated distinct perfusion of the left upper lung field (a reverse mismatch in the area). (Courtesy of Spencer RP: Ventilation/perfusion reverse mismatch in septic pulmonary emboli. *Clin Nucl Med* 21:328–329, 1996.)

probable cavitation. Bacteremia and endocarditis were diagnosed. A pulmonary ventilation study done after inhalation of technetium-99m–DTPA aerosol showed nearly absent ventilation of the left lung with minor entry into the lower segments (Fig 1). A perfusion study with IV 99mTc-macroaggregated albumin showed distinct perfusion of the left upper lung field, indicating a reverse mismatch.

Conclusion.—In this IV drug abuser with tricuspid valve vegetations, evolving lung lesions were most likely associated with septic pulmonary emboli. A distinct reverse mismatch was demonstrated on lung scans. Septic pulmonary emboli should be part of the differential diagnosis in patients with a ventilation-perfusion reverse mismatch.

▶ This case raises an interesting point. Is there something unique to septic emboli from drug abuse that causes reverse mismatch? Frankly, I doubt it. I have always associated reverse mismatch with significant atelectasis. Unfortunately, a chest film was not shown in this case and, therefore, I cannot decide whether that is relevant here. Then Dr. Spencer cites a publication suggesting that reverse mismatch is an indication of pulmonary infection.[1] It seems to me that pulmonary infection is a common cause of pulmonary atelectasis, so I have yet to be dissuaded of the idea that pulmonary atelectasis is not the overriding physiologic factor in all these cases.

A. Gottschalk, M.D.

Reference

1. Li DJ, Stewart I, Miles KA, et al: Scintigraphic appearances in patients with pulmonary infection and lung scintigrams of intermediate or low probability for pulmonary embolism. *Clin Nucl Med* 19:1091, 1994.

Idiopathic Peripheral Pulmonary Artery Stenosis: An Unusual Cause of Ventilation-Perfusion Mismatch

Giuliano V, Dadparvar SM, Velez-Rivera C (Hahnemann Univ, Philadelphia)
J Nucl Med 36:1608–1610, 1995   1–10

Introduction.—Peripheral pulmonary artery stenosis (PPS) is a condition that occurs in children, typically in association with other congenital cardiac anomalies. The case reported here is unusual in that an adult initially treated for pulmonary embolism was found to have idiopathic PPS.

> *Case Report.*—Man, 39, sought treatment after 3 months of progressive dyspnea and vague bilateral pleuritic chest pain. A nonsmoker in good health, his fitness regimen included 6 miles of jogging each day. The patient was found to have moderate hypoxia by arterial blood gas analysis. Results of 2-dimensional echocardiography suggested pulmonary hypertension. A technetium-99m–macroaggregated albumin perfusion scan yielded findings compatible with pulmonary embolism, and anticoagulation therapy was started. When 6 weeks of treatment brought about no improvement, the patient underwent pulmonary angiography.
>
> This examination showed branch stenoses of the right upper lobe pulmonary artery and basilar segmental left lower lobe branches. Pulmonary artery pressures were elevated. The patient then underwent elective percutaneous transluminal balloon angioplasty therapy. The clinical response was excellent, and follow-up pulmonary scintigraphy revealed an improved ventilation-perfusion (V/Q) mismatch pattern.

Discussion.—Pulmonary hypertension is an uncommon cause of V/Q mismatch; even rarer causes are pulmonary artery agenesis and stenosis. Although scintigraphic findings in this case were similar to those of pulmonary embolism, the patient's clinical course and lack of response to anticoagulation therapy were atypical. The use of pulmonary angiography to obtain the diagnosis of PPS was essential in determining the patient's need for surgical management. Idiopathic pulmonary artery stenosis should be considered in cases of V/Q mismatch.

▶ If you want to start a violent argument sometime, get a group of world-class pulmonologists, pulmonary surgeons, and pulmonary pathologists together and ask them the cause of idiopathic PPS. At least one of your pros is certain to argue that it is chronic pulmonary embolism and, of course, will not respond to acute therapy because all clots are organized, etc. At any rate, one of the key lessons from this case is that when you have what appears to be a pulmonary embolism that clinically does not act like one, get an angiogram—a far out pulmonary embolism mimic may be lurking around somewhere. This is certainly such an example.

A. Gottschalk, M.D.

Staging of Non-small-cell Lung Cancer by Whole-body Fluorine-18 Deoxyglucose Positron Emission Tomography
Bury T, Dowlati A, Paulus P, et al (CHU Sart Tilman, Liege, Belgium)
Eur J Nucl Med 23:204–206, 1996   1–11

Background.—The evaluation of patients with non–small-cell cancer who are candidates for surgical treatment includes clinical staging of the disease. Uncontrolled cellular proliferation and increased metabolic activity generally characterize malignant tumors. The increase in metabolic activity can be evaluated by PET. The accuracy of whole-body FDG-PET and conventional imaging in staging non–small-cell lung cancer were compared.

Methods.—Whole-body FDG-PET and conventional imaging were performed in 61 patients between 44 and 83 years of age with non–small-cell lung cancer. Conventional imaging included chest and abdomen CT scan-

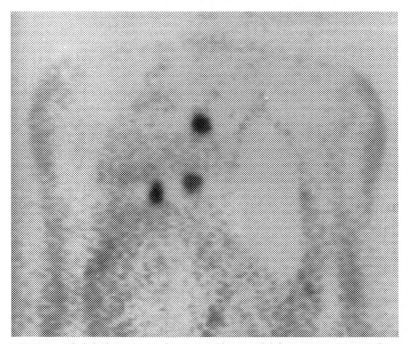

FIGURE 2.—Whole-body PET scan of a 54-year-old man with left pneumonectomy, an adenocarcinoma in the right lower lobe, and 2 metastatic bone lesions. Note the tracer accumulation in the left urinary tract. (Courtesy of Bury T, Dowlati A, Paulus P, et al: Staging of non-small-cell lung cancer by whole-body fluorine-18 deoxyglucose positron emission tomography. *Eur J Nucl Med* 23:204–206, 1996. Copyright Springer-Verlag.)

ning and bone scintigraphy. When imaging indicated metastatic disease, biopsy or follow-up was used to confirm the diagnosis.

Results.—Positron emission tomography correctly identified all primary tumors and correctly changed the N stage, determined by CT, in 13 patients. Positron emission tomography also increased the stage in 6 patients and decreased the stage in 7 patients, compared with conventional imaging. There were 3 false positive and no false negative distant PET findings. The presence of metastatic lesions was confirmed by biopsy or follow-up in 19 patients (Fig 2).

Discussion.—These findings confirm the usefulness of PET for evaluating solitary pulmonary nodules and staging non–small-cell lung cancer. Whole-body FDG-PET is more accurate than conventional imaging in thoracic and extrathoracic staging of non–small-cell lung cancer. The diagnostic accuracy of FDG-PET in detecting metastases at each distant site cannot be determined at this time. Positron emission tomography imaging changed the management of more than 20% of these patients. Seven patients underwent surgery with curative intent; in 3 patients, treatment was modified; and in 5 patients, a more curative treatment approach was adopted.

▶ I am not convinced that you can win many gold stars by showing that PET is better than conventional imaging methods for staging lung cancer. Conventional imaging methods for staging lung cancer are lousy. The internationally famous thoracic surgeons I listen to (e.g., Dr. J. Cooper) would not dream of operating on a patient without obtaining mediastinal tissue from mediastinoscopy. This is because conventional imaging methods are known to be very bad. Recently, however, significant excitement regarding PET imaging for staging lung cancer and finding recurrence has developed. The reason for this is also pointed out by these authors. There seems to be general agreement that although false positive sites can be found (particularly with inflammatory changes such as those caused by histoplasmosis or sarcoid), false negative cases are rare.

A. Gottschalk, M.D.

Decision Logic for Retreatment of Asymptomatic Lung Cancer Recurrence Based on Positron Emission Tomography Findings

Frank A, Lefkowitz D, Jaeger S, et al (Creighton Univ, Omaha, Neb)
Int J Radiat Oncol Biol Phys 32:1495–1512, 1995   1–12

Background.—Poor local control is a major contributor to treatment failure in patients with lung neoplasms of any cell type. The use of CT and chest radiography for monitoring treatment response often is inadequate because these modalities cannot distinguish necrotic tumor or fibrosis from recurrent tumor. The efficacy of PET-FDG imaging in detecting subclinical local lung cancer recurrence was investigated. The value and feasibility of re-treating these recurrences also were studied.

TABLE 1.—Individual Patient Characteristics and Treatment Data

PT No.	Age/Sex	Hist. + stage	Treatment	RT dose (Gy)	No. PET exams	SER CT	SR x-ray	RE-TX	RE-TX dose (Gy)	FU months	Status
1	67-year-old male	Recurrent ACA MD I	Chemo/XRT	59.40 1.80 QD	4	3	Yes	No	—	29	NED
2	75-year-old male	SCC I	XRT	55.80 1.80 QD	5	4	Yes	Yes	2880 QD	40	Died loc. Rec.
3	70-year-old male	SCC, WD II	XRT	64.80 1.80 QD	4	2	Yes	Yes	6400 QD	20	Died BO
4	54-year-old female	ACA, PD II	Surgery/XRT	45.00 3.00 QD	3	3	Yes	No	—	34	NED
5	76-year-old male	SCC I	XRT	59.40 1.80 QD	4	4	Yes	No	—	33	AWD
6	72-year-old female	SmC III-A	Chemo/XRT	50.40 1.80 QD	2	2	Yes	No	—	6	Died METS
7	64-year-old male	ACA III-B	Chemo/XRT	59.40 1.80 QD	2	2	Yes	No	—	12	Died METS
8	67-year-old male	SCC, PD II	Surgery/XRT	55.80 1.80 QD	2	2	Yes	No	—	5	Died METS
9	78-year-old female	SCC, PD I	XRT	54.00 1.80 QD	4	5	Yes	Yes	2200 QD	28	NED
10	74-year-old female	SmC III-A	Chemo/XRT	50.40 1.80 QD	3	3	Yes	No	—	24	NED

(Continued)

TABLE 1 (cont.)

11	80-year-old female	ACA, PD II	XRT	61.10 1.80 QD	2	1	Yes	Yes	4600 QD	6	Died MI
12	72-year-old male	ACA, MD III-A	XRT	66.00 1.80 QD	4	4	Yes	No	—	21	NED
13	58-year-old female	SCC, MD III-A	Chemo/XRT	60.00 1.50 BID	4	4	Yes	Yes	2160 QD	20	NED
14	67-year-old male	SmC, UD III-A	Chemo/XRT	50.40 1.80 QD	1	1	Yes	No	—	3	Died PNX, sepsis
15	66-year-old male	SmC, UD III-A	Chemo/XRT	50.40 1.80 QD	3	2	Yes	No	—	7	Died PN, CHF
16	57-year-old male	ACA, PD III-A	Chemo/XRT	60.00 1.50 BID	1	1	Yes	No	—	2.5	Died PE
17	64-year-old male	ACA, MD III-A	Chemo/XRT	60.00 1.50 BID	3	4	Yes	No	—	11	Local recurrence, distant METS
18	65-year-old female	SCC, MD III-A	XRT	60.00 1.50 BID	3	3	Yes	No	—	13	NED
19	78-year-old female	SCC, MD III-A	Chemo/XRT	60.00 1.50 BID	4	4	Yes	No	—	9	Local recurrence, distant METS
20	64-year-old male	SCC, PD II	Chemo/XRT	60.00 1.50 BID	2	2	Yes	No	—	8	NED

Abbreviations: AJCC, American Joint Committee on Cancer; *NED,* no evidence of disease; *SCC,* squamous-cell carcinoma; *AWD,* alive with disease; *ACA,* adenocarcinoma; *QD,* once daily fraction; *SmC,* small-cell carcinoma; *BID,* twice daily fractions; *WD,* well differentiated; *MD,* moderately differentiated; *CHF,* congestive heart failure; *PD,* poorly differentiated; *Loc Rec,* local recurrence; *RT,* radiation therapy; *TX,* treatment; *PNX,* pneumothorax; *BO,* bowel obstruction; *SER,* serial; *FU,* follow-up; *PT,* patient; *XRT,* external radiation; *RE-TX,* retreatment; *PT No.,* patient number.

(Reprinted from *Int J Radiat Oncol Biol Phys,* Frank A, Lefkowitz D, Jaeger S, et al: Decision logic for retreatment of asymptomatic lung cancer recurrence based on positron emission tomography findings. Vol 32, pp 1495–1512, Copyright 1995, with kind permission from Elsevier Science Ltd, The Boulevard, Langford Lane, Kidlington OX5 1GB, UK.)

TABLE 2.—Discordant PET-CT Findings After Therapy in Regard to Evidence of Tumor Progression

Pt No.	Cell type	PET results	CT results
2	SCC	Increased FDG activity at primary site 9 months P XRT. Positive study	Decrease in original size of tumor from 23 to 11.5 cm^3. Negative study
2	SCC	Decreased FDG activity of tumor mass P re-rt. Negative study	Interval increased size of mass from 11.5 cm^3 to 31 cm^3. Positive study.
9	SCC	Tissue changes negative for increased FDG. Negative study	Tissue changes suspicious for tumor 12 months P XRT. Positive study
10	SmC	Increased FDG uptake at primary site 3 months P chemo. Positive study	Complete regression of tumor after chemo. Negative study
13	SCC	Increased FDG activity at primary site 12.6 months P XRT. Positive study	Stable appearance of soft tissue density along posterior aortic arch 5.1 cm^3. Negative study
13	SCC	Decreased FDG activity of retreated site 5.6 months P RE-XRT. Negative study	Increased tissue density along posterior aspect of aortic arch 5.1 cm^3 to 13.6 cm^3. Positive study
15	SmC	Persistent increased FDG at primary site 3 months P chemo. Positive study	Complete regression of tumor P chemo. Negative study
17	ACA	Increased FDG activity in hilar mass 13.5 months P XRT. Positive study	Persistent mass decreased in size 45 cm^3 to 37 cm^3. Negative study
18	SCC	Increased FDG activity in area of fibrosis 13 months P XRT. Positive study	Radiation fibrosis. Negative study

Abbreviations; SCC, squamous-cell carcinoma; *SmC*, small-cell carcinoma; *ACA*, adenocarcinoma; *PT No.*, patient number; *P XRT*, after irradiation; *P Chemo*, after chemotherapy; *P Re-XRT*, retreatment with external irradiation;

(Reprinted from *Int J Radiat Oncol Biol Phys*, Frank A, Lefkowitz D, Jaeger S, et al: Decision logic for retreatment of asymptomatic lung cancer recurrence based on positron emission tomography findings. Vol 32, pp 1495–1512, Copyright 1995, with kind permission from Elsevier Science Ltd, The Boulevard, Langford Lane, Kidlington OX5 1GB, UK.)

Methods.—Twenty patients underwent PET during a 4-year period (Table 1). All had biopsy-proven lung cancer. Treatment consisted of or included external radiation. Baseline PET and CT scans were available for 20 patients. Survivors had a total of 40 sequential PET scans and 35 CT scans. Follow-up after the completion of treatment ranged from 5 to 40 months. The differential uptake ratio was determined for increased FDG uptake for certain areas.

Findings.—The 20 baseline PET scans had a median differential uptake ratio of 5.59. A value of more than 3 was chosen empirically as an indicator of tumor. Baseline PET and CT findings were 100% correlated in detecting the site of primary tumor involvement. Regions of discordance in the mediastinal and hilar regions were evident on initial PET and CT scans in 4 of these 20 patients. Discordant posttreatment PET-CT results were documented in 7 of 17 patients (Table 2). Two false positive results on PET scans were caused by radiation pneumonitis and 1 by macrophage glycolysis in tumor necrosis. Analysis of sequential PET and CT examinations, biopsy findings, and patients' clinical course suggested that PET detected asymptomatic tumor recurrence with a 100% sensitivity, 89.3% specificity, and 92.5% accuracy. The sensitivity was 67%, specificity was 85%, and accuracy of CT was 82% for detecting early recurrences. On the basis of PET findings, 5 patients underwent additional treatment with external irradiation. Four of these patients had biopsy specimens corroborating the positive PET findings. Two of the 5 patients undergoing additional treatment were alive with no evidence of disease up to 34 months after initial treatment.

Conclusions.—The use of PET scanning in the follow-up of patients treated for lung cancer appears to be an effective method for detecting recurrent disease. In selected patients in the current study, additional treatment of asymptomatic recurrent tumor resulted in decreased or absent FDG activity.

▶ The PET pulmonary people are very enthusiastic about their ability to detect recurrent lung cancer after surgery. They have used many words (this paper is 17 pages long) to describe very few patients. This experience, together with the Duke experience,[1] includes fewer than 15 proven cases. In short, we applaud the enthusiasm, but we worry about the numbers.

A. Gottschalk, M.D.

Reference

1. Duhaylongsod FG, Lowe VJ, Patz EF, et al: Detection of primary and recurrent lung cancer by means of F-18 fluorodeoxyglucose positron emission tomography (FDG PET). *J Thorac Cardiovasc Surg* 110:130–140, 1995.

Regional 2-[18F]Fluoro-2-deoxy-D-glucose Uptake Varies in Normal Lung

Miyauchi T, Wahl RL (Univ of Michigan, Ann Arbor)
Eur J Nucl Med 23:517–523, 1996   1–13

Introduction.—Positron emission tomography using FDG produces metabolic information that can help in tissue characterization in patients being evaluated for primary or metastatic lung cancer. It has been noted that some small tumors in the lower lobes of the lungs (close to the diaphragm and liver) have been missed with this approach. Regional uptake of FDG in varying regions of clinically normal lungs was retrospectively reviewed to determine whether these tumors were occasionally missed because of increased background fluorine-18 activity in the lower lungs.

Methods.—Sixteen patients with newly diagnosed and untreated lung lesions strongly suspected to be non–small-cell lung cancers underwent measurement of standardized uptake values (SUVs) for FDG of normal lung distant from the nodular lesion. Fifteen patients with known or suspected primary breast cancers without pulmonary lesions or cardiovascular disease acted as controls. About 370 MBq of FDG was administered intravenously after PET transmission images of the thorax were obtained. Patients remained supine throughout. The FDG SUVs were determined for images that were taken 50–70 minutes after FDG injection. Each patient had as many as eighteen 6 × 6-pixel regions of interest positioned over normal lung in anterior, mid, and posterior portions of the upper, middle, and lower lung fields.

Results.—The mean SUVs of the entire population were significantly higher for the posterior lung portion, compared with the anterior and mid portions. The mean SUV of the lower lung field was determined to be significantly higher, compared with the upper and middle lung fields. These findings were observed in both patient groups.

The highest SUVs in normal lung for the study group and control group were 1.418 and 1.576, respectively. The mean SUV for primary lung cancer lesions is 9.44 for the ECAT 921/EXACT PET scanner used. The recover coefficient for a spherical lesion of 5 mm in diameter with a true SUV of 9.44 and a reconstructed system resolution of 1 cm would be about 0.05. The measured SUV for this lesion would be 0.472. This SUV of 0.472 is lower than normal lung SUVs of patients in this cohort.

Conclusion.—Background ^{18}F activity in the posterior and lower lungs is significantly increased, compared with the upper and anterior portions of the lungs. This increased background could contribute to occasional false negative findings in posterior and lower lungs, particularly for small lesions. Factors such as increased blood flow, FDG delivery, and scatter from the heart and liver may add to increased lung background activity. These regional differences in normal FDG lung uptake should be considered when interpreting PET studies in patients with suspected primary or metastatic lung carcinoma. If a high-resolution PET scanner is not used, the regional variation in ^{18}F uptake may be crucial in evaluating small lower lobe pulmonary lesions. Further investigation should be done to determine whether lower lung lesions are more difficult to detect than those located more cranially in the upper lung.

▶ I think the key point in this paper is that you not only need to know how big a lesion is before it becomes detectable with whatever system you use (your eyes or 1 of the common quantitative schemes currently in use), you also need to know how big it must be for the region of lung you are looking at. This will be particularly important for those doing FDG SPECT imaging of the lung.

A. Gottschalk, M.D.

Prediction of Pulmonary Function After Resection of Primary Lung Cancer: Utility of Inhalation-Perfusion SPECT Imaging
Imaeda T, Kanematsu M, Asada S, et al (Gifu Univ, Gifu City, Japan)
Clin Nucl Med 20:792–799, 1995   1–14

Introduction.—The search continues for accurate ways of predicting postoperative lung function for patients undergoing pneumonectomy or lobectomy. Preoperative technetium-99m–macroaggregated albumin (MAA) and ^{99m}Tc Technegas inhalation SPECT images were evaluated for their usefulness in predicting postoperative lung function in patients with primary lung cancer who were scheduled for pulmonary resection.

Methods.—Thirty-three patients with primary lung cancer underwent routine pulmonary function tests, CT scans, and ^{99m}Tc-MAA perfusion SPECT imaging. Six patients also underwent ^{99m}Tc Technegas inhalation SPECT imaging. The percentage vital capacity, forced vital capacity (FVC), and forced expiratory volume in 1 second were considered reliable indices for overall pulmonary function. Surgical procedures included 10 right upper lobectomies, 5 right middle lobectomies, 7 right lower or lower and middle lobectomies, 1 left pneumonectomy, 6 left upper lobectomies, and 4 left lower lobectomies. Predicted postoperative values for lung function were compared with the measured 3-month and 6-month postoperative values.

Results.—All predicted postoperative values for lung function were more closely correlated with the measured 6-month than the measured 3-month values. The highest correlation was seen between the predicted postoperative FVC value and the measured 6-month postoperative FVC value. The measured postoperative lung function improved more at 6 months postoperatively, compared with 3 months after surgery. There was no significant difference in 3-month and 6-month radioactivity on the operated side of the lung, as determined by ^{99m}Tc-MAA SPECT images. This suggests that pulmonary blood flow on the operated side had completely recovered within 3 months of operation. Radioactivity in both the upper and lower lobes on the nonoperated lung increased shortly after surgery and had not returned to preoperative levels at the 6-month evaluation. The predicted postoperative values for both SPECT imagings were similar in all except 1 patient. It could not be determined which SPECT imaging findings were superior. The lowest limit value for adaptability was estimated to be 1.1 L for FVC and 900 mL for forced expiratory volume in 1 second.

Conclusion.—The measured 6-month postoperative values indicated greater improvement than did the 3-month values. There were no significant differences in 3-month and 6-month radioactivity values on the operated side of the lung in most patients. It may be that the alveolus-airway system had completely recovered by 3 months and that the greater improvement in the measured 6-month postoperative lung function, compared with the measured 3-month postoperative lung function, was caused by recovery of the thoracic system from decreased muscle strength and pain on the operative side. It was difficult to determine which SPECT imaging was superior because values from both perfusion and inhalation analysis were similar.

▶ These authors have gone to a lot of work to define precisely the potential area of surgical resection, using both perfusion and Technegas ventilation images to estimate postoperative lung function. What I get from these data and all this hard work is that the old method of looking at the MAA perfusion scan with simple planar technique was pretty damn good; these authors did not do significantly better than we used to do with our crude method. Furthermore, the macroaggregate perfusion scan seems to be an excellent surrogate for ventilation in that these authors could do no better using Technegas than with the macroaggregate study. Therefore, if you want to try these elegant, precise techniques, be my guest. If, however, you are using the old-fashioned planar methods, don't stop. You will continue to do quite well.

A. Gottschalk, M.D.

A Pulmonary Metastasis From Renal Cell Carcinoma Seen on a Lung Perfusion Scan
Boutselis AG, Zu'bi S (Baystate Med Ctr, Springfield, Mass; Tufts Univ, Boston)
Clin Nucl Med 20:1084–1085, 1995   1–15

Introduction.—Representing about 3% of all adult malignancies, renal cell carcinoma is most commonly metastasized to the lungs, although it can also metastasize to bone, regional lymph nodes, the liver, adrenals, and the brain. Chest radiographs identify most pulmonary metastases, with chest CT being advocated as a secondary test. Little is reported on lung perfusion scans used to evaluate patients with renal cell carcinoma.

Case Report.—Man, 75, with pulmonary metastases from renal cell carcinoma had ventilation and perfusion imaging to rule out pulmonary embolism. He was admitted for dehydration and hypercalcemia. Areas of increased tracer uptake were seen on his technetium-99m–macroaggregated albumin perfusion scan, corresponding to the metastatic lesions seen on his chest radiographs. A defect at the left base was shown on the ^{133}Xe ventilation scan.

Results.—An area of decreased activity, which corresponded to the location of a metastatic lesion seen on the patient's chest radiograph, was seen on the ventilation scan. The perfusion scan revealed large areas of increased activity and a central area of decreased activity, which may have represented tumor necrosis.

Conclusion.—Tumor metastases may have invaded the pulmonary artery and caused shunting of the tumor vessels with the pulmonary artery. The increased tracer uptake seen on his lung perfusion scan may have been caused by the resultant shunt vascularity.

▶ The authors present an unusual case. When someone mentions a lung lesion that perfuses on a perfusion lung scan, I usually think of bronchoalveolar carcinoma. Other unusual cases I came across included asymmetric pulmonary thallium uptake in sarcoidosis[1] and the diagnosis of pulmonary arteriovenous malformation diagnosed by radionuclide angiography.[2] The latter case also reminds me to remind you that right/left shunts—particularly in younger patients—may show a lot of thyroid uptake as well as the expected renal and brain uptake.

References

1. Schraml FV, Turton DB, Bakalar RS, et al: Persistent asymmetric pulmonary T1-201 uptake in type III sarcoidosis. *Clin Nucl Med* 20:1093–1094, 1995.
2. Ünal SA, Mudun A, Ertugrul E, et al: Pulmonary arteriovenous malformation diagnosed with radionuclide angiography. *Clin Nucl Med* 20:1097–1099, 1995.

Radiation Pneumonitis Imaged With Indium-111-Pentetreotide
Olmos RAV, van Zandwijk N, Boersma LJ, et al (The Netherlands Cancer Inst, Amsterdam)
J Nucl Med 37:584–588, 1996   1–16

Purpose.—When radiation pneumonitis is recognized early, adequate treatment can be offered and the chances of late sequelae reduced. Although gallium-67 citrate scanning is sensitive, normal radiotracer uptake by the sternum and spine may hinder the determination of lung injury. The use of the somatostatin analogue indium-111–pentetreotide for detecting and monitoring radiation pneumonitis was studied.

Methods.—The study included 11 patients with cancer who had received radiotherapy to the chest, all but 1 of whom had clinical evidence

TABLE 2.—Scintigraphic and Radiographic Results

Lung uptake ^{111}In-Pentetreotide (INIA uptake ratio)*

Patient no.	Right anterior	Left anterior	Right posterior	Left posterior	V/Q scan abnormalities	Chest radiography/CT scan abnormalities
1	−(1.22)	−(1.18)	−(1.11)	−(1.13)	No	No
2	+++(1.74)		++(1.54)		Right lung (slightly)	Right upper field
3	+(1.33)	−(1.19)	−(1.21)	−(1.10)	Both lungs	Both sides (R>L)
4	+++(1.99)	+++(1.94)	+++(1.82)	+++(1.98)	Both lungs	Both sides
5	−(1.15)	−(1.17)	−(1.02)	−(1.01)	Both lungs	Equivocal
6	++(1.43)	++(1.50)	++(1.42)	++(1.54)	Both lungs	Both sides
7		++(1.75)		++(1.38)	Left lung	No
8	−(1.12)		−(1.12)		Right lung (Equivocal)	Pleural effusion
9	++(1.37)	++(1.29)	++(1.39)	++(1.34)	Both lungs	Both sides
10	+++(1.91)	+++(2.02)	+++(2.15)	+++(1.64)	Both lungs	Both sides
11		+++(2.16)		++(1.54)	Left lung	Left lung

Abbreviations: INIA ratio, irradiated-to-nonirradiated area uptake ratio; +++, strongly positive; ++, moderately positive; −, negative.
(Reprinted by permission of the Society of Nuclear Medicine, from Olmos RAV, van Zandwijk N, Boersma LJ, et al: Radiation pneumonitis imaged with indium-111-pentetreotide. *J Nucl Med* 37:584–588, 1996.)

of radiation pneumonitis. Planar imaging was done 24 hours after IV administration of ^{111}In-pentetreotide, 110–130 MBq. Lung uptake was graded visually and assessed quantitatively using the irradiated-to-nonirradiated area (INIA) ratio. The findings were checked against the radiation field for each patient, and compared with the V/Q images, radiographs, or CT scans. The distribution of lung uptake was mapped by complementary SPECT studies.

Results.—The results of ^{111}In-pentetreotide scanning were positive in 9 of the 10 symptomatic patients. Eight patients had strongly or moderately positive results, including 1 patient who was not responding to steroid therapy. The ninth patient, who was responding well to steroid therapy, had a weakly positive result. The ^{111}In-pentetreotide scan results were negative in 1 symptomatic patient who proved to have nonspecific viral pneumonitis and in 1 asymptomatic patient. The areas of radiation pneumonitis depicted by positive scans corresponded to areas of decreased ventilation/perfusion and to radiographic abnormalities (Table 2). The lowest INIA ratio recorded in an irradiated lung area with visible uptake was 1.29, with a range of 1.01–2.16. For patients treated with mantle irradiation fields, SPECT studies demonstrated lung uptake in both the superficial and deep areas. For those receiving internal mammary lymph node chain irradiation, uptake was seen only in anterior areas.

Conclusions.—In symptomatic patients who have received chest radiotherapy, ^{111}In-pentetreotide scanning can detect areas of radiation pneumonitis. This study may be useful in detecting and differentiating radiation pneumonitis. In patients undergoing ^{111}In-pentetreotide scanning for tumor detection, it is important to remember that irradiated lung areas may produce false positive results. The findings in patients treated with steroids support the theory that radiation injury involves enhanced production and release of cytokines from alveolar macrophages.

▶ I am not sure this suggestion will go far as a diagnostic test. If you look at the data, the pentetreotide did better in 1 case and lost out to the standard radiographic imaging techniques in 2 others. The bulk of the cases (8 patients) had comparable results with both the tracer and conventional radiographic imaging studies. Furthermore, one of the key problems with the radiation pneumonitis is in determining which of these patients will have pulmonary fibrosis develop, which is not necessarily related to acute radiation pneumonitis. If there is a prognostic feature with pentetreotide uptake, it was not presented here. However, this series has merit because it points out a cause of uptake that you need to be familiar with if you are using this tracer to avoid making a false positive diagnosis of neoplastic uptake in the lungs.

A. Gottschalk, M.D.

Technetium-99m-MIBI Scintigraphy in Pulmonary Tuberculosis

Önsel Ç, Sönmezoglu K, Çamsari G, et al (Cerrahpasa Med Facility, Istanbul, Turkey; Yedikule Chest Clinic, Istanbul, Turkey)

J Nucl Med 37:233–238, 1996
1–17

Background.—Tuberculin skin testing and clinical features are of little value in diagnosing active pulmonary tuberculosis, especially in certain populations such as the elderly and immunocompromised individuals. In 50% of patients, identification of acid-fast bacilli by staining is not useful,

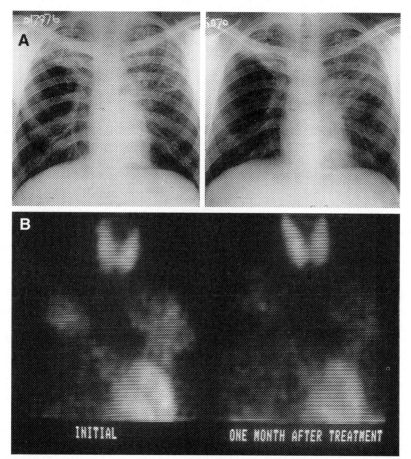

FIGURE 1.—Imaging in a man, 26, with active, localized pulmonary tuberculosis in both lungs. A, posteroanterior chest roentgenogram on the left side demonstrates focal infiltration with some cavitation in both upper lung fields, being more prominent on the left side. Despite exposure differences, partial regression of the lesions is seen on the right radiograph obtained 1 month after chemotherapy. B, abnormal focal accumulations of technetium-99m–methoxyisobutylisonitrile on 1-hour scan in both upper lungs, and partial diminution after chemotherapy can be easily seen in the corresponding scintigraphs. (Reprinted by permission of the Society of Nuclear Medicine, from Önsel Ç, Sönmezoglu K, Çamsari G, et al: Technetium-99m-MIBI scintigraphy in pulmonary tuberculosis. *J Nucl Med* 37:233–238, 1996.)

radiographic findings may be unremarkable, and results of sputum examination and chest roentgenogram may conflict. A definitive diagnosis may be made by transbronchial biopsy, an invasive procedure, or by culturing of sputum, which can take between 2 and 8 weeks. Various radiopharmaceuticals have been used in evaluating tuberculosis. Technetium-99m–methoxyisobutylisonitrile (MIBI) has been shown to accumulate in lung and other tumors, and in pulmonary tuberculosis during thyroid tumor imaging. The effectiveness of ^{99m}Tc-MIBI imaging in evaluating pulmonary tuberculosis was investigated.

Methods.—Scanning was performed in 36 patients between 13 and 59 years of age with proven or suspected pulmonary tuberculosis. Before scanning, patients received IV injections of 370 Mbq (10 mCi) of ^{99m}Tc-MIBI. Anterior and posterior images were obtained 15 and 60 minutes after injection. When there was no abnormality on early images, additional oblique-lateral views or SPECT images were obtained after late planar imaging. Patients were not receiving chemotherapy at this time. In 12 patients, scintigraphy with ^{99m}Tc-MIBI was repeated between 1 and 3 months after chemotherapy was started.

Results.—Increased focal uptake of ^{99m}Tc-MIBI was seen in 92% of patients with active localized pulmonary tuberculosis (Fig 1). There was no accumulation of ^{99m}Tc-MIBI in 2 patients with minimal infiltration on chest radiographs. Diffuse uptake was seen in the 2 patients with miliary pulmonary tuberculosis. The ^{99m}Tc-MIBI scans were true positive in 4 of 5 patients with culture-proven tuberculosis; scans were false positive in 2 of 5 patients with negative sputum cultures. In 6 of 10 patients with active localized pulmonary tuberculosis, repeat imaging showed reduced uptake of ^{99m}Tc-MIBI that correlated with findings on chest radiographs; in 1 of these 10 patients, there was increased uptake that correlated with clinical and radiographic findings and that indicated resistance to first-line chemotherapy, and in 3 of these 10 patients, there were no significant scintigraphic changes in spite of clinical and partial radiologic regression.

Discussion.—Because of its good imaging characteristics and shelf availability, ^{99m}Tc-MIBI is superior to other radionuclide techniques in evaluating pulmonary tuberculosis. Clinicians should be aware of ^{99m}Tc-MIBI uptake in patients with pulmonary tuberculosis as a nonspecific event. This scintigraphy is useful in diagnosing chronic pulmonary tuberculosis because of its high sensitivity.

▶ These strike me as interesting, though last ditch type, data. If I want to know whether pulmonary tuberculosis is active, I will get a repeat chest radiograph in 2 weeks. However, if for some management reason you need to know the same day, then ^{99m}Tc-MIBI could be a useful option. If you have a little more time, gallium-67 works quite well; and, of course, thallium (also a potassium analogue) should work as well as ^{99m}Tc-MIBI, except that the counts would be somewhat limited. However, by far the cheapest option is a repeat chest film.

A. Gottschalk, M.D.

Lung Uptake on Technetium-99m-MDP Bone Scan in Wegener's Vasculitis

Kuyvenhoven JD, Ommeslag DJ, Ackerman CM, et al (Univ Ziekenhuis Gent, Belgium; Algemeen Ziekenhuis Heilige Familie, Gent, Belgium)
J Nucl Med 37:857–858, 1996   1–18

Introduction.—Most causes of soft-tissue uptake on bone scans result from heterotopic calcification, either metastatic or dystrophic. Lung uptake on bone scans is often caused by metastatic calcification, fibrothorax, metastasis, pleural fluid, primary lung tumors, or radiation therapy. The case of a patient with Wegener's vasculitis with significant lung uptake not caused by any known condition was presented.

Case Report.—Woman, 65, was referred because of knee and elbow pain and a complaint of sore throat, bloody nose, shortness of breath, persistent cough, and weight loss. No structural lesions were seen on a chest radiograph (Fig 1). A bone scan with technetium-99m–methylene diphosphonate (MDP) showed significant uptake in both lungs, particularly at the basis (Fig 2). Although major pathology was suspected, the patient refused further tests.

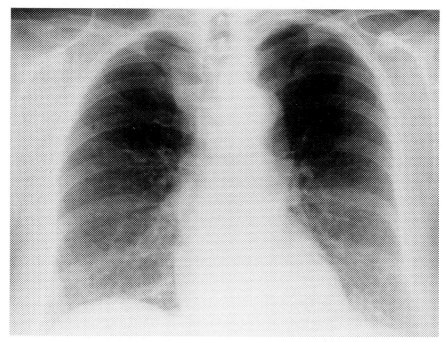

FIGURE 1.—Chest radiograph shows posteroanterior view without definite abnormalities. (Reprinted by permission of the Society of Nuclear Medicine, from Kuyvenhoven JD, Ommeslag DJ, Ackerman CM, et al: Lung uptake on technetium-99m-MDP bone scan in Wegener's vasculitis. *J Nucl Med* 37:857–858, 1996).

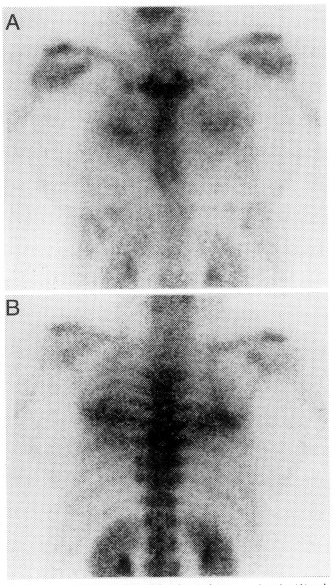

FIGURE 2.—Technetium-99m–methylene diphosphonate bone scan. Anterior (**A**) and posterior (**B**) views of the thorax show bilateral, mainly basal, lung uptake (Reprinted by permission of the Society of Nuclear Medicine, from Kuyvenhoven JD, Ommeslag DJ, Ackerman CM, et al: Lung uptake on technetium-99m-MDP bone scan in Wegener's vasculitis. *J Nucl Med* 37:857–858, 1996).

She was admitted 6 days later with severe dyspnea and fulminant hemoptysis. A chest radiograph showed bilateral basal infiltrates. Wegener's vasculitis was diagnosed. After 1 month of treatment with cyclophosphamide and glucocorticoid, the patient improved dramatically. At 4 months, there were no perinuclear antineutrophil cytoplasmic antibodies and no abnormalities on chest radiographs.

Discussion.—Wegener's granulomatosis is marked by granulomatous inflammation and necrotizing vasculitis. The combined lung and kidney involvement and presence of perinuclear antineutrophil cytoplasmic antibodies made a diagnosis of Wegener's vasculitis fairly certain. Wegener's vasculitis should be included in the differential diagnosis of lung uptake on ^{99m}Tc-MDP bone scan. Clinicians should be aware that patients with this condition may deteriorate rapidly.

▶ I suspect that the only reason the authors find this to be the first case of lung uptake in Wegener's vasculitis is that nobody has bothered to report it before. As the authors point out, this is a *necrotizing* vasculitis. I believe any type of necrotic tissue is highly likely to take up a bone tracer. For example, we see it in necrotic heart (myocardial infarction), we see it in necrotic brain (stroke), we see it in necrotic soft tissue (postoperative incisions), and in necrotic kidney (after irradiation vasculitis and ischemia). Therefore, I am not amazed to find that it occurs in necrotic vasculitis.

A. Gottschalk, M.D.

The Radionuclide Salivagram in Children With Pulmonary Disease and a High Risk of Aspiration

Bar-Sever Z, Connolly LP, Treves ST (Children's Hosp, Boston; Harvard Med School, Boston)
Pediatr Radiol 25:S180–S183, 1995   1–19

Background.—Aspiration of saliva can cause significant pulmonary morbidity. The radionuclide salivagram can detect the aspiration of saliva. This technique was used in a series of pediatric patients with conditions predisposing them to aspiration or with a history of recurrent pneumonia or chronic lung disease.

Methods.—Thirty-one patients aged 3 weeks to 16.7 years underwent study with 34 salivagrams. All the patients had either recurrent pneumonia or unexplained chronic lung disease. Of the 31 patients, 25 had neurologic conditions associated with a predisposition for aspiration and 16 required enteric tube feedings. Sublingual technetium-99m was administered at a dose of 300 µCi (11.1 MBq) in a drop of saline, after which serial posterior images were obtained for 1 hour.

Results.—Eight of the 31 patients (26%) had demonstrated aspiration passing beyond the level of the carina. Five of those patients had a major clinical diagnosis of cerebral palsy with psychomotor retardation, and 3 patients had congenital malformations with associated CNS involvement.

Conclusions.—The radionuclide salivagram provides useful information for assessing suspected aspiration. It is recommended for use in the evaluation of any patient with recurrent pneumonia or unexplained chronic lung disease and a condition predisposing to aspiration. The technique is also useful in determining the penetration of aspirated saliva and the patient's ability to clear aspirated tracer.

▶ The authors describe a nice simple technique with an easy-to-read end point. This should be a very useful test that you can easily adapt to your practice when the appropriate patient presents to you.

A. Gottschalk, M.D.

Utility of Technetium-99m-DTPA in Determining Regional Ventilation
Cabahug CJ, McPeck M, Palmer LB, et al (State Univ of New York at Stony Brook)
J Nucl Med 37:239–244, 1996   1–20

Background.—Pulmonary scintigraphy is used to evaluate patients with suspected pulmonary embolism. The deposition of radiolabeled aerosols in the lungs may be an index of regional ventilation. Nebulized technetium-99m–DTPA aerosols are useful in diagnosing embolism in patients who breathe spontaneously. The value of radiolabeled aerosols in evaluating ventilated lung regions in patients receiving mechanical ventilation was investigated.

Methods.—Three radioaerosol nebulizer kits were used to evaluate the nebulizer efficiency and particle distribution of ^{99m}Tc-DTPA aerosols. A gamma camera was used to study patients who had tracheotomy and were receiving mechanical ventilation. Regional ventilation with krypton-81m gas and ^{99m}Tc-DTPA aerosol were simultaneously measured. The distribution of radioactivity in computer-generated images was compared.

Results.—The smallest particles were produced by the UltraVent nebulizing system, compared with the Aero Tech I and Venti-Scan II systems. Images of ^{99m}Tc-DTPA deposition using the UltraVent nebulizer did not accurately represent regional ventilation as measured by ^{81m}Kr equilibrium. Visual inspection showed significant particle deposition in the trachea region that decreased, but was not eliminated, after the tracheotomy tube inner cannula was replaced. Regional analysis showed a poor correlation between radioactivity distributions of both isotopes. Segmental analysis indicated that residual tracheal activity significantly affected the upper and middle regions of the lung.

Conclusion.—The lungs of patients receiving mechanical ventilation can be imaged after inhalation of ^{99m}Tc-DTPA, but there is poor correlation between aerosol deposition and regional ventilation. When a gas such as ^{81m}Kr is used, the definition of ventilated lung segments is improved because tracheal activity with the radiolabeled gas is lowered.

▶ These data confirm my own personal bias that when an aerosol study shows significant central ventilation, the smartest thing you can do with it is to throw it away. Do not use it in your diagnostic analysis. In these instances, I believe there are not enough aerosolized particles delivered to the periphery of the lung to get good statistical analysis of what is going on—comparable to using too few particles of macroaggregates for the perfusion scan.

People frequently show me (usually in scan-reading panels, etc.) cases with fouled up aerosol studies. I simply disregard the aerosol study and read the case, using the chest radiograph and perfusion scan. This technique has been used in a very large series obtained in Pizza, Italy (they call it Pizza-PED). The investigators have obtained excellent results using only a chest radiograph and a perfusion scan. Therefore, when you see a rotten aerosol study, I suggest you forget it and use the Italian technique. Their data certainly support this concept.

A. Gottschalk, M.D.

Evaluation of Lung Ventilation and Alveolar Permeability in Cirrhosis
Kao C-H, Huang C-K, Tsai S-C, et al (Taichung Veterans Gen Hosp, Taiwan, Republic of China)
J Nucl Med 37:437–441, 1996   1–21

Background.—Impaired pulmonary function is associated with severe hepatic disease. However, the physiologic mechanism of this impairment is not well understood. An investigation was made of technetium-99m–DTPA radioaerosol lung scintigraphic changes in lung ventilation and alveolar permeability (AP) in patients with liver cirrhosis.

Methods.—Twenty-nine patients were assessed by ^{99m}Tc-DTPA aerosol inhalation lung scintigraphy. Equilibrium lung ventilation images were interpreted visually, based on the presence or absence of inhomogeneous distribution, inverted base-to-apex gradient, and segment defects. A control group consisted of 12 healthy nonsmokers.

Findings.—None of the patients had significantly abnormal lung ventilation findings. However, decreased lung ventilation in the basilar lung zone was noted in 13 patients. Twenty percent of patients with no ascites, 50% with slight-to-moderate ascites, and 88% with moderate-to-severe ascites had lung ventilation abnormalities. Patients had higher time-activity curve slopes on AP studies than did control subjects. The slopes for the right total lung were comparable among patients with cirrhosis of differing severity. However, the slopes for right upper and right lower lung differed significantly between some subgroups. Also, albumin and bilirubin levels were not correlated significantly with slope values (Fig 2).

Conclusion.—Lung ventilation appears to be normal in most patients with cirrhosis of the liver. However, the disease may predispose patients to AP damage. The extent of the damage is unassociated with disease severity.

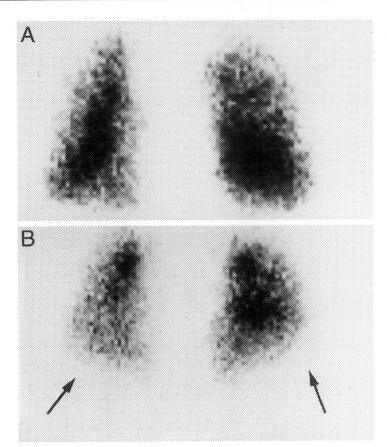

FIGURE 2.—Normal (**A**) and abnormal (**B**) lung ventilation patterns. Reduced ventilation is seen in the basilar zone of the right lung (*arrows*). (Reprinted by permission of the Society of Nuclear Medicine, from Kao C-H, Huang C-K, Tsai S-C, et al: Evaluation of lung ventilation and alveolar permeability in cirrhosis. *J Nucl Med* 37:437–441, 1996).

▶ As I look at Figure 2, I am conflicted. I do not know whether this is just a patient who has normal ventilation but cannot push his diaphragm down because there is extensive ascites present or whether this is truly a patient who has basilar hypoventilation. These studies were done with the patient in the supine position, which further confounds this problem. To convince me, these authors would have to do a transmission image indicating that there is more lung available to ventilate than is seen on this aerosol image. My guess is that they would not find it.

A. Gottschalk, M.D.

Comparison of Iodine-123-Disintegrins for Imaging Thrombi and Emboli in a Canine Model

Knight LC, Maurer AH, Romano JE (Temple Univ, Philadelphia)
J Nucl Med 37:476–482, 1996   1–22

Background.—There are numerous limitations to the radiopharmaceuticals that have been tested for use in imaging deep vein thrombosis and pulmonary embolism. For example, radiolabeled platelets and fibrinogen display slow blood clearance and poor binding to mature thrombi. The short, synthetic peptides with a binding site for activated platelets that have been tested have shown poor binding to preexisting thrombi. Disintegrins are peptides found in snake venom that bind well to activated platelets at the glycoprotein IIb-IIIa receptor. The value of various radiolabeled disintegrins in imaging thrombi and emboli were evaluated.

Methods.—The following 8 disintegrins were purified from snake venom: bitistatin, albolabrin, echistatin, eristostatin, kistrin, mambin, halysin, and barbourin. These disintegrins were radiolabeled with iodine-123 and tested in dogs for the ability to image 24-hour-old deep vein thrombi and pulmonary emboli. Labeled fibrinogen and platelets served as controls.

Results.—The highest uptake in deep vein thrombi was displayed by ^{123}I-bitistatin (Table 3). Bitistatin had higher deep vein thrombi-to-blood ratios than all other disintegrins, ^{125}I-fibrinogen, or technetium-99m–hexamethylpropyleneamine oxime (HMPA) platelets. Within 1 hour, images of deep vein thrombi with ^{123}I-bitistatin were focally positive and had improved by 4 hours. The highest uptake in pulmonary emboli was also displayed by ^{123}I-bitistatin (Table 4). The uptake of barbourin was moderate. In pulmonary emboli, the uptake of bitistatin was superior to ^{125}I-fibrinogen and ^{99m}Tc-HMPAO platelets. The embolus-to-blood ratios of ^{123}I-bitistatin averaged 27; this was higher than platelets, fibrinogen, echistatin, mambin, and halysin. In lungs, liver, and heart, ^{123}I-bitistatin background was low, which allowed pulmonary emboli to be visualized between 2 and 4 hours after injection.

TABLE 3.—Uptake of Various Compounds in Venous Lesions 4 Hours After Injection

Compound	No.	%ID/g	DVT-to-Blood	DVT-to-Muscle
Bitistatin	6	0.21 ± 0.06	9.8 ± 2.5	125 ± 41
Albolabrin	3	*0.036 ± 0.018	*4.5 ± 2.7	*19 ± 12
Echistatin	3	*0.009 ± 0.001	*1.0 ± 0.2	*3.3 ± 0.7
Eristostatin	3	*0.030 ± 0.014	*2.0 ± 1.1	*9.6 ± 5.6
Kistrin	4	*0.018 ± 0.005	*2.5 ± 0.6	*9.2 ± 2.8
Mambin	3	*0.028 ± 0.003	*4.5 ± 0.8	*16 ± 1
Barbourin	3	*0.028 ± 0.008	*4.2 ± 1.5	*26 ± 18
Halysin	2	*0.029 ± 0.005	*3.9 ± 0.5	25 ± 9
Fibrinogen	27	0.18 ± 0.02	*2.8 ± 0.4	83 ± 11
Platelets	4	0.15 ± 0.06	*5.0 ± 2.3	*230 ± 73

*$P < 0.05$ vs. bitistatin.

TABLE 4.—Uptake of Various Compounds in Pulmonary Emboli 4 Hours After Injection

Compound	No.	%ID/g	PE-to-Blood	PE-to-Muscle	PE-to-Lung
Bitistatin	11	0.64 ± 0.17	27 ± 7	360 ± 109	46 ± 16
Albolabrin	4	*0.12 ± 0.05	14 ± 5	*65 ± 31	*12 ± 4
Echistatin	4	*0.009 ± 0.001	*1.0 ± 0.03	*3.3 ± 0.3	*2.5 ± 1.8
Eristostatin	5	*0.21 ± 0.06	12 ± 4	*56 ± 18	*15 ± 5
Kistrin	8	*0.11 ± 0.05	20 ± 11	*53 ± 23	*10 ± 6
Mambin	5	*0.070 ± 0.022	*12 ± 4	*38 ± 10	*11 ± 6
Barbourin	6	*0.23 ± 0.11	16 ± 8	*105 ± 71	26 ± 12
Halysin	4	*0.034 ± 0.003	*4.5 ± 0.5	*28 ± 5	*5.1 ± 0.5
Fibrinogen	35	*0.18 ± 0.02	†*2.7 ± 0.3	*88 ± 16	*11 ± 3
Platelets	2	*0.14 ± 0.02	*4.1 ± 0.7	249 ± 62	9

*$P < 0.05$ vs. bitistatin.
†$P < 0.05$ vs. barbourin.
(Reprinted by permission of the Society of Nuclear Medicine, from Knight LC, Maurer AH, Romano JE: Comparison of iodine-123-disintegrins for imaging thrombi and emboli in a canine model. *J Nucl Med* 37:476–482, 1996.)

Conclusion.—The characteristics of the disintegrin bitistatin were very favorable for imaging deep vein thrombi and pulmonary emboli in the canine model. Further research in humans is recommended.

▶ An imaging technique for reliably detecting deep vein thrombosis or pulmonary embolism as a "hot spot" has been described as the "holy grail" of the thromboembolism business. Finding pulmonary emboli is particularly difficult for reasons that make a lot of sense if you think about them. Do you perfuse the region of the pulmonary embolus? By definition, you do not. If you do not, how do you deliver the tracer you are interested in to the clot that is the target? The answer is "with great difficulty." If you are lucky, the surface of some of the clot may get some perfusion if it is adjacent to a patent branch vessel, but the signal-to-noise ratio you get when just a surface of your target is perfused is often minimal and, therefore, the image does not succeed.

Finally, if you cannot image a coil (and these authors use coils), you will never image anything. In my view, imaging coils have always been successful, probably because they may enlarge the vessel and keep it open to some degree or possibly because there is continual formation of acute clot in and around the coils. I have been involved with experimented systems that worked with coils that did not work when autologous thrombus was used instead to create the embolus.

The above are discouraging comments, but I think the authors are to be commended. They have developed a tracer that looks 5 times more promising than platelets, and platelets worked from time to time. I would like to see them try bitistatin in an autologous clot canine model to see how it compares to the coil clots they are now using. To me, that would be the next step in the quest for the "holy grail."

A. Gottschalk, M.D.

2 Hematology and Oncology

Introduction

Nuclear medicine has passed through the "decade of the heart," is fast completing the "decade of the brain," and seems to have already entered a phase of incredible activity related to the scintigraphy and radiotherapy of tumors. A plethora of articles was published this past year detailing the efforts being made to impact positively on the diagnosis and treatment of patients with cancer. This chapter is so large for that reason. Much of the work involves new receptor-ligand systems thought to be excellent for the development of tumor-specific radiopharmaceuticals. Another large body of work seeks to extend the PET methodology to tumor diagnosis, staging, and, perhaps, to evaluation of cancer treatments. We also may have a role in tumor treatment and the treatment of tumor-associated morbidity such as bone pain. Instrumentation developments are ongoing to extend the use of PET radiopharmaceuticals into clinics without the financial resources to purchase cyclotrons and dedicated PET cameras.

All of this nuclear oncology research activity is reflected in the series of representative papers that follow.

Ronald Neumann, M.D.

Vasoactive Intestinal Peptide Receptor Scintigraphy
Virgolini I, Kurtaran A, Raderer M, et al (Univ of Vienna; Research Ctr Seibersdorf, Austria)
J Nucl Med 36:1732–1739, 1995   2–1

Purpose.—There is growing interest in the clinical use of peptide receptor–specific radioligands, such as somatostatin analogues and vasoactive intestinal peptide (VIP). High expression of VIP receptors on various tumor cells has been demonstrated, suggesting that radiolabeled VIP could be useful for in vivo localization of intestinal adenocarcinomas and endocrine tumors. Vasoactive intestinal peptide receptor imaging has compared favorably with octreotide receptor imaging in patients with adenocarcinomas. The biodistribution, safety, and absorbed dose of iodine-123–VIP were investigated in patients.

Methods.—The study included 18 patients with intestinal adenocarcinomas or endocrine tumors. High specific activity ^{123}I-VIP was prepared through purification by high-performance liquid chromatography. The patients were given a mean 172-MBq IV dose of ^{123}I-VIP, amounting to less than 300 pmole per patient. For the first 30 minutes, sequential images were obtained; whole-body images in anterior and posterior views were then obtained at various intervals. The gamma camera data were used, together with measured activities in urine, feces, and blood, for dosimetry calculations.

Results.—The primary site of ^{123}I-VIP uptake was the lung. Within 0.7 hour, peak lung activity accounted for a mean of 40% of the injected dose; this figure fell to 21% at 3.5 hours, 14% at 7 hours, and 8% at 22 hours. Radioactivity in the urine accounted for 37% of the injected dose at 4 hours, 68% at 8 hours, 82% at 16 hours, and 93% at 24 hours. The labeled peptide had a mean effective half-life of 2.2 hours in the lungs and 6 hours in the bladder. The calculated radiation-absorbed dose was 67 μGy/MBq in the lung, 77 μGy/MBq in the bladder, and 104 μGy/MBq in the thyroid, with an effective dose of 28 μSv/MBq. The ^{123}I-VIP scans detected pancreatic adenocarcinoma in 2 patients, an ileocecal carcinoid tumor in 1 patient, lymph node metastases in 2 patients, and liver metastases in 2 of 3 patients.

Conclusion.—The dosimetric findings of HPLC-purified ^{123}I-VIP suggest that it is a safe and promising tracer for localization of tumors expressing VIP receptors. This peptide tracer has a unique biodistribution, with high affinity for normal lung tissue and for different types of tumor cells. The molecular basis of VIP receptor scanning remains to be determined.

In Vitro Identification of Vasoactive Intestinal Peptide Receptors in Human Tumors: Implications for Tumor Imaging
Reubi JC (Univ of Berne, Switzerland)
J Nucl Med 36:1846–1853, 1995   2–2

Background.—Many tumors overexpress neuropeptide receptor, suggesting the use of radioactive neuropeptide receptor imaging to localize tumors. Somatostatin receptor (SS-R) has proven its value for this purpose, although it cannot visualize certain common types of cancers, such as colonic adenocarcinomas and non–small-cell lung cancers. Vasoactive intestinal peptide (VIP) has emerged as a potentially valuable new imaging agent. Vasoactive intestinal peptide receptor (VIP-R) autoradiography was performed to assess the VIP-R content of various human tumors, including a comparison of VIP-R and SS-R content.

Methods.—The study included tissue sections of 339 human tumors of various types. All were studied by in vitro receptor autoradiography using iodine-125–VIP to determine their VIP-R content. Adjacent tissue sections were studied with [125]I-[Tyr3]-octreotide to determine their SS-R content.

Findings.—Many different types of cancer cells were found to express VIP-R, including most breast cancers and their metastases; endometrial, prostate, bladder, and colon carcinomas; and both small-cell and non–small-cell lung cancers (Table 1). All undifferentiated neuroendocrine tumors expressed VIP-R, as did about half of undifferentiated tumors. Tumors expressed VIP-R much more often than SS-R. However, some tumors expressed VIP-R less often or not at all, including growth hormone–producing adenomas, medullary thyroid carcinomas, and Ewing sarcomas. The tumors showed high-affinity VIP-R specific for both VIP and pituitary adenylate cyclase–activating peptide. There was no apparent cross-competition between VIP and SS (Table 2).

Conclusion.—In vitro receptor autoradiography demonstrates VIP-R expression in most human carcinomas. These receptors are frequent among breast, ovarian, endometrial, prostate, bladder, lung, esophageal,

TABLE 1.—Percentage of Vasoactive Intestinal Peptide Receptor–expressing Tumors Measured With In Vitro Autoradiography: Comparison with Somatostatin Receptor Status

Tumor	Type	VIP-R-positive tumors (% Incidence)	SS-R-positive tumors* (% Incidence)
Breast ca	P	24/24 (100)	14/24 (58)
	M	15/15 (100)	6/15 (40)
Ovarian ca		20/24 (83)	0/24 (0)
Endometrial ca		12/12 (100)	NT
Prostate ca	P	25/25 (100)	0/25 (0)
	M	7/7 (100)	NT
Bladder ca		4/4 (100)	0/4 (0)
Colon ca		21/21 (100)	7/21 (33)†
Pancreatic ca		9/12 (75)	0/12 (0)
Esophageal ca		4/4 (100)	0/4 (0)
Lung cancers			
nSCLC		9/12 (75)	1/12 (8)†
SCLC		3/4 (75)	3/4 (75)
Brain tumors			
Astrocytomas		13/13 (100)	10/13 (77)
Glioblastomas		12/16 (75)	1/16 (6)†
Meningiomas		15/16 (94)	16/16 (100)†
Neuroendocrine tumors			
GEP tumors			
Differentiated		11/11 (100)	11/11 (100)
Undifferentiated		3/6 (50)	0/6 (0)
Pheochromocytomas		10/18 (55)	13/18 (72)
MTC		0/14 (0)	6/14 (43)
Neuroblastomas		8/14 (57)	12/14 (86)
Pituitary adenomas			
GH producing		5/19 (26)	19/19 (100)†
Inactive		16/19 (84)	8/19 (42)
Lymphomas		11/19 (58)	17/19 (89)
Ewing's sarcoma		0/10 (0)	0/10 (0)†

*Somatostatin receptor (*SS-R*) measured with ^{125}I-[Tyr3]-octreotide.

†These results were taken from previous studies.

Abbreviations: VIP-R, vasoactive intestinal peptide receptor; *ca,* carcinoma; *P,* primary; *M,* metastasis; *GH,* growth hormone; *NT,* not tested; *nSCLC,* non–small-cell lung cancer; *SCLC,* small-cell lung cancer; *GEP,* gastroenteropancreatic; *MTC,* medullary thyroid carcinomas.

(Reprinted by permission of the Society of Nuclear Medicine, from Reubi JC: In vitro identification of vasoactive intestinal peptide receptors in human tumors: Implications for tumor imaging. *J Nucl Med* 36:1846–1853, 1995.)

TABLE 2.—Lack of Cross-competition Between Vasoactive Intestinal Peptide and Somatostatin

Tissue*	^{125}I-[Tyr3]-octreotide binding		^{125}I-VIP binding	
	IC$_{50}$ for VIP (nM)	IC$_{50}$ for PACAP (nM)	IC$_{50}$ for SS-14 (nM)	IC$_{50}$ for octreotide (nM)
Tumoral				
Carcinoids, colon ca, islet cell ca, breast ca, neuroblastomas, pheochromocytomas, prostate ca, ovarian ca, endometrial ca, astrocytomas, pituitary adenomas	> 1000	> 1000	> 1000	> 1000
Nontumoral				
Gut mucosa, gut vessels, prostate, peritumoral vessels	> 1000	> 1000	> 1000	> 1000

*Three to 8 different samples of each tissue type listed were investigated for somatostatin receptor (SS-R) or vasoactive intestinal peptide receptor (VIP-R) binding. IC$_{50}$ values for the 4 peptides were calculated. In these experiments, the displacement capacity of each peptide was compared with the 5- to 7-point displacement curve of the radioligand by its corresponding unlabeled analogue. Nonspecific binding: 10^{-6} M of unlabeled octreotide and VIP, respectively.

Abbreviations: ca, carcinoma; *IC$_{50}$,* peptide dose required for 50% binding inhibition; *PACAP,* pituitary adenylate cyclase–activating polypeptide; *SS-14,* somatostatin analogue.

(Reprinted by permission of the Society of Nuclear Medicine, from Reubi JC: In vitro identification of vasoactive intestinal peptide receptors in human tumors: Implications for tumor imaging, *J Nucl Med* 36:1846–1853, 1995.)

colonic, and pancreatic cancers, as well as in neuroendocrine and brain tumors. Labeled VIP analogues are of great potential value for in vivo tumor localization.

Neuropeptide Receptors in Health and Disease: The Molecular Basis for In Vivo Imaging

Reubi JC (Univ of Berne, Switzerland)
J Nucl Med 36:1825–1835, 1995   2–3

Introduction.—Spurred by the development of somatostatin, interest in neuropeptides among nuclear medicine physicians has grown in recent years. Interpretation of neuropeptide imaging data requires a basic under-standing of the somatostatin receptors (SS-Rs) and the conditions under which they are expressed. Current knowledge of the biology of SS-Rs under normal and pathologic conditions was reviewed, including a com-parison of the in vitro and in vivo data. Some newer neuropeptides were discussed as well.

Neuropeptides and In Vitro Detection.—The neuropeptides are synthe-sized primarily in the brain, although there is growing evidence that they are also synthesized in nonneuronal tissues. Their multiple production sites reflect their many actions in regulating essential biological processes (Table 1). Current knowledge regarding the neuropeptide receptors comes from in vitro studies using biochemical, molecular biological, in situ hy-bridization, and immunologic techniques. In normal tissues, the actions of somatostatin are mediated by specific membrane receptors on the target cells. Cells in many different areas have been found to express SS-Rs, from

TABLE 1.—Major Neuropeptides (Including Gut and Pituitary Peptides and Hypothalamic Releasing Hormones)

Opioid peptides	Bradykinin
Substance P	Bombesin/Gastrin-releasing peptide
Gastrin	Neuropeptide Y
Cholecystokinin	Galanin
Vasoactive intestinal peptide	Atrial natriuretic factor
Pituitary adenylate cyclase activating peptide	Neurotensin
Alpha-melanocyte-stimulating hormone	Secretin
Arginine-vasopressin	Melatonin
Oxytocin	Somatostatin
Angiotensin	Thyrothropin-releasing hormone
Insulin	Luteinizing hormone-releasing hormone
Calcitonin	Corticotropin-releasing factor
Endothelin	Growth hormone-releasing factor

(Reprinted by permission of the Society of Nuclear Medicine, from Reubi JC: Neuropeptide receptors in health and disease: The molecular basis for in vivo imaging. *J Nucl Med* 36:1825–1835, 1995.)

the brain to the gastrointestinal mucosa, the peripheral nervous system, and the immune and vascular systems. In tumors originating from somatostatin target tissues, SS-Rs are often expressed at a high density (Table 3). These tumors sometimes express differing SS-R subtypes; the most frequent of these is SSTR2, which also has the highest affinity for octreotide. So far, however, little is known regarding the effects of octreotide therapy on the growth of SS-R-positive tumors. The in vitro data on SS-Rs in nontumoral diseases were reviewed as well.

In Vitro/In Vivo Correlations.—Correlative studies in patients with cancer suggest that the results of in vivo SS-R imaging match up well with the in vitro SS-R status of resected tissues. The correlation is especially good for tumors with a high density and homogeneous distribution of SS-Rs. Substantial discrepancies are noted in some tumor types, including breast tumors, non–small-cell lung cancers, and glioblastomas. The reasons for false negative and false positive in vitro and in vivo studies were discussed (Table 4), as were the in vitro/in vivo correlations in nontumoral tissues and normal tissues.

Emerging Neuropeptides.—Some types of tumors do not express SS-Rs, leading to the search for other neuropeptide receptors. Some of these have shown potential value for in vivo imaging, such as vasoactive intestinal peptide receptors. These receptors occur in a wide range of cancer cell types and are found more frequently than SS-Rs (Fig 5). Other studies have looked at the potential of substance P receptor and alpha-melanocyte–stimulating hormone receptor imaging.

Summary.—In vitro studies of neuropeptide receptors play a key role in the development of neuropeptide analogues for imaging purposes. Further advances will require in vitro studies of the disease conditions in which neuropeptide receptors are expressed, the development of stable neuropeptide analogues with adequate circulatory clearance, and direct comparisons of the in vitro and in vivo findings. Somatostatin receptor imaging has become a standard procedure in nuclear medicine, and vasoactive intesti-

---

TABLE 3.—Human Tumors That Express Somatostatin Receptors

Neuroendocrine tumors	High incidence
Pituitary adenomas, islet cell tumors, carcinoids, paraganglioma(s), medullary thyroid carcinomas, pheochromocytomas, small-cell lung cancers	
Tumors of the nervous system	High incidence
Astrocytomas, neuroblastomas, medulloblastomas, meningiomas	
Renal cell carcinomas	High incidence
Malignant lymphomas	High incidence
Breast cancers	About 50%
Ovarian and colonic cancers	Low incidence

Note: Data were obtained with in vitro ligand binding and autoradiographic studies with radiolabeled Tyr^3-octreotide.

(Reprinted by permission of the Society of Nuclear Medicine, from Reubi JC: Neuropeptide receptors in health and disease: The molecular basis for in vivo imaging. *J Nucl Med* 36:1825–1835, 1995.)

TABLE 4.—List of Potential Reasons for False Somatostatin Receptor Tumor Status In Vitro or In Vivo

False negative in vitro status
Tumors with low cellularity and low SS-R density
Tumors with high endogenous SS production (SSoma, MTC, pheo)
Tumors with SS-R subtypes, not recognized by certain ligands (i.e., octreotide)
Tumors with nonhomogeneous SS-R distribution (breast tumors)
Technical
  Loss of SS-R
  Long delay between removal and freezing of sample
  Uncontrolled thawing of frozen sample
Tumors with high nonspecific binding
Poorly representative sample
  Low tumor-to-stroma ratio
  Metastasis rather than PT
Patient undergoing drug therapy (i.e., corticosteroid)

False positive in vitro status
SS-R analysis with tissue homogenates (uncontrolled contamination with nontumoral SS-R-positive tissues)

False negative in vivo status
Tumors with low cellularity and low SS-R density
Tumors with high endogenous SS production (SSoma, MTC, pheo)
Tumors with SS-R subtypes, not recognized by certain ligands (i.e., octreotide)
Tumors located in region with high background
Tumors located inside intact blood-brain barrier (poor ligand permeability)

False positive in vivo status
Tumors located inside disturbed blood-brain barrier (nonspecific trapping of ligand)
Identification of nontumoral SS-R-positive tissues (activated lymphocytes, vessels and granulomas)
Binding to antibodies against chronically injected octreotide (seldom)

Abbreviations: SS-R, somatostatin receptor; *SSoma,* somatostatinoma; *MTC,* medullary thyroid cancers; *pheo,* pheochromocytomas; *PT,* primary tumor.
(Reprinted by permission of the Society of Nuclear Medicine, from Reubi JC: Neuropeptide receptors in health and disease: The molecular basis for in vivo imaging. *J Nucl Med* 36:1825–1835, 1995.)

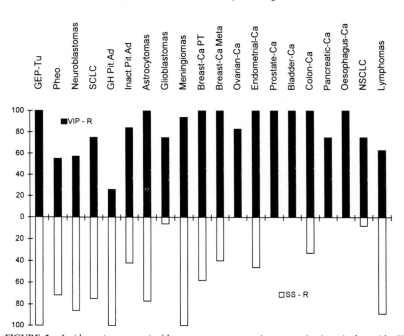

Incidence (%) of human tumors expressing VIP - R or SS - R

FIGURE 5.—Incidence (percentage) of human tumors expressing vasoactive intestinal peptide (*VIP*) receptors (in comparison with somatostatin receptors [SS-Rs] identified in the same tumors). *Abbreviations: GEP*, gastroenteropancreatic tumor; *Pheo*, pheochromocytoma; *SCLC*, small-cell lung cancer; *GH Pit. Ad*, growth hormone pituitary adenoma; *CA*, cancer; *PT*, primary tumor; *Meta*, metastasis; *NSCLC*, non–small-cell lung cancer. (Adapted from Reubi JC: In vitro identification of vasoactive intestinal peptide receptors in human tumors: Implications for tumor imaging. *J Nucl Med* 36:1846–1853, 1995. Reprinted by permission of the Society of Nuclear Medicine, from Reubi JC: Neuropeptide receptors in health and disease: The molecular basis for in vivo imaging. *J Nucl Med* 36:1825–1835, 1995.)

nal peptide receptor imaging may be developed along the same lines. Other neuropeptides may soon become target candidates for in vivo imaging.

▶ Tumor scintigraphy is becoming increasingly sophisticated as the result of new knowledge of surface receptors present on tumor cells. The best known example is, of course, gallium-67 scintigraphy, which depends, in large part, on the presence of transferrin receptors. The newer agent indium-111–octreotide is useful because it binds to some of the somatostatin receptors. Understanding these mechanisms enables one to pick the best radiopharmaceutical for a particular patient's tumor imaging needs. Abstracts 2–1 to 2–3 present the story of yet another cell receptor, VIP, including the results of an early scintigraphy study using a radiopharmaceutical created particularly to bind to the VIP receptor and an excellent review of the field of the so-called neuropeptide receptors from the standpoint of imaging.

R. Neumann, M.D.

Radiolocalization of Squamous Lung Carcinoma With ^{131}I-labeled Epidermal Growth Factor

Cuartero-Plaza A, Martínez-Miralles E, Rosell R, et al (Universitat Autònoma de Barcelona; Hosp Universitari del Mar, Barcelona; Hosp Germans Trias i Pujol, Badalona, Spain)
Clin Cancer Res 2:13–20, 1996   2–4

Introduction.—In Western countries, non–small-cell lung carcinomas constitute more than 70% of all lung cancers. New opportunities for improved diagnosis or therapy are provided by the recognition of the molecular abnormalities that participate in the development of tumors. In squamous carcinomas, there has been a demonstration of overexpression of epidermal growth factor receptor. Radiolabeled anti-epidermal growth factor receptor monoclonal antibodies have been shown to localize to these tumors. The tolerance, pharmacokinetics, and radiolocalization properties of iodine-131–labeled epidermal growth factor were determined in patients with advanced squamous cell carcinoma.

Methods.—Iodine-131–labeled epidermal growth factor was administered IV over 4 hours to 9 patients with advanced squamous cell carcinoma. For 3 days, their vital signs were monitored and daily scintigrams and biological samples for pharmacokinetic analysis were taken. Patients with positive tumor scans had technetium-99m–labeled human serum albumin administered.

Results.—Positive tumor scans were seen in 6 patients and 4 had received more than 1 mg of epidermal growth factor. Tumors were visualized the same day of the infusion; however, the best images were obtained at 50–74 hours. No false positive images were found. With increasing epidermal growth factor doses, whole-body radioactivity retention rose significantly. Urinary excretion eliminated most epidermal growth factor. During the course of the study, tumor:normal tissue uptake ratios increased. There were self-limited, dose-related gastrointestinal adverse effects with all patients.

Conclusion.—Recombinant epidermal growth factor can localize to non–small-cell lung carcinoma efficiently. It has more favorable pharmacokinetic properties than monoclonal antibodies and can be administered safely to patients. To examine the potential of epidermal growth factor and epidermal growth factor–related peptides in the imaging and/or therapy of epidermal growth factor receptor–overexpressing human cancers, more studies are needed.

▶ In addition to the large group of neuropeptide receptors described in the earlier papers, tumor cells have a myriad of other cell-membrane receptors that in theory at least could be targeted by radioligands developed as radiopharmaceuticals for scintigraphy and/or therapy. For example, epidermal growth factor receptor is overexpressed (expressed far in excess of normal) by many squamous-cell carcinomas. In this paper, a radioiodinated form of the natural ligand epidermal growth factor was used in patients with non–small-cell lung cancers in a phase I study. The investigators report that this recombinant radioiodine-labeled epidermal growth factor was safe to administer, localized in squamous lung cancers efficiently, and had better pharmacokinetic properties than radiolabeled monoclonal antibodies.

The rising incidence of lung cancers worldwide will require inexpensive, accurate staging techniques for this disease. Perhaps radiopharmaceuticals of this type will find broad application.

R. Neumann, M.D.

Technetium-99m-Sestamibi Scintimammography of Breast Lesions: Clinical and Pathological Follow-up

Khalkhali I, Cutrone J, Mona I, et al (Univ of California, Los Angeles, Torrance)
J Nucl Med 36:1784–1789, 1995   2–5

Objective.—Because mammography has low positive predictive values for both palpable and nonpalpable breast lesions, expensive biopsies with significant concomitant morbidity are frequently necessary. The effectiveness of technetium-99m–labeled sestamibi scintimammography as a complementary technique to mammography for the detection of breast cancer was studied, and a preliminary report of the status of axillary metastasis in patients with breast cancer was reviewed.

Methods.—Mammography and scintimammography after an injection of 20 mCi of ^{99m}Tc-labeled sestamibi were done in 100 women (mean age, 48 years) with 85 palpable and 21 nonpalpable lesions. All nonpalpable lesions were excised, and fine-needle aspiration was done on palpable lesions. Results were correlated and images were evaluated by 2 blinded investigators. An area of increased focal uptake on scintimammography was considered to be carcinoma.

Results.—There were 28 palpable and 2 nonpalpable lesions pathologically confirmed to be carcinoma. Mammography showed abnormal masses in 20 lesions, microcalcification without masses in 3, asymmetric density in 6, and no abnormal findings in 1. Scintimammography showed increased focal uptake in all malignant lesions. In the 65 lesions confirmed pathologically to be nonmalignant, 49 were palpable and 16 were nonpalpable. Mammography showed abnormal masses in 41 lesions, microcalcification in 4, asymmetric density in 7, and no findings in 13. Scintimammographic findings were negative in all cases. Scintimammography findings of focal areas of increased uptake proved to be benign in 9 lesions (7 palpable and 2 nonpalpable). Mammography showed 7 abnormal masses and 2 lesions with microcalcifications. Scintimammography gave false negative results for 2 malignant lesions, 1 a nonpalpable cluster of microcalcifications with no mass. This latter lesion was visualized by mammography. Scintimammography had a sensitivity of 93.7%, a specificity of 87.8%, a positive predictive value of 76.9%, and a negative predictive value of 97%. Its sensitivity for palpable lesions was 96.5% and its specificity was 87.5%; for nonpalpable lesions, sensitivity was 66.6% and specificity was 88.8%

Conclusion.—Scintimammography, because it has a higher sensitivity and specificity for detecting breast cancer than does conventional mammography, reduces the need for breast biopsies.

Technetium-99m-MIBI Scintimammography for Suspicious Breast Lesions
Palmedo H, Schomburg A, Grünwald F, et al (Univ of Bonn, Germany)
J Nucl Med 37:626–630, 1996   2–6

Objective.—Conventional mammography has a low positive predictive value for breast cancer and a low sensitivity in patients with dense breasts. In some studies, technetium-99m–labeled sestamibi has been shown to distinguish between benign and malignant breast tumors, although it appears to be less sensitive for small tumors. The diagnostic accuracy of ^{99m}Tc-labeled sestamibi in primary breast cancer and lymph node metastases comparing SPECT with planar imaging was studied.

Methods.—Planar and SPECT imaging studies were done in 54 women aged 22–81 years with suspicious lesions, after injection of 740 MBq of ^{99m}Tc-labeled sestamibi into the arm contralateral to the involved breast. Focal accumulation of tracer was considered abnormal. All lesions were excised.

Results.—Adenocarcinoma was diagnosed pathologically in 24 women. Scintigraphy found 21 malignancies, 20 of them palpable. For planar imaging, the overall sensitivity was 88% and overall specificity was 83%. For SPECT, corresponding values were 83% and 80%. Forty lesions were palpable and 14 were nonpalpable. Tumor diameters ranged from 6 to 90 mm. Sensitivity and specificity of ^{99m}Tc-labeled sestamibi for palpable lesions were 100% and 80% and for nonpalpable lesions were 25% and 90%. There were 3 false negative results with normal planar and SPECT images. Conventional mammography was normal for 1 of these tumors, and MRI was equivocal. Five patients had false positive findings on planar and SPECT images. The smallest tumor detected, 9 mm, was seen on planar imaging only. One patient with fibrocystic disease also had a false positive finding on SPECT image. Scintimammography detected cancer in 2 patients with dense breasts whose mammograms were equivocal. Nine of 11 patients with axillary lymph node metastases had positive findings on scintigrams, for a sensitivity of 82%. There were 2 false positive findings on axillary SPECT images but no false positive findings on planar images. Specificities were 100% for axillary SPECT images and 94% for planar images.

Conclusion.—Scintimammography with ^{99m}Tc-labeled sestamibi is a sensitive method for detecting palpable breast cancer. Single-photon emission CT and planar images are equally accurate.

Dynamic Indium-111-Pentetreotide Scintigraphy in Breast Cancer

Bajc M, Ingvar C, Palmer J (Lund Univ, Sweden)
J Nucl Med 37:622–626, 1996   2–7

Objective.—Because some breast cancers may express somatostatin receptors, such expression may be useful as a tumor regulator and a prognostic factor. The efficacy of indium-111–pentetreotide breast imaging and whether breast cancer expresses somatostatin receptors were evaluated in a study that also examined the relation of the somatostatin receptor to the histopathology and to estrogen (ER) or progesterone receptor (PgR).

Methods.—After an IV injection of 110 MBq of ^{111}In-pentetreotide, whole-body scintigraphy was done in 24 patients (2 men) aged 36–83 years with confirmed invasive breast cancer, and in 8 controls at 0.5, 5, and 24 hours after injection. Anterior and posterior images were obtained simultaneously. Increased uptake of tracer was considered abnormal. Estrogen receptor and PgR were detected using an enzyme immunoassay.

Results.—Twenty patients had 21 confirmed infiltrative ductal carcinomas, and 4 had confirmed infiltrative lobular carcinomas. Tumor size ranged from 7 to 90 mm. There was increased uptake of tracer in all 19 specimens (18 patients) studied. Somatostatin receptors were found in all specimens but intensity distribution varied. Scintigraphy allowed visualization of 16 ductal carcinomas and 3 lobular carcinomas at 0.5 hour. Single-photon emission CT provided additional information in 1 patient who had increased liver uptake. Whereas 8 patients with positive scans had increased uptake in the uninvolved breast at each study point and 2 other patients with positive scans had increased uptake in the uninvolved breast at 5 hours, only 1 patient had bilateral breast cancer. Scintigraphy made it possible to locate the tumor in a specific quadrant in all patients with positive scans. Scintigraphy showed increased axillary uptake in 7 of 14 patients with lymph node involvement. Nodes in 8 patients were negative by pathology. Four of 8 control patients had increased tracer uptake in both breasts at 5 hours. Patients with breast cancer had a significantly higher breast index compared with control patients. Findings in 11 patients were positive for ER, and findings in 12 patients were positive for PgR. There was no relation between ER or PgR and somatostatin receptors.

Conclusions.—A higher incidence of somatostatin receptor expression was found in patients with breast cancer than in controls. Early pentetreotide scintigraphy selectively visualizes masses in patients with high somatostatin density. Bilateral uptake increases with time even in patients with unilateral disease.

The Use of Thallium-201 in the Preoperative Detection of Breast Cancer: An Adjunct to Mammography and Ultrasonography
Cimitan M, Volpe R, Candiani E, et al (Centro di Riferimento Oncologico-IRCCS, Aviano, Italy)
Eur J Nucl Med 22:1110–1117, 1995   2–8

Objective.—Because mammography can give false negative results in women with dense or dysplastic breasts and ultrasonography is unable to distinguish benign from malignant lesions, there is interest in developing thallium-201 scintigraphy to differentiate benign and malignant disease. A ^{201}Tl scintigraphy study of a large number of patients to complement mammography and ultrasonography in the assessment of breast abnormalities and an analysis of various pathologic features of malignant lesions to determine a possible association with ^{201}Tl uptake by tumor cells was reviewed.

Methods.—After the injection of 110 MBq of ^{201}Tl chloride, scintigraphy was done in 72 patients, aged 31–82 years, with suspicious breast abnormalities, at 10 minutes and 3 hours. Results were interpreted by 3 blinded nuclear medicine physicians. After surgical excision of the lesions, pathologic features, including estrogen and progesterone receptor status, were determined.

Results.—Of the 76 lesions examined, 56 were malignant, ranging in size from 0.6 to 6 cm. Mammography gave 7 false negative results, but on ultrasonography, 87% of images were abnormal. In 51 of 56 tumors, ^{201}Tl uptake was greater than in surrounding normal tissue. Optimal visualization was achieved at 3 hours for 17 tumors. The 20 benign lesions, including 1 ductal hyperplasia and 6 atypical lesions, yielded negative results on ^{201}Tl scan, with 1 exception that showed a tumor-to-background ratio of 1.33. Mammography results were suspicious in 60% of these lesions and ultrasonography in 70%. Sensitivity and specificity for ^{201}Tl were 91% and 95%; for mammography, 87% and 40%; and for ultrasonography, 94% and 26%. Accuracy was 92% for ^{201}Tl imaging, 74% for mammographic imaging, and 75% for ultrasonography. Thallium intensity varied between 1.2 and 2.5. Four of 5 false negative ^{201}Tl scans were of lesions smaller than 1.5 cm; none of these patients had lymph node involvement. There was no association between ^{201}Tl uptake and tumor grade, invasiveness, or receptor status. Thallium imaging allowed visualization of only 6 of 22 cases of axillary lymph node involvement, whereas 7 of 31 patients without lymph node involvement had false positive scans.

Conclusions.—Thallium-201 breast scans are a useful adjunct to mammography and ultrasonography. Sensitivity of thallium scans for malignant lesions greater than 1.5 cm was 97%; for lesions 1.5 cm or less, it was 80%. The accuracy was 92% for ^{201}Tl imaging, 74% for mammographic imaging, and 75% for ultrasonography.

▶ The problems with primary breast cancer detection by x-ray mammography usually occur in patients with extensive fibrocystic disease, which results in "dense" mammograms capable of "hiding" the small changes typical of early cancers. For this reason, there is extensive work under way to validate scintimammography. The most promising results are highlighted by these 4 papers (Abstracts 2–5 to 2–8), which report on the use of ^{99m}Tc-sestamibi, ^{111}In-pentetreotide, and ^{201}Tl chloride. In addition, particular methods and gamma camera modifications have been reported to increase the likelihood that nuclear medicine can make a significant contribution in detecting this disease at an early stage.

R. Neumann, M.D.

Positron Tomographic Assessment of Estrogen Receptors in Breast Cancer: Comparison With FDG-PET and In Vitro Receptor Assays
Dehdashti F, Mortimer JE, Siegel BA, et al (Washington Univ, St Louis; Univ of Illinois, Urbana)
J Nucl Med 36:1766–1774, 1995   2–9

Background.—The findings of a recent experimental study suggested that FDG uptake may serve as an index of the level of functional stimulation of tumor estrogen receptors (ERs) in some circumstances. Tumor FDG uptake determined by PET also has been found to correlate well with the aggressiveness of several types of tumors, such as primary brain tumors, malignant lymphomas, and breast cancer. Thus, the ER status of breast cancer may be associated with its FDG tumor uptake. It was hypothesized that ER-positive tumors, with a better prognosis, would have lower tumor FDG uptake than more aggressive ER-negative tumors.

Methods.—Thirty-two patients with primary breast masses and 21 with clinical or radiologic evidence of recurrent or metastatic breast carcinoma were studied. Twenty-four primary, 15 metastatic, and 4 recurrent carcinomas subsequently were diagnosed. Estrogen receptor status in 40 malignancies was known. Both 16α-[^{18}F]fluoro-17β-estradiol (FES) and FDG PET were performed. The uptake of each tracer in each lesion was assessed qualitatively and semiqualitatively.

Findings.—The overall agreement between in vitro ER assays and FES PET was 88%, which is similar to that among replicate in vitro assays. However, no significant associations were found between tumor FDG uptake and ER status or between tumor FDG and tumor FES uptake.

Conclusions.—In agreement with previous findings, FES PET reliably determines ER status in breast tumors. Changes in ER-positive tumors that are useful for assessing tumor response to treatment may occur in FDG uptake after hormonal treatment. Further research is needed to test this hypothesis.

Investigations of Breast Tumors With Fluorine-18-fluorodeoxyglucose and SPECT
Holle L-H, Trampert L, Lung-Kurt S, et al (Univ Clinics of Saarland, Hamburg/ Saar, Germany)
J Nucl Med 37:615–622, 1996   2–10

Background.—Because of the cost and limited availability of PET, alternatives have been sought for imaging FDG. The efficacy of a commercially available dual-head gamma camera with specially designed high-energy collimators in the assessment of breast tumors of unknown histology was investigated.

Methods and Findings.—Fifty women 20–82 years of age with breast tumors of unknown histology were included. A combined FDG SPECT and whole-body technique was used. Malignancy was identified accurately in all patients with tumors of more than 2.3 cm. The smallest FDG-positive lesion was 1.4 cm. In a subgroup of patients, adding quantitative assessment improved sensitivity. Lymph node metastases were identified accurately in 9 of 13 patients. The detection of distant metastases depended on lesion size and location. False positive FDG findings were obtained in inflamed tissue, in a rapidly growing phyllodes tumor, and in supposedly healthy breast tissue.

Conclusions.—The combined whole-body FDG scans and FDG SPECT with a dual-head gamma camera can image primary and metastatic breast cancer, providing added information in uncertain cases. Thus, FDG SPECT and whole-body image acquisition may be adequate for meeting the increasing demand for FDG examinations.

Fluorine-18-Fluorodeoxyglucose-guided Breast Cancer Surgery With a Positron-sensitive Probe: Validation in Preclinical Studies
Raylman RR, Fisher SJ, Brown RS, et al (Univ of Michigan, Ann Arbor)
J Nucl Med 36:1869–1874, 1995   2–11

Background.—The use of PET with FDG has recently been found to be successful in the imaging of many breast tumors and tumor-involved lymph nodes. The feasibility of using FDG with a positron-sensitive intraoperative probe to guide breast tumor excision was explored further.

Methods.—The probe consisted of a plastic scintillator tip coupled with a photomultiplier tube with fiberoptic cable. Anticipated resolution degradation was assessed by measuring line spread functions in the presence of background radiation. A human torso phantom and cardiac insert were used to simulate realistic photon background distributions. Optimal discriminator settings were based on measures of the relationship between resolution and energy threshold. Probe sensitivity as a function of energy threshold was determined for simulated tumors of various sizes. Breast cancer localization in vivo was assessed in a rodent model.

Findings.—Resolution was maximized in a realistic background photon environment by increasing the energy threshold to levels at or above the Compton continuum edge. At this setting, the sensitivity of the probe was 58 cps/μmCi for simulated tumors of 3.18 mm in diameter and 11 cps/μmCi for simulated tumors of 6.35 mm in diameter. Probe readings were well correlated with histologic findings. In general, the probe could discriminate between tumor and normal tissue.

Conclusions.—A β-sensitive probe using energy thresholding seems appropriate for FDG-guided breast cancer surgery. Patient trials are now needed to confirm its suitability for surgical excision guidance.

▶ Breast cancer is receiving increasing attention, and certainly nuclear medicine is no exception. We are suddenly developing the radiopharmaceuticals, instruments, and methodologies to detect and monitor both primary and metastatic breast cancers.

The paper by Dehdashti et al. (Abstract 2–9) reports their work using both ^{18}F-FDG and ^{18}F-fluoro-17-estriol, which they developed as a PET method to determine the estrogen receptor status of breast cancers. Wahl [1] postulated that changes may occur in breast cancer FDG uptake after hormonal treatment of estrogen receptor–positive tumors; these changes may be useful as an assessment of tumor response to treatment. Now the stage is set for such studies.

The paper by Holle and associates (Abstract 2–10) examines the efficacy of a commercially available dual-head SPECT camera with specially designed high-energy collimators for the assessment of breast tumors. Handheld intraoperative detectors are also under development for PET energies. The paper by Raylman et al. (Abstract 2–11) reports on the feasibility of using FDG with such a probe to guide breast cancer excisional surgery.

R. Neumann, M.D.

Reference

1. Wahl RL, Zasadny K, Helvie M, et al: Metabolic monitoring of breast cancer chemotherapy using positron emission tomography: Initial evaluation. *J Clin Oncol* 11:2101–2111, 1993.

Detection of Malignancies With SPECT Versus PET, With 2-[Fluorine-18] Fluoro-2-deoxy-D-glucose
Martin WH, Delbeke D, Patton JA, et al (Vanderbilt Univ, Nashville, Tenn)
Radiology 198:225–231, 1996   2–12

Background.—Increasing evidence suggests that FDG PET may be more accurate than CT and other imaging modalities in selected patients with suspected malignancies, especially those with indeterminate lesions in the lung, liver, or pancreas. However, FDG PET is costly and not widely available. The diagnostic accuracy of FDG SPECT was compared with that of FDG PET in the assessment of malignancies.

Methods.—Twenty-four patients aged 28–77 years with known or suspected malignancies underwent sequential FDG PET and FDG SPECT. The studies were performed with fluorine-18 sodium fluoride in a cylindric phantom containing different-sized spheres with activity ratios of 5:1, 10:1, and 15:1.

Findings.—The volume sensitivity of PET was 2.238 cpm/μmCi and of SPECT, 270 cpm/μmCi. The SPECT spatial resolution was 17 mm at full width at half maximum, whereas the spatial resolution for PET was 6.5 mm. In the phantom studies, a ratio of 5:1 detected a lesion 1.5 cm or more in diameter, and a ratio of 10:1 detected a lesion 1.3 cm or more in diameter, with an information density of 150 counts/cm^2. In patients, 46 hypermetabolic lesions consistent with tumor were visualized by FDG PET, compared with 36 by FDG SPECT. The sensitivity of FDG SPECT was 92% for detecting malignancies of 1.8 cm or more in diameter visualized by FDG PET.

Conclusions.—According to these limited study data, FDG SPECT can provide diagnostic data comparable to those of FDG PET for malignancies 1.8 cm or more in diameter, particularly in patients who are not undergoing concurrent chemotherapy. This modality may detect smaller lesions if the lesion-to-background ratio is 5.1 or greater or the tumor is superficial.

Phase I Study of Rhenium-186-HEDP in Patients With Bone Metastases Originating From Breast Cancer

de Klerk JMH, van het Schip AD, Zonnenberg BA, et al (Univ Hosp Utrecht, The Netherlands)
J Nucl Med 37:244–249, 1996   2–13

Objective.—Bone pain associated with metastatic breast cancer is a serious and common symptom. Palliative treatment by localized external-beam therapy or hemibody irradiation is complicated by the presence of multiple pain sites. Targeted radionuclide therapy offers many advantages. The maximum tolerated dose of rhenium-186 in patients with symptomatic bone metastases originating from breast cancer was determined.

Methods.—Rhenium-186–hydroxyethylidene diphosphonate (HEDP) was administered in escalating doses, beginning at 1,295 MBq and increasing in increments of 555 MBq, to 12 patients aged 36–64 years, with at least 4 bone metastases each. Toxicity, pharmacologic effects, bone scan index, leukocyte count, platelet count, and alkaline phosphatase levels were determined.

Results.—Patients reported no acute side effects, but 6 had a transient pain flare lasting 1–3 days. Platelet and leukocyte toxicity was limited to grade 2 for patients receiving doses of 2,385 MBq or less. Patients receiving 2,960 MBq had grade 3 and 4 platelet toxicity. Bone scan indices ranged from 8 to 48. No renal or hepatic toxicity was observed. Seven patients with elevated alkaline phosphatase levels before treatment had a transient decline during the first 4 weeks of treatment.

Conclusion.—The maximum tolerated dose of [186]Re-HEDP in patients with symptomatic bone metastases was 2,405 MBq. Thrombocytopenia was a serious side effect at higher doses.

Radioiodine Breast Uptake in Nonbreastfeeding Women: Clinical and Scintigraphic Characteristics

Hammami MM, Bakheet S (King Faisal Specialist Hosp, Riyadh, Saudi Arabia)
J Nucl Med 37:26–31, 1996   2–14

Objective.—Radioiodine breast uptake has been studied in breast-feeding women but not in non–breast-feeding women being treated for differentiated thyroid cancer. The scintigraphic characteristics of radioiodine breast uptake in nonlactating women and the prevalence of galactorrhea and elevated prolactin levels were prospectively studied.

Methods.—Whole-body radioiodine scans were obtained for 23 nonlactating women with radioiodine breast uptake 24 hours after administration of 185 MBq of iodine-123 and 3 days after administration of a therapeutic dose of iodine-131 for postablation scans. Although uptake was not quantified, breast intensity was related to residual thyroid intensity. Levels of thyroid-stimulating hormone, thyroglobulin, prolactin, and free T4 were determined.

Results.—The incidence of radioiodine breast uptake in nonlactating women was estimated to be at least 6%. Patterns of breast uptake included full, focal, crescentic, and irregular. Two patients had unilateral uptake. Although pattern and location of uptake were characteristic in most women, uptake resembled lung metastasis in 9. Ten of 21 patients had galactorrhea and 4 of 17 patients had elevated prolactin levels. No consistent differences were found in either uptake patterns or intensity between patients with normal or elevated prolactin levels or between patients with and without expressible galactorrhea and patients not checked for galactorrhea. On follow-up scans, only 1 of 14 patients showed no breast uptake, suggesting that uptake was not related to time elapsed since discontinuing breast-feeding. Approximately 75% of patients had uptake in both ^{123}I and ^{131}I scans, but no consistent uptake patterns were observed.

Conclusion.—Although the reason for breast uptake in nonlactating women is unknown, breast uptake should be investigated, even in the absence of breast-feeding, if accumulation of radioiodine is found in scans of patients being treated for thyroid cancer.

Radioactive Iodine Treatment and External Radiotherapy for Lung and Bone Metastases From Thyroid Carcinoma

Schlumberger M, Challeton C, De Vathaire F, et al (Institut Gustave-Roussy, Villejuif, France)

J Nucl Med 37:598–605, 1996   2–15

Objective.—Retrospective studies provide indirect evidence that iodine-131 treatment improves the survival of patients with distant metastases of differentiated thyroid carcinoma. To follow up on results of a study of 394 patients with lung and bone metastases showing that administration of ^{131}I is beneficial, other treatment modalities for patients with massive metastatic dissemination were studied.

Methods.—The median follow-up was 50 months. A whole-body scan was done once a year for 2 years and then every 5 years unless uptake indicated residual metastatic disease. The scan was repeated in 3–6 months. Each scan was performed 5 days after administration of 100 mCi of ^{131}I to adults or 1 mCi of ^{131}I per kg to children.

Results.—Metastases were found in 47% of patients at the beginning of treatment and in the other 53% after 6 months to 41 years later. Twenty-two percent of the latter patients had a neck relapse before metastatic disease was discovered. Bone metastases only were found in 27% of patients, and bone and lung metastases were seen in 18%. Lung metastases only were found in 75% of patients with papillary carcinoma and in 41% with follicular carcinoma. Lung metastases only were found in 94% of patients younger than 20 years and in 30% of patients older than 60 years. Whole-body scans found metastases in 67% of patients. After treatment, 124 patients had a complete response, and 108 of these had lung metastases only. The other 16 patients had a single localized bony metastasis. Prognostic survival factors were younger age, ^{131}I uptake by metastases, and limited extent of disease. The survival rates for complete response were 96% at 5 years, 93% at 10 years, and 89% at 15 years. The corresponding survival rates for patients who did not achieve a complete response were 37%, 14%, and 8%. Nineteen secondary malignancies were found in 16 patients with metastatic differentiated thyroid carcinoma.

Conclusions.—Patients with thyroid carcinoma who are treated for early discovered distant metastases have improved survival if their metastases accumulate ^{131}I. Prognostic survival factors also include younger age and limited extent of disease.

Fluorine-18 Fluorodeoxyglucose Positron Emission Tomography in the Follow-up of Differentiated Thyroid Cancer

Grünwald F, Schomburg A, Bender H, et al (Univ of Bonn, Germany)

Eur J Nucl Med 23:312–319, 1996   2–16

Background.—Most patients with differentiated thyroid cancer have a very good prognosis, particularly those with primary tumor stages 1 through 3. Because of the relative "benignness" of this malignancy, relatively low FDG PET sensitivity may be expected, especially in highly differentiated thyroid carcinomas. The clinical use of whole-body FDG PET imaging in the follow-up of patients treated with iodine-131 for differentiated thyroid cancer was examined and compared with the findings of other imaging modalities.

Methods and Findings.—Thirty-three patients with differentiated thyroid cancer underwent whole-body FDG PET imaging during follow-up. Twenty-six patients had papillary tumors and 7, follicular tumors. Primary tumor stages were stage 1 in 6 patients, stage 2 in 8, stage 3 in 3, and stage 4 in 14. In 18 patients, FDG PET findings were normal. Three had a slightly increased metabolism in the thyroid bed, assumed to be associated with remnant tissue. Findings from FDG PET showed a local recurrence in 1 patient, lymph node metastases in 10, and distant metastases in 3. There were many discrepancies between imaging results and whole-body scintigraphy (WBS) with [131]I. Three patients had distant metastases proven by ^{131}I and a normal FDG PET, and 4 had ^{131}I-negative lymph node metastases on PET. Differences in lesion localization also were evident, even in patients with concordant staging. The correlation of FDG PET was stronger with technetium-99m MIBI scinitigraphy than with ^{131}I-WBS.

Conclusions.—In the routine follow-up of differentiated thyroid cancer, serum thyroglobulin measurement and ^{131}I-WBS appear sufficient. However, in patients with metastases proven by ^{131}I, a PET scan also should be obtained to localize coexisting ^{131}I-negative metastases, especially in those with poorly differentiated tumors. This is particularly important for the mediastinum, which cannot be examined sonographically. However, a PET scan is not needed when all other imaging and serum thyroglobulin findings are normal.

Early Stage Melanoma: Lymphoscintigraphy, Reproducibility of Sentinel Node Detection, and Effectiveness of the Intraoperative Gamma Probe
Mudun A, Murray DR, Herda SC, et al (Emory Univ, Atlanta, Ga; Veterans Affairs Med Ctr, Atlanta, Ga)
Radiology 199:171–175, 1996   2–17

Objective.—Because of the success of lymphoscintigraphy and gamma probe localization of sentinel nodes (SNs) using large radiolabeled colloids, the reproducibility of the technique in detecting SNs in patients with early-stage malignant melanoma using a modified technetium-99m sulfur colloid preparation and the intraoperative gamma probe was evaluated.

Methods.—Four to six 0.25–0.50-mL intradermal injections of 0.25–0.50 mCi of technetium-99m sulfur colloid were administered to 25 patients (11 men), aged 24–75 years, with malignant melanoma. All patients had had biopsies; 23 had clinical stage I or II melanoma and 2 had recurrent disease. Dynamic images were obtained every 10 seconds for 10 minutes after injection, and static images were obtained thereafter every 5 minutes, for as long as 2 hours. Sentinel node location was marked on the skin with ink in patients undergoing surgical biopsy. Histopathology evaluation was done on biopsy samples. Imaging studies were conducted twice in 13 patients to determine reproducibility.

Results.—Primary melanoma sites were found in the trunk in 12 patients, in the limbs in 9 patients, and in the head and neck in 4 patients. All patients had at least 1 SN. Eight had more than 1 node, and 3 of the 8 had bilateral axillary SNs. The intraoperative gamma probe identified SNs in all patients, and 6 patients were found to have metastatic lymph node disease. In the reproducibility study, SNs were visualized in all 13 patients, and the same SN was found in 11 of the 13. In 3 patients, the number of lymph nodes visualized was not the same in both studies. Ten studies were completely reproducible, including identity and location of SNs and number of drainage pathways.

Conclusion.—Lymphoscintigraphy is a reliable technique for visualizing SNs, and the gamma probe is an effective aid in the surgical management of patients with malignant melanoma.

The Impact of Dynamic Lymphoscintigraphy and Gamma Probe Guidance on Sentinel Node Biopsy in Melanoma
Pijpers R, Collet GJ, Meijer S, et al (Free Univ Hosp, Amsterdam)
Eur J Nucl Med 22:1238–1241, 1995   2–18

Objective.—Identifying the sentinel node (SN), the first tumor-draining lymph node in patients with malignant melanoma, using vital dyes fails in 20% of cases. The usefulness of lymphoscintigraphy and the gamma probe in locating deep-seated nodes was investigated.

Methods.—Immediately after technetium-99m colloidal albumin was injected, lymphoscintigraphy was done in 41 consecutive patients (19 males) aged 17–76 years. The camera followed the flow from the injection site, and the first focal accumulation was assumed to be the SN. After dynamic lymphoscintigraphy, patients were divided into 3 groups. In group A (12 patients), imaging was done 2 hours after injection and, on day 2, 1–2 hours before operation without imaging. The 14 group B patients had static imaging after 18 hours, just before surgery. The 15 group C patients had static imaging 2 hours after dynamic imaging, followed by surgery within 1 day.

Results.—In 39 patients, the SN was visualized within 20 minutes after injection. In 2 patients, SNs were located 2 hours later, after static imaging. Dynamic imaging enabled the visualization of multiple lymphatic channels in 11 of 41 patients. The SN retained the highest fraction of tracer for at least 18 hours. The gamma probe facilitated the location of the best incision site and the location of deep-seated nodes, particularly in the cervical and axillary areas. The most highly radioactive nodes were dye-positive in 53 of 75 biopsies. Nonstained nodes were found in 4 patients, 1 from group B and 3 from group C.

A total of 85 nodes were excised, and 8 were found to contain microscopic metastases. Elective lymph node dissection revealed that the SN was the only cancer-containing node in 4 of the 8 patients in whom it was done.

Conclusions.—Dynamic lymphoscintigraphy successfully localized the SN. The tracer was retained for a sufficient time to permit flexible scheduling of surgery. The gamma probe was useful in locating deep-seated nodes and in helping to determine the optimal excision site. The technique is minimally invasive and easily learned.

Antibody-dependent Signal Amplification in Tumor Xenografts After Pretreatment With Biotinylated Monoclonal Antibody and Avidin or Streptavidin
Kassis AI, Jones PL, Matalka KZ, et al (Harvard Med School, Boston)
J Nucl Med 37:343–352, 1996   2–19

Introduction.—The ability of radiolabeled monoclonal antibodies (MAb) to bind to tumor-associated antigens has been useful in targeting various radionuclides to tumors in both diagnostic and therapeutic settings. One of the biggest limitations in doing this is the low percentage of injected dose per gram of targeted tumor. Target-signal augmentation has recently been used in several systems in which a pair of polymeric molecules with no affinity for each other are bridged with a polymeric molecule with high affinity for both of the other molecules. The abilities of avidin (Av) and streptavidin (SAv) were examined and compared for their ability to amplify the targeted signal after administration of biotinylated MAb.

Methods.—The murine anti-human mammary cancer MAb B72.3 (100 µg) was injected in nude mice. Three days later, mice bearing around 200–300 mg of tumor were used to compare uptake of about 10–500 µg iodine-125–labeled Av or SAv in tumor and normal tissues. Mice were killed 24 hours later to determine the biodistribution of ^{125}I.

Results.—For Av, the percentage of injected dose per gram of tumor was constant throughout a range of injected doses. It varied for SAv. The number of moles of Av and SAv in tumor and normal tissues rose with higher doses of administered Av and SAv. The absolute values of SAv were about 10–20 times those observed for Av. The number of biotin receptor sites for which radiolabeled antibody molecules could bind within the tumor was about 1.8 times higher with SAv than with Av. The tumor-to-normal tissue ratios rose with injections of larger doses of Av but not SAv.

Conclusion.—Streptavidin is the preferred "second-step" reagent in tumor localization analyses. At a dose of 2.5 mg of streptavidin per kilogram, the number of receptors available for targeting by radiolabeled biotin derivatives was around 1.8 times the number of antigen-binding sites available for targeting by the radiolabeled antibody. Findings suggest the possibility of target amplification in vivo. Further signal augmentation is likely to be achieved by the successive repeated administration of polymeric reagents because of their high affinity for forming a specific binding pair with the last-targeted molecule.

Pilot Radioimmunotherapy Trial With ¹³¹I-Labeled Murine Monoclonal Antibody CC49 and Deoxyspergualin in Metastatic Colon Carcinoma
Divgi CR, Scott AM, Gulec S, et al (Mem Sloan-Kettering Cancer Ctr, New York; Natl Cancer Inst, Bethesda, Md)
Clin Cancer Res 1:1503–1510, 1995   2–20

Introduction.—An inevitable host immune response occurs when murine antibodies are used. The result is faster serum and whole-body clearance and decreased or absent targeting with repeat administration. To evaluate the effect on the immune response, cumulative toxicity, and efficacy, 6 patients with metastatic colon cancer received repeated outpatient infusions of iodine-131–labeled CC49 and deoxyspergualin (DSG).

Methods.—Patients received 20 mg of CC49 labeled with 15 mCi/m² of ¹³¹I biweekly with concurrent DSG, 200 mg/m² daily for 5 days. The maximum number of courses for both was 4. Anterior and posterior whole-body ¹³¹I images were taken at varying time points to approximate biodistribution after each antibody infusion. Human antimouse antibody (HAMA) titers were measured.

Results.—Targeting to known tumor was observed in all 6 patients after the first radioantibody infusion. There was comparable targeting of radioactivity to tumor after repeat ¹³¹I-labeled CC49 administration in 4 of the 6 patients. Four patients received all 4 courses of therapy. Of these, 3 did not experience acute side effects. Two patients had grade II or less anaphylactoid reactions that were treated without sequelae. One patient with an anaphylactoid reaction had faster serum clearance of radioactivity after repeat infusions of ¹³¹I-labeled CC49.

The HAMA titers in patients receiving concurrent CC49 with DSG were significantly lower than those in patients receiving CC49 without DSG. No correlation was observed between the HAMA titer and serum clearance of tumor targeting of ¹³¹I-labeled CC49. No patients had clinical responses.

Conclusion.—Deoxyspergualin can reduce the human immune response to murine monoclonal antibody. Multiple infusions of ¹³¹I-labeled CC49 were administered safely with no change in serum or whole-body kinetics in half the patients treated biweekly for metastatic colon cancer.

Phase I Study of Intravenous ¹⁷⁷Lu-labeled CC49 Murine Monoclonal Antibody in Patients With Advanced Adenocarcinoma

Mulligan T, Carrasquillo JA, Chung Y, et al (Natl Cancer Inst, Bethesda, Md; NIH, Bethesda, Md; Dow Chemical Company, Midland, Mich)

Clin Cancer Res 1:1447–1454, 1995   2–21

Introduction.—The value of radioimmunoconjugates in cancer therapeutics depends on the preferential expression of tumor-associated antigens by tumor cells compared with normal cells, the effective delivery and penetration of the radioimmunoconjugate into the tumor, prolonged retention of the isotope within the tumor site, and high-energy deposition from the radionuclide to kill tumor with minor damage to normal tissues. The murine monoclonal antibody CC49 was conjugated to the chemical chelate 1,4,7,10-tetraaza-1-(1-carboxy-3-(4-aminophenyl)propyl)-tris-4,7,10-((carboxy)methyl)cyclododecane that was labeled with a β-emitter, lutetium-177. The ¹⁷⁷Lu-labeled CC49 had already shown regression of human colon adenocarcinoma xenographs in nude mice. Patients with histologically confirmed recurrent metastatic adenocarcinoma refractory to standard therapy and whose tumors expressed the tumor-associated glycoprotein 72 antigen were evaluated for determination of the maximum tolerated dose of ¹⁷⁷Lu-labeled CC49 in a phase I investigation.

Methods.—The starting dose of ¹⁷⁷Lu was 10 mCi/m². It was escalated to 15 mCi/m² in cohorts of 3 patients until dose-limiting toxicity was detected. The dose of CC49 was held constant at 20 mg. Patients underwent pharmacokinetic sampling and immunoscintigraphy at appropriate intervals.

Results.—Of a total of 9 patients, 5 had metastatic breast cancer, 3 had colorectal cancer, and 1 had lung cancer. Tumor localization in the predominant site of metastatic disease was effective for all 9 patients. Bone marrow toxicity developed in 3 patients at the second ¹⁷⁷Lu; dose level of 25 mCi/m²; 2 patients had grade 4 thrombocytopenia, and grade 3 thrombocytopenia developed in 1 patient.

The plasma half-life of the immunoconjugate was 67 hours. Wholebody retention was prolonged and had a biological half-life of 258 hours. Prolonged ¹⁷⁷Lu retention was observed in the reticuloendothelial system. The dosimetry estimates were consistent with the clinical dose-limiting toxicities observed on imaging and biopsy. Most of the ¹⁷⁷Lu was localized in the cellular compartment, not in the bone. There were no antitumor responses.

Conclusion.—Dose escalation above 25 mCi/m² caused bone marrow toxicity, limiting the delivery of potentially therapeutic doses of ¹⁷⁷Lu to metastatic tumor sites outside the bone.

Targeting of Small-cell Lung Cancer Using the Anti-GD2 Ganglioside Monoclonal Antibody 3F8: A Pilot Trial
Grant SC, Kostakoglu L, Kris MG, et al (Mem Sloan-Kettering Cancer Ctr, New York)
Eur J Nucl Med 23:145–149, 1996   2–22

Introduction.—Small-cell lung cancer (SCLC) has been shown to be relatively sensitive to immune-mediated killing mechanisms in vitro. It is considered an excellent model with which to investigate the use of immunotherapy. The ability of the anti-GD2 ganglioside monoclonal antibody 3F8 to target tumor sites was studied in patients with SCLC.

Methods.—Of 12 patients with pathologically confirmed SCLC and no previous exposure to mouse antibodies, 2 had a positive skin test to iodine and were not tested further. The other 10 patients received 3F8 labeled with 2 or 10 mCi of IV iodine-131. Whole-body radionuclide scans were completed on postinfusion days 1, 2, and 3 in 5 patients and days 1, 2, 3, and 7 in 5 patients. Single-photon emission CT was done on day 3 as needed in 4 patients.

Results.—Five patients had recurrent disease and 5 patients had a new diagnosis of SCLC. Patients with a new diagnosis received 3F8 before initial chemotherapy. Localization to tumor sites was shown in all patients. Radionuclide imaging of ^{131}I-labeled 3F8 identified all previously identified sites of systemic disease. Multiple small brain metastases were not imaged by 3F8 in 1 patient. This finding was consistent with the known behavior of large molecules and the blood-brain barrier. One patient died of unrelated causes 6 days after administration of 3F8. No significant toxicity occurred. The mean serum half-life was 64.2 hours.

Conclusion.—The use of 3F8 to target GD2 on tumor cells in patients with SCLC was well demonstrated. Further investigation should be directed toward the therapeutic application of anti-GD2 in SCLC, optimal doses of antibody and radionuclide, the choice of radionuclide, and the use of chimeric or humanized antibodies.

Detection of Pelvic Recurrence of Colorectal Carcinoma: Prospective, Blinded Comparison of Tc-99m-IMMU-4 Monoclonal Antibody Scanning and CT
Stomper PC, D'Souza DJ, Bakshi SP, et al (Roswell Park Cancer Inst, Buffalo, NY; State Univ of New York, Buffalo)
Radiology 197:688–692, 1995   2–23

Introduction.—Few prospective, blinded investigations have compared monoclonal antibody scanning with CT of the pelvis in the detection of pelvic recurrences of colorectal carcinoma. The role of monoclonal antibody scanning techniques in conjunction with or in place of CT scanning and MRI for the detection of recurrent colorectal carcinoma has not been defined. The accuracy of imaging with technetium-99m–labeled Fab' fragment of the anticarcinoembryonic antigen antibody (CEA) IMMU-4 was prospectively compared with CT for detection of pelvic recurrence of colorectal carcinoma.

Methods.—Blinded interpretations of pelvic CT and ^{99m}Tc IMMU-4 antibody scanning were done in 61 patients with suspected recurrence of previously treated colorectal carcinoma. Findings were correlated with surgical-pathologic data in 23 patients or with clinical and CT follow-up results in 38 patients. Sensitivity, specificity, and positive and negative predictive values were calculated.

Results.—Twenty-nine (48%) of 61 patients had recurrent colorectal carcinoma. The overall accuracy of antibody screening alone in detecting pelvic recurrence was 82%. This was identical to the accuracy of CT alone and combined CT and antibody scanning. For antibody scanning for pelvic recurrence, sensitivity was 79%, specificity was 84%, positive predictive value was 82%, and negative predictive value was 82%. These values were not significantly different from those of CT alone or CT and antibody scanning combined. Without decreasing specificity, the sensitivity of antibody scanning for pelvic recurrence was significantly increased with larger size of recurrent tumors (less than 2 cm vs. 2 cm or more), higher levels of serum anticarcinoembryonic antigen antibody (2.5 or less vs. more than 2.5 ng/mL), and combined planar and SPECT antibody scanning, compared with planar scanning alone. Antibody scanning was useful in clarifying recurrent tumor from fibrosis.

Conclusion.—The ^{99m}Tc IMMU-4 antibody scanning does not improve sensitivity or specificity of pelvic CT in the detection of recurrent pelvic colorectal carcinoma. It can help differentiate recurrent tumor from fibrosis.

Radioimmunoscintigraphy in Patients With Early Stage Cutaneous Malignant Melanoma
Blend MJ, Hyun H, Patel B, et al (Univ of Illinois Hosp and Med Ctr, Chicago; Michael Reese Hosp and Med Ctr, Chicago; NeoRx Corp, Seattle)
J Nucl Med 37:252–257, 1996   2–24

Objective.—Prophylactic lymphadenectomy in patients with cutaneous malignant melanoma with no evidence of lymph node metastasis is a controversial practice. Neither CT nor MRI has shown sufficient sensitivity in the staging of the disease. The sensitivity of a noninvasive imaging procedure using a technetium-99m Fab fragment of monoclonal antibody NR-ML-05 for staging early-stage metastatic disease was studied.

Methods.—Unlabeled monoclonal antibody and then labeled antibody were infused in normal saline into 26 patients (10 women) with malignant melanoma. Ten patients had suspected local disease, 12 had suspected regional disease, and 4 had suspected distant disease. Radioimmunoscintigraphy was performed 6–9 hours later. Patients were followed for 6–60 months. At the time of the study, 20 patients had had their primary lesions excised and 12 had simultaneous regional lymph node dissection.

Results.—All infusions were well tolerated. One man with a supposed normal pelvic examination—after a cutaneous lesion was removed from his right lower leg—was found to have a 1.1-cm lesion on radioimmunoscintigraphy that was shown to be malignant by surgical pathology. Examination and other diagnostic modalities located 18 lesions before radioimmunoscintigraphy imaging. The monoclonal antibody identified 8 of these lesions as malignant and 8 as benign. It failed to identify 2 lesions that were later determined to be malignant, for a sensitivity of 86%. Of 15 patients determined by this technique to have localized disease, only 10 had a clinical diagnosis of localized disease. Radioimmunoscintigraphy results correctly identified 14 patients as having stage I/II disease, misdiagnosed 1 patient with stage I/II disease as having stage III disease, and misdiagnosed 1 patient with stage III disease as having stage I/II disease. Radioimmunoscintigraphy results correctly diagnosed stage III disease in 1 patient who had a clinical diagnosis of stage IV disease.

Conclusion.—Radioimmunoscintigraphy results led to correct staging of 93% of patients, whereas clinical and radiologic examinations led to correct staging in 73% of patients.

▶ The use of radiolabeled monoclonal antibodies for radioimmunoscintigraphy (RIS) and radioimmunotherapy (RIT) is now a well-established part of the overall portfolio of research in nuclear medicine. After about 15 years of study, the first few diagnostic products finally have been approved for clinical use. Research in this area is still ongoing at all levels of product development, so I've tried to choose several articles that illustrate the various foci of this research (Abstracts 2–19 to 2–24). The papers selected run the gamut in answering still-undecided questions regarding RIS and RIT:

1. Are there ways to overcome the low percent of injected dose per gram of tumor target through the use of signal amplifiers?

2. Can we pharmacologically reduce the inevitable host immune response that occurs when murine or even chimeric and humanized forms of the antibody are administered?

3. Can we create useable radiopharmaceuticals for solid tumor therapy without bone marrow toxicity limiting the radiation dose before the cancer is treated sufficiently?

4. Can we produce an antibody-based treatment breakthrough for those cancers that currently have no good treatments?

5. How well will RIS fare in nonresearch applications for staging cancers when compared with current clinical practices such as CT?

R. Neumann, M.D.

Leakage Measurement During Selective Limb Perfusion Using a Gamma Probe

Sandrock D, Horst F, Gatzemeier W, et al (Georg-August Univ, Göttingen, Germany; Humboldt Univ, Berlin)
Eur J Nucl Med 23:534–538, 1996   2–25

Introduction.—Treatment of a malignant melanoma of the upper or lower limbs without regional or distant metastases involves removing the lesion and administering regional chemotherapy with alkylating substances during hyperthermic perfusion of the limb. Leakage from the limb to the rest of the body must be monitored. Different lightweight probe systems have been introduced to monitor leakage from limbs. The sensitivity of a commercial probe system in a phantom model simulating the blood pool of the heart was studied and validated with 20 patients.

Methods.—A portable gamma probe was used with digital display. The physical properties were investigated in a phantom study simulating blood pool activity at different angles of the probe to the surface and at different distances. For the patient studies, the limb circulation was surgically separated from the systemic blood circulation in 20 patients, the limb was selectively perfused for 60 minutes. Fifteen MBq of technetium-99m–labeled autologous red blood cells was injected into the limb circulation. As a standard, an equal amount was kept. Blood samples were drawn from the systemic circulation every 10 minutes and simultaneous count rates were measured by the probe system at the lower end of the sternum.

Results.—The conventional blood sampling method found leakage values between 0% and 86% for the 20 patients; leakage increased over the time the perfusion system was running. During perfusion, count rates of the probe ranged from 0 to 73 counts per second. The count rate of the probe system correlated strongly with the results of the conventional measurement.

Conclusion.—This probe system will allow the oncologic surgeon to know whether there is leakage from the limb to the rest of the body when administering regional chemotherapy. For selective limb perfusion, the probe system represents a simple approach to leakage quantification.

Continuous Intraoperative External Monitoring of Perfusate Leak Using Iodine-131 Human Serum Albumin During Isolated Perfusion of the Liver and Limbs

Barker WC, Andrich MP, Alexander HR, et al (NIH, Bethesda, Md; Natl Cancer Inst, Bethesda, Md)
Eur J Nucl Med 22:1242–1248, 1995   2–26

Introduction.—In early isolated regional chemotherapy perfusions, leaks into the systemic circulation ranging from 40% to 80% were not uncommon and were considered acceptable because the dose levels were not severe. The use of limb perfusion–delivered tumor necrosis factor in the treatment of melanoma and sarcoma requires doses that are 10 times the maximally tolerated systemic levels. Even a leakage of more than 10% could result in systemic complications. Thus, there is a need for an external real-time leak monitoring system.

Methods.—Fifty-three isolated limb perfusions were given to 48 patients with melanoma or sarcoma of the extremity. The patients were randomly assigned to receive melphalan alone or a combination of melphalan, tumor necrosis factor, and interferon-γ. To track the leakage of blood from the isolated perfusion circuit into the general systemic vascular space, human serum albumin labeled with iodine-131 was used with an externally mounted and collimated NaI(Tl) detector. To validate this external monitoring method, blood samples were obtained from the systemic and limb perfusion circuits at the start of the treatment period and at the 15-, 30-, 60-, and 90-minute treatment time points.

Results.—In the 54 limb perfusions monitored, all but 1 had no more than 8% total systemic leak during the treatment period. The patient with the greatest leak had received melphalan alone and had a calculated leak of 14%. Treatment was continued because melphalan toxicities are less severe if released into the systemic circulation and the 10% leakage rule for tumor necrosis factor was not observed. For leak estimation, there is a very good correlation between the conventional and experimental models. Leaks that were greater than 2% had excellent correlation with the measured systemic blood sample data.

Conclusion.—There was a good demonstration for the use of external monitoring. Variability in leak estimates of 2% or less may be caused by incomplete mixing of isotope throughout the perfusion circuit, or extraction processes, which decrease the amount of circulating human serum albumin. This method can be used with multi-isotope monitoring as well as with alternative tracers, such as technetium-99m–labeled red blood cells or ^{99m}Tc human serum albumin.

▶ Regional chemotherapy has the advantage of permitting higher doses of the drug(s) to be delivered to the tumor bed while hopefully avoiding the systemic toxicities often found with effective chemotherapy drugs. However, when isolated perfusion is chosen as the method to deliver the drugs, conventional or experimental, the surgical oncologist needs to know in real time whether leaks to the systemic circulation are occurring. Abstracts 2–25 and 2–26 give possible solutions by using portable gamma probes; one was derived from a commercially available thyroid uptake system from Germany to count ^{99m}Tc-labeled autologous red blood cells. Both systems appear to work well in solving a real clinical problem associated with regional chemotherapy.

R. Neumann, M.D.

Noninvasive Monitoring of Tumor Metabolism Using Fluorodeoxyglucose and Positron Emission Tomography in Colorectal Cancer Liver Metastases: Correlation With Tumor Response to Fluorouracil

Findlay M, Young H, Cunningham D, et al (Royal Marsden Hosp, Surrey, England)
J Clin Oncol 14:700–708, 1996   2–27

Background.—Although clinical applications of PET are increasing, especially in the fields of neurology and cardiology, its role in oncology is less well defined. Positron emission tomographic studies in patients with gastrointestinal malignancies have been done mainly in patients with colorectal cancer and using FDG. In the current study, the metabolism of colorectal cancer liver metastases using FDG PET before and during the first month of chemotherapy was investigated.

Methods.—Twenty patients were enrolled in the study. Fluorouracil was administered in a protracted venous infusion with or without interferon-α 2b for two 10-week intervals separated by a 2-week break. Scans were obtained before treatment and 1–2 and 4–5 weeks after the start of treatment. Intravenous FDG was injected after fasting, and scanning was performed with a large-area positron camera. Results were compared with the findings of CT performed 12 weeks after the initiation of chemotherapy.

Findings.—Eighteen of the 20 patients had evaluable liver metastases. Eleven patients had objective partial responses. A total of 27 metastatic lesions could be examined. Pretreatment ratios of FDG uptake in the tumor and normal liver (T:L) and standardized uptake values were unassociated with lower 1- to 2-week and 4- to 5-week T:L ratios and 4- to 5-week standard uptake values. Responding lesions had greater decreases in metabolism. The T:L ratio at 4–5 weeks discriminated response from nonresponse in a lesion-by-lesion and overall patient response assessment with a 100% sensitivity and a specificity of 90% (for lesion by lesion) and 75% (for overall).

Conclusions.—Positron emission tomographic assessment of FDG tumor uptake yields data that correlate with the antitumor effect of chemotherapy in patients with liver metastases from colorectal cancer. The potential of FDG PET extends beyond assessment of early response of colorectal liver metastases to a variety of clinical investigational settings.

Metabolic Imaging of Untreated Prostate Cancer by Positron Emission Tomography With [18]Fluorine-labeled Deoxyglucose

Effert PJ, Bares R, Handt S, et al (RWTH Univ of Aachen, Germany)
J Urol 155:994–998, 1996   2–28

Background.—The role of PET in the assessment of prostate cancer is not well documented. The value of this modality with FDG for metabolic grading of untreated primary prostate cancer and for differentiating between benign and malignant prostatic disease was investigated.

Methods.—Forty-eight patients with different stages of untreated prostate cancer and 16 with histologically confirmed benign prostatic hyperplasia (BPH) were included. Static PET was performed after IV injection of 150–300 MBq of FDG. Accumulation of the tracer was quantitated by determining differential uptake ratios and prostate-to-skeletal muscle ratios.

Findings.—Low FDG uptake was observed in 81% of the primary tumors. Tracer accumulation was unassociated with increasing tumor grade or stage. Uptake values in patients with BPH and in those with malignant disease overlapped significantly. There was a trend toward lower prostate-to-skeletal muscle ratios in patients with BPH. Increased FDG accumulation was found in some patients with BPH and malignant prostatic disease and in patients with lymph node and bone metastases from prostate cancer.

Conclusions.—In most patients with untreated primary prostate cancer, FDG PET is not useful for metabolic labeling. In addition, this technique does not reliably distinguish between BPH and primary prostate cancer. Increased FDG accumulation can be observed in some primary prostate tumors and metastatic deposits of prostate cancer.

Thoracic Nodal Staging With PET Imaging With ¹⁸FDG in Patients With Bronchogenic Carcinoma

Patz EF Jr, Lowe VJ, Goodman PC, et al (Duke Univ, Durham, NC)
Chest 108:1617–1621, 1995   2–29

Background.—Computed tomography is only 60% sensitive in detecting nodal metastases of bronchogenic carcinoma, and it is not very specific. In addition, CT does not reliably predict the histologic type of cancer. Positron emission tomography using FDG provides both anatomical and physiologic information.

Patients.—Positron emission tomography was performed in 42 adult patients with newly diagnosed bronchogenic carcinoma before planned sampling of the thoracic nodes. Adenocarcinomas were most prevalent. A total of 62 node stations—40 in the hilar/lobar region and 22 mediastinal sites—were sampled. In 14 cases, thoracic CT scanning with IV contrast enhancement was also performed.

Findings.—The PET imaging was 83% sensitive and 82% specific in detecting thoracic node metastases. The respective figures for CT were 43% and 85%. The PET imaging accurately predicted the presence or absence of metastases in 75% of hilar/lobar node stations. There were 7 false positive node stations, 3 of which were normal on CT scanning. None of the 3 false negative stations were positive on CT. There was only 1 false negative PET study of the mediastinal nodes. In contrast, CT was only 58% sensitive in detecting mediastinal metastases.

Conclusion.—An FDG-PET study with normal results nearly eliminates the need to sample the mediastinal nodes preoperatively. A study with abnormal results probably indicates spread of bronchogenic cancer to the mediastinum.

Fluorine-18-Fluorodeoxyglucose PET Imaging of Soft-tissue Sarcoma
Nieweg OE, Pruim J, van Ginkel RJ, et al (Univ Hosp Groningen, The Netherlands; The Netherlands Cancer Inst, Amsterdam)
J Nucl Med 37:257–261, 1996   2–30

Background.—Because FDG is concentrated in various types of tumor tissue and PET enables analysis of tumor biology, PET may be useful in the treatment of soft-tissue sarcomas. The current study determined FDG uptake in soft-tissue sarcoma, its sensitivity, the correlation between histologic grade and glucose consumption, and whether FDG PET can differentiate benign from malignant lesions.

Methods.—Eighteen patients with soft-tissue sarcoma and 4 with a benign soft-tissue lesion underwent PET imaging. Glucose tumor consumption was calculated using Patlak's graphic analysis, with the lumped constant assumed.

Findings.—Positron emission tomography with FDG clearly visualized all soft-tissue sarcomas. Glucose consumption was a median of 13 μmol/ 100 g/min. Glucose metabolism was correlated with the histopathologic malignancy grade. No association with standardized uptake values was found. Among those with benign lesions, FDG PET visualized a lesion in 1 patient, was equivocal in 1 patient, and did not visualize in 2 patients. Although benign lesions were distinguished from high-grade malignant lesions, they were not consistently differentiated from lesions with low or intermediate malignancy grades.

Conclusions.—Positron emission tomography with FDG effectively visualizes soft-tissue sarcomas. Its sensitivity is 100%. Glucose metabolic rate is associated with tumor malignancy grade. However, FDG is apparently not appropriate for discriminating benign lesions from soft-tissue sarcomas with low or intermediate malignancy grades.

Carbon-11-Methionine PET Imaging of Malignant Melanoma
Lindholm P, Leskinen S, Någren K, et al (Univ of Turku, Finland)
J Nucl Med 36:1806–1810, 1995   2–31

Introduction.—Of all the nuclear medicine techniques for assessing the extent of metastatic melanoma, whole-body FDG PET seems best. Amino acids and their analogues may be useful for specific imaging of melanoma, and PET imaging with L-[methyl-carbon-11]methionine (^{11}C-methionine) has been successfully used in imaging several types of cancer. A preliminary study of ^{11}C-methionine PET imaging of malignant melanoma was reported.

Methods.—The study included 10 patients with melanoma but no liver metastasis. Eight had metastatic melanoma of the skin and 2 had primary melanoma. Carbon-11–methionine PET scanning was performed in all patients before they started treatment for their melanoma. Seven patients underwent dynamic scanning for 40 minutes and the other 3 for 10–20 minutes. Scanning was performed 25–45 minutes after ^{11}C-methionine injection. The PET findings were compared with those of clinical and imaging follow-up and autopsy.

Results.—The ^{11}C-methionine PET technique detected 22 of 22 melanoma lesions measuring greater than 1.5 cm in diameter. However, it missed 5 smaller areas of pulmonary involvement. The untreated melanoma lesions had an average standardized uptake value of 6.3, with an uptake rate of 0.085/min. The quality of the PET scans was good. They effectively imaged metastatic melanoma of the inguinal and iliac nodes, and there was no problem in demonstrating tumors close to the bladder.

Conclusion.—This technique demonstrates all melanoma metastases measuring larger than 1.5 cm in diameter and may also be of value in measuring in vivo tumor metabolic activity. It may also be possible to predict the response to treatment on the basis of early changes in ^{11}C-methionine uptake.

▶ Dr. Henry N. Wagner's summary of the 1996 Society of Nuclear Medicine annual meeting[1] reports that 88 presentations involved FDG oncology studies, and he has named FDG the "molecule of the century"! So, it is no surprise that there was already a plethora of reports on PET FDG studies of various cancers. I've selected some of those for you to review and threw in one concerned with ^{11}C-methionine PET imaging of malignant melanoma, just so you know that there are other molecules!

R. Neumann, M.D.

Reference

1. Wagner HN Jr: 1996 SNM annual meeting: Medical problem solving. *J Nucl Med* 37:11N–14N, 17N, 26N, 1996.

Comparative Study of Body Composition by Dual-energy X-ray Absorptiometry
Aloia JF, Vaswani A, Ma R, et al (Winthrop-Univ Hosp, Mineola, NY; Brookhaven Natl Lab, Upton, NY)
J Nucl Med 36:1392–1397, 1995   2–32

Background.—Several methods of determining body composition have been developed, but all have drawbacks. Dual-energy x-ray absorptiometry (DEXA) has been recommended as a generally available, relatively inexpensive, and precise method of determining fat and lean tissue mass, which is associated with little radiation exposure. Determinations of fat mass (FM) and fat-free mass (FFM) with DEXA were compared with those obtained with 4 other techniques of body composition measurement.

Methods.—Healthy women (127 white women and 38 black women) with a body mass index of 18–30 were evaluated with DEXA, total-body potassium (by counting the radioactive isotope potassium-40), total-body nitrogen (determined by prompt γ neutron activation), total-body carbon (determined by an inelastic neutron-scattering system), and total-body water (determined with tritiated water dilution) to calculate FM and FFM.

Results.—Fat-free mass measurements obtained with the 5 methods all were significantly different from each other. The FM measurements obtained with DEXA and with total-body potassium were similar, as were FM measurements obtained with total-body nitrogen and total-body carbon. There were statistically significant differences in FM measurements with all other pairings. Dual-energy x-ray absorptiometry was more accurate in determining FM than in determining FFM. However, DEXA consistently overestimated FM and underestimated FFM, compared with the other methods. The differences between DEXA FM values and the FM values with other methods were constant, but the differences between DEXA and other methods in FFM values increased with increasing body mass index.

Conclusions.—The greater differences between FFM values obtained with DEXA compared with other methods at high values of FFM suggest that DEXA is measuring something different than the other methods. Adjustment of the DEXA program for separating bone and soft tissue and separating fat and lean in soft tissue may be needed.

A Correlative Study of Ultrasound Calcaneal and Dual-energy X-ray Absorptiometry Bone Measurements of the Lumbar Spine and Femur in 1000 Women

Rosenthall L, Tenenhouse A, Caminis J (McGill Univ, Montreal; Montreal Gen Hosp)
Eur J Nucl Med 22:402–406, 1995   2–33

Background.—Ultrasound devices have been manufactured to evaluate bone quality at peripheral sites. However, the spine and proximal femur are sites of more clinical interest because they are sites of low-trauma fracture secondary to osteopenia. The ability of ultrasound parameters to predict bone mineral density (BMD) of the lumbar spine and proximal femur in women was studied.

Methods.—Ultrasound determinations of the speed of sounds (SOS), broadband ultrasound attenuation (BUA), and stiffness were determined for the left and right heels of 1,000 women. Young adult *t*-scores were calculated for stiffness. The ultrasound heel parameters were correlated with the corresponding lumbar and femoral BMDs. Analyses were done for the entire cohort and for 3 age subgroups: those younger than 45 years, those 45–55 years, and those older than 55 years.

Results.—The correlation coefficients between ultrasound calcaneus and the other sites varied between 0.53 and 0.60 in the entire cohort and between 0.53 and 0.55 in the age subgroups. The *t*-scores of the lumbar spine and femoral neck had a correlation coefficient of 0.70 in the entire cohort and between 0.62 and 0.69 in the age subgroups. Correlation coefficients between calcaneal SOS, BUA, and stiffness and the BMDs of the lumbar spine, femoral neck, and Ward's triangle varied between 0.54 and 0.61. A 0.64 correlation was found between the left and right SOS and BUA. The accuracy of the prediction of abnormalities at 1 site by abnormalities of another site ranged from 58.2% to 85.9% in the total cohort.

Conclusions.—The bone status of one site cannot be predicted by the bone status at another site with a clinically significant level of accuracy. Bone mineral density may not be the sole determinant of bone strength. Ultrasonography, as a measure of bone quality related to components of bone other than mineral density, may therefore yield important information related to fracture risk.

▶ Dual-energy x-ray absorptiometry (DEXA) has become a big part of our nuclear medicine practice at the NIH for bone mineral measurement and body composition studies. We are solely a research hospital, and reimbursement is not a part of our daily concerns, but I have been amazed at the interest in these techniques by our clinical research colleagues. Abstracts 2–32 and 2–33 provide some comparative prospectives.

Rosenthall et al. compared the DEXA technique with ultrasound calcaneal measurements of bone mineral density in 1,000 women. They found the ultrasound transmission test still unproven as a predictor of fracture risk. A second goal was to examine the accuracy of the various site-specific measurements in predicting each other. They conclude that no site can predict the status of another site with sufficiently high accuracy to be clinically useful.

If you have a DEXA machine, you can also use it to obtain certain measures of body composition. We have added this to our practice as well, and I was glad to see the report comparing the DEXA measurements to older techniques that measure total-body potassium, nitrogen, water, and carbon. Their findings suggest that at high fat-free mass values, DEXA differs significantly, so some adjustments in technique may be needed.

R. Neumann, M.D.

Comparison of Nuclear Bone and Gallium Scans in the Therapeutic Evaluation of Bone Lymphoma

Moon T-Y, Kim EE, Kim Y-C, et al (Pusan Natl Univ, Korea; Univ of Texas, Houston; Korea Univ, Seoul)
Clin Nucl Med 20:721–724, 1995   2–34

Introduction.—The functional status of a tumor, not just its morphology, is important in evaluating therapeutic response or recurrence. In recent years, gadolinium-enhanced MRI, FDG, contrast-enhanced CT scans, and nuclear medicine studies, such as PET scans, have been used to monitor the effects of cancer therapy. The accuracy of nuclear bone scans was compared with that of gallium-67 scans for demonstration of the therapeutic response in bone lymphoma.

Methods.—Forty patients with bone lymphoma lesions had bone and ^{67}Ga whole-body scans obtained within 2 weeks of each other. The scans were graded visually from 1 to 4. Grade 3 signifies a similar count density to that of normal iliac alar activity on bone scans and normal liver activity on ^{67}Ga scans. The patients were clinically free of disease for 1.5–6.8 years. A retrospective comparison was made of 40 technetium-99m methylene diphosphonate (MDP) bone scans with ^{67}Ga scans before therapy, 29 bone scans and 13 ^{67}Ga scans during therapy, and 33 bone scans and 15 ^{67}Ga scans after therapy.

Results.—Before therapy, the incidence of abnormal findings of bony lymphoma was 87.5% with bone scans and 80% with ^{67}Ga scans. Lesion improvement was found in 66% of bone scans during therapy and in 72.7% of bone scans after therapy. Lesion improvement was found in 84.6% of ^{67}Ga scans during therapy and in 86.7% of ^{67}Ga scans after therapy. Before therapy the mean grade of ^{99m}Tc MDP uptake was 3.06 and was considered a successful therapeutic response. It was 2.34 during therapy and 1.75 after therapy. Before therapy, the mean grade of ^{67}Ga uptake was 3.22. It was 1.42 during therapy and 1.30 after therapy.

Conclusion.—In evaluation of the therapeutic response of bone lymphoma, ^{67}Ga scans appear to be more reliable than nuclear bone scans. Both types of scans are helpful in evaluating whole-bony structures or soft-tissue abnormalities.

Comparison of Gallium-67-citrate and Thallium-201 Scintigraphy in Peripheral and Intrathoracic Lymphoma
Waxman AD, Eller D, Ashook G, et al (Cedars-Sinai Med Ctr, Los Angeles)
J Nucl Med 37:46–50, 1996   2–35

Introduction.—Gallium-67-citrate has been extensively used in evaluating patients with lymphoma. Little is known about the sensitivity or specificity of ^{67}Ga-citrate by tumor grade or type or about thallium-201 accumulation in lymphoma. The differences in ^{67}Ga uptake as a function of tumor grade and type were investigated, and the sensitivity of ^{201}Tl uptake in Hodgkin's and non-Hodgkin's lymphoma was determined.

Methods.—Gallium-67 and ^{201}Tl scintigraphy were performed on 36 patients: 9 with low-grade lymphoma, 11 with intermediate-grade lymphoma, 4 with high-grade lymphoma, and 12 with Hodgkin's disease. All patients had biopsies. Statistical comparisons were made for ^{201}Tl and ^{67}Ga scans in all lymphoma subgroups using a semiquantitative rating system.

Results.—In patients with low-grade lymphoma, ^{67}Ga sensitivity was only 56% and site sensitivity was 32%. Thallium-201 sensitivity, however, was 100% for these patients and sites. Thallium-201 was more avid for low-grade lymphoma than for intermediate-grade, high-grade, or Hodgkin's lymphoma when ^{201}Tl was compared to itself in lymphoma subgroups. There was significantly less ^{67}Ga sensitivity for low-grade lymphoma than for intermediate-grade and Hodgkin's lymphomas. When ^{201}Tl and ^{67}Ga were compared in the intermediate-grade, high-grade, or Hodgkin's disease groups, there were no significant differences.

Conclusion.—Compared to ^{67}Ga citrate, ^{201}Tl demonstrates significantly greater tumor avidity in the low-grade lymphoma group, and ^{67}Ga-citrate apppears relatively nonavid for low-grade lymphoma. In evaluating patients with low-grade lymphoma, ^{67}Ga-citrate should not be considered dependable. Within the abdomen, neither ^{201}Tl nor ^{67}Ga is dependable in the evaluation of low-grade lymphoma. Gastrointestinal excretion of ^{201}Tl is unpredictable as it did not clear on multiple delayed images obtained up to 7 days after injection. In the intermediate-grade and high-grade lymphoma groups, ^{67}Ga imaging appeared to be a superior technique.

Utility of Gallium-67 Scintigraphy in Low-grade Non-Hodgkin's Lymphoma

Ben-Haim S, Bar-Shalom R, Israel O, et al (Rambam Med Ctr, Haifa, Israel; Technion-Israel Inst of Technology, Haifa, Israel)
J Clin Oncol 14:1936–1942, 1996   2–36

Introduction.—Gallium-67 scintigraphy has an important role in monitoring response to therapy in patients with lymphoma and in early detection of disease recurrence. Patients with low-grade non-Hodgkin's lymphoma have traditionally been considered non–gallium-avid. This investigation was conducted to determine the sensitivity of gallium-67 scintigraphy in these patients when using modern equipment and techniques.

Methods.—Gallium-67 scintigraphy was performed on 57 patients with low-grade non-Hodgkin's lymphoma. Forty patients had the procedure at presentation, 3 during treatment, and 14 at suspected disease recurrence after clinical remission. Using a large field-of-view or dual-head digital camera, planar and tomographic images were obtained. Thirty of the 45 patients with gallium-avid low-grade non-Hodgkin's lymphoma had 93 follow-up scans. Correlations were made between clinical findings, CT scans, and outcomes.

Results.—In 45 of 57 patients and in 113 of 164 disease sites, ^{67}Ga scintigraphy showed positive findings. In the more common types of low-grade non-Hodgkin's lymphoma, the sensitivity was higher: 84% for patients with follicular, predominantly small cleaved cell type; 91% for patients with follicular, mixed small cleaved and large cell types. In patients with mucosa-associated lymphoid tissue lymphoma and small lymphocytic lymphoma, the sensitivity was lower. The ^{67}Ga scans were positive for 25 of 28 patients with disease recurrence after clinical remission, with a sensitivity of 89%.

Conclusion.—In patients with low-grade non-Hodgkin's lymphoma, ^{67}Ga scintigraphy has good sensitivity when modern technology is used. In these patients, ^{67}Ga scintigraphy can be used to provide early detection of disease recurrence and to monitor response to therapy.

Predicting Malignancy Grade With PET in Non-Hodgkin's Lymphoma
Rodriguez M, Rehn S, Ahlström H, et al (Univ of Uppsala, Sweden)
J Nucl Med 36:1790–1796, 1995   2–37

Background.—Non-Hodgkin's lymphoma (NHL) is divided into high- and low-grade disease. Because treatment decisions are based on grade, differentiating between them is important. Positron emission tomography studies to detect and grade malignant lymphomas and/or predict prognosis are limited in number. The value of PET with carbon-11–methionine and FDG in determining NHL grade was studied.

Methods.—Twenty-three patients with high-grade, low-grade, or transformed low-grade NHL were included. Standardized uptake values, transport rate, and mass influx values were determined for the whole tumor and the tumor area with the highest activity levels, comprising 4 contiguous pixels in each tumor and designated as a hot spot.

Findings.—All tumors were detected by both tracers. However, FDG discriminated between high- and low-grade NHL, whereas ^{11}C-methionine did not. Three transformed low-grade NHLs were intermediate according to FDG. All quantitative uptake values were associated with each other for both tracers, except for the mean regions of interest standardized uptake value and transport rate of ^{11}C-methionine. Mean regions of interest uptake was highly correlated with hot spots.

Conclusions.—The grade of NHL can be predicted by FDG but not ^{11}C-methionine. Future studies should focus on the development of more specific tracers and on clinically important issues in evaluating the disease in patients with malignant lymphoma.

Can Positron Emission Tomography (PET) Be Used to Detect Subclinical Response to Cancer Therapy?
Price P, for the EC PET Oncology Concerted Action and the EORTC PET Study Group (Royal Postgraduate Med School, London)
Eur J Cancer 31A:1924–1927, 1995   2–38

Background.—Recent advances in PET open the way to in vivo investigations of anticancer therapy in humans. The radiopharmaceutical FDG has been used in imaging studies of several different types of cancer. In vivo functional imaging with PET could be useful in staging, detection of subclinical disease, identification of unknown primary tumors, and differentiation of recurrent tumors from fibrosis. A European workshop was convened to discuss the potential of FDG-PET scanning as a way of assessing response to cancer therapy.

Findings.—Fifteen European centers presented data on the use of PET for this purpose; 12 were investigating tumor responsiveness to chemotherapy and 3 to radiotherapy. Four groups were studying brain tumors; 3, lymphomas; 3, colonic metastases; 3, breast cancer; and 1 each, soft-tissue sarcomas, germ-cell tumors, and thyroid cancer. Study methods and data interpretation varied; however, assessment of tumor FDG metabolic rate was thought to be a promising technique for measuring tumor response. In general, the experience suggested a relationship between the changes in tumor FDG uptake after 1 or 2 cycles of chemotherapy and the ultimate clinical response, responses being best for patients with the greatest reductions in FDG uptake. Some of the data shed light on the effects of chemotherapy on normal tissues and on tumor response to chemotherapy.

Discussion.—Experience to date suggests that PET with FDG could provide useful information on clinical and subclinical responses to anticancer therapy. In the future, functional imaging with PET could be of value in assessing the early response to therapy and the presence of residual disease. Even more accurate information could be obtained by the use of more specific markers of cellular proliferation. Toward further studies of the use of PET imaging in clinical oncology, a new study group was formed to facilitate PET/clinical collaborations in the European research community.

Whole-body PET: Physiological and Artifactual Fluorodeoxyglucose Accumulations
Engel H, Steinert H, Buck A, et al (Univ Hosp, Zurich, Switzerland)
J Nucl Med 37:441–446, 1996   2–39

Background.—Whole-body PET scanning with FDG is now a clinical reality. When reading such scans, physiologic and artifactual FDG accumulations must be distinguished from abnormal accumulations. The occurrence and appearance of "normal" activity accumulations in nonattenuation-corrected whole-body FDG PET scans were investigated in many organ sites.

Methods.—Fifty patients, aged 18–80 years, who were referred for tumor staging of malignant melanoma underwent whole-body PET scanning. Patients were asked about their physical activities before FDG injection. All were instructed to have nothing by mouth for at least 4 hours before the study.

Findings.—Viscera showed mean uptake grades between 1.7 and 2.05 on a grading scale of 0–6. The activity was homogeneously distributed in all organs but the intestines. Various muscle groups, especially the orbital musculature, had relatively high mean uptake values of 2–4.2. Ninety percent of the scans showed myocardial uptake. Reconstruction artifacts were present around the bladder and the renal collecting system.

Conclusions.—Most normal accumulations of FDG in nonattenuation corrected whole-body PET are easy to recognize and distinguish from the typically focal FDG accumulation associated with metastatic disease. Muscular FDG uptake, correlated with physical activity before and immediately after injection, can be minimized through correct positioning and explicit patient instruction.

Standardized Uptake Values of Fluorine-18 Fluorodeoxyglucose: The Value of Different Normalization Procedures

Schomburg A, Bender H, Reichel C, et al (Univ of Bonn, Germany)
Eur J Nucl Med 23:571–574, 1996   2–40

Background.—Although static image analyses of FDG PET studies do not equal absolute metabolic rate determinations, various algorithms have been developed for normalizing static FDG uptake. Different normalization procedures were compared to determine their relative dependence on individual patient characteristics.

Methods.—One hundred twenty-six patients underwent whole-body FDG PET. Standard FDG uptake values (SUVs) were calculated for liver and lung tissue. These values were normalized for total body weight, lean body mass, and body surface area.

Findings.—Standardized FDG uptake values normalized for body surface area were clearly better than SUV parameters normalized for total body weight and lean body mass. Compared with SUV parameters derived from the other normalization procedures, variation and correlation coefficients of body surface area–normalized uptake values were minimal. After normalizing for total body weight, uptake values still depended on body weight and blood sugar levels. Normalizing for lean body mass did not affect the positive association with lean body mass and patient height.

Conclusions.—Normalizing FDG uptake values for body surface area depends less on individual patient characteristics than do FDG uptake values normalized for other parameters. Thus, the former appear more useful for FDG PET oncologic studies.

Quantification of Serial Tumor Glucose Metabolism

Wu H-M, Hoh CK, Huang S-C, et al (Univ of California, Los Angeles)
J Nucl Med 37:506–513, 1996   2–41

Background.—Studies have suggested that FDG PET imaging may be used as a tumor localization technique. The total-lesion evaluation method generates a correlation coefficient (*r*) constrained Patlak parametric image of the lesion with 3 calculated glucose metabolic indices: (1) the total-lesion metabolic index (K_{T_tle}, mL/min per lesion), (2) the total-lesion voxel index (V_{T_tle}, voxels per lesion), and (3) the global average metabolic index

(K_{V_tle}, mL/min per voxel). A method of improving the precision of FDG PET scans in patients with cancer was developed, and this total-lesion evaluation method was tested.

Methods.—In 4 patients with metastatic melanoma, computer simulations before and after chemotherapy were evaluated. To assess the accuracy of this new method, the glucose metabolic indices from conventional region of interest and multiplane evaluation were used as standards.

Results.—The total-lesion evaluation method improved precision and accuracy of FDG PET scans compared with the conventional region of interest method. Using the total-lesion evaluation method, excellent correlations to the corresponding values from region of interest methods and multiplane evaluation and CT lesion volume measurements were seen in the K_{T_tle} and V_{T_tle} indices from human FDG PET scans.

Conclusions.—The total-lesion evaluation method is a reliable way of measuring FDG tumor uptake. The advantages of this method over conventional region of interest methods include less sensitivity to the region of interest definition, no need for image registration of serial scan data, and incorporated tumor volume changes in the global tumor metabolism.

Analysis of 2-Carbon-11-Thymidine Blood Metabolites in PET Imaging
Shields AF, Mankoff D, Graham MM, et al (Univ of Washington, Seattle; Veterans Affairs Med Ctr, Seattle)
J Nucl Med 37:290–296, 1996   2–42

Background.—Carbon-11–labeled thymidine and PET currently are being used to identify tumors and evaluate tumor proliferation in vivo. Because ^{11}C-labeled thymidine in the ring-2 position is rapidly degraded in vivo to thymine, CO_2, and other compounds, the kinetics and distribution of these metabolites must be considered when modeling the uptake of thymidine. The time course of the metabolites in the blood must first be measured. The best way to measure these metabolites and mathematically model their generation was determined.

Methods and Findings.—Arterial blood samples were obtained from 14 patients and processed to obtain 3 input curves, including the total activity, the activity with CO_2 removed, and the fraction of CO_2 free activity in intact thymidine. Within 11 minutes of thymidine injection, CO_2 reached a plateau of 65% of total blood activity. When a 1-minute infusion of labeled thymidine was used, the mean time to degradation to thymine and non-CO_2 metabolites was 2.9 minutes. When the findings of the blood metabolism were fitted with a compartmental model, the fraction of CO_2 free activity in intact thymidine curve could be determined accurately with as few as 3 measured points with a root mean square error of 2% in the integrated curve, compared with the curve including all blood samples. The integral of thymidine blood activity was the input to thymidine models; thus, similar errors could be expected in calculating DNA synthetic rates. Determining CO_2 could be achieved with as few as 5 samples with a root mean square error of 4% in plateau $\%CO_2$ value.

Conclusions.—Although metabolites must be considered when interpreting the findings of ^{11}C-thymidine PET, the reproducibility of the degradation curves may permit the use of a limited number of samples to measure the catabolic products of thymidine. Data from the blood are needed along with kinetic models to determine DNA synthetic rates.

▶ Positron emission tomography, like all nuclear medicine procedures, requires particular attention to quality control and methodology. I've included these 4 papers (Abstracts 2–39 to 2–42) to provide you with needed information about FDG and ^{11}C-thymidine studies as tumor detection or monitoring procedures.

R. Neumann, M.D.

Technetium-99m Labeling of DNA Oligonucleotides

Hnatowich DJ, Winnard P Jr, Virzi F, et al (Univ of Massachusetts, Worcester; Boston Univ)
J Nucl Med 36:2306–2314, 1995   2–43

Objective.—Results of conjugating single-stranded DNA with hydrazino nicotinamide and diethylenetriamine-pentaacetic acid (DTPA) and labeling with technetium-99m and indium-111 were reviewed.

Background.—Deoxyribonucleic acid and RNA may have potential as radiopharmaceuticals. If DNA and RNA were radiolabeled, they may carry radioactivity to target cells or tissues. However, methods for radiolabeling them with diagnostic and therapeutic radionuclides must be developed. Depending on the particular oligonucleotide, ^{99m}Tc may be the preferred imaging radionuclide. A method of radiolabeling DNA with ^{99m}Tc using a derivative of DTPA attached to the DNA to form chelates with reduced ^{99m}Tc has been described. It has been shown that a hydrazino nicotinamide moiety can form stable complexes with ^{99m}Tc when conjugated to antibodies.

Methods.—The previously developed hydrazino nicotinamide moiety was used to radiolabel DNA with [99m]Tc. For comparison, DNA with ^{111}In was labeled with the DTPA chelate. Complementary 22-base, single-stranded oligonucleotides with a primary amine attached to the 3' or 5' end and a biotin moiety on the opposite end also were obtained. Deoxyribonucleic acid was conjugated with hydrazino nicotinamide by an N-hydroxysuccinimide derivative and with DTPA by the cyclic anhydride.

Results.—Analysis was done with reversed-phase high-performance liquid chromatography. In both cases, conjugation was essentially complete. Purified hydrazino nicotinamide–DNA was radiolabeled with ^{99m}Tc by transchelation from glucoheptonate at up to 60% efficiency. The DTPA-DNA was radiolabeled with ^{111}In acetate at up to 100% efficiency. Analysis by size-exclusion high-performance liquid chromatography showed that for both radiolabels, the DNAs retained their ability to bind to streptavidin through the biotin moieties and their ability to hybridize with their complementary DNA in saline. High-performance liquid chromatography radiochromatograms of serum incubates showed a change in ^{99m}Tc to a high molecular weight, strongly indicating serum protein binding; this was not true for ^{111}In. With ^{111}In, but not ^{99m}Tc, low–molecular weight degradation products were observed. This may have resulted from the use of phosphodiester-linked oligonucleotides. The DNAs were then bound to streptavidin-conjugated magnetic beads and incubated in fresh 37°C human serum. After 24 hours, less than 4% of ^{99m}Tc and 14% of ^{111}In was lost.

Conclusions.—Amino-modified, single-stranded DNA can be conjugated with hydrazino nicotinamide and stably radiolabeled with ^{99m}Tc. The stability of the label is similar to that for ^{111}In radiolabeled by DTPA. An interesting note is that the labeled ^{99m}Tc-DNA binds to serum proteins. Such binding was not observed in ^{111}In-DNA. This binding may be related to the hydrazino nicotinamide moieties.

Monitoring Gene Therapy With Cytosine Deaminase: In Vitro Studies Using Tritiated-5-Fluorocytosine

Haberkorn U, Oberdorfer F, Gebert J, et al (German Cancer Research Ctr, Heidelberg, Germany; Univ of Heidelberg, Germany)
J Nucl Med 37:87–94, 1996   2–44

Objectives.—Uptake parameters for 5-fluorocytosine were assessed in vitro, and information that may help develop additional PET measurements was sought.

Background.—Suicide genes code for nonmammalian enzymes that convert nontoxic prodrugs into toxic metabolites. The active drug is produced at the tumor site after systemic application of the nontoxic prodrug. Cytosine deaminase converts 5-fluorocytosine into 5-fluorouracil, which is highly toxic. No anabolic pathway is known to exist in mammalian cells that results in incorporation of 5-fluorocytosine into the nucleic acid fraction. Pharmacologic effects are, therefore, moderate, and high therapeutic doses can be used. 5-Fluorocytosine is uniformly distributed in mammalian tissues. Tissue-specific accumulation and significant binding to plasma proteins have not been observed. 5-Fluorouracil interferes with DNA and protein synthesis because uracil is substituted by 5-fluorouracil in RNA, and because of inhibition of thymidylate synthetase by 5-fluorodeoxyuridine monophosphate. This results in impaired DNA biosynthesis.

Methods.—A human glioblastoma cell line was stably transfected with the cytosine deaminase gene from *Escherichia coli*. High-performance liquid chromatography was done after lysates of cytosine deaminase–expressing cells and control cells with ^{3}H-5-fluorocytosine were incubated. Various incubation times were used with therapeutic quantities of 5-fluorocytosine, and uptake of fluorocytosine was measured.

Saturation and competition experiments with 5-fluorocytosine and 5-fluorouracil were conducted. Efflux also was measured.

Results.—Cytosine deaminase–expressing cells produced ^{3}H-5-fluorouracil. Only ^{3}H-5-fluorocytosine was produced in control cells. There were significant quantities of 5-fluorouracil in the medium of cultured cells. This may be responsible for the bystander effect seen in previous studies. Uptake measurements showed a moderate and nonsaturable accumulation of radioactivity in tumor cells. This suggests that 5-fluorocytosine enters cells through diffusion only. There was a significant difference in uptake of 5-fluorocytosine between cytosine deaminase–positive cells and control cells after incubation for 48 hours. No difference in uptake was found after incubation for 2 hours. A rapid efflux was noted.

Conclusions.—5-Fluorocytosine transport may be the limiting factor for therapeutic application of this procedure, even though enzyme activity sufficiently inhibited growth of tumor cells in vitro. Further studies are needed to determine whether PET can measure in vivo cytosine deaminase activity in solid tumors and whether modulation of 5-fluorouracil transport metabolism can improve tracer accumulation.

▶ Genes, gene therapy, and nucleic acid–based radiopharmaceuticals are finally making appearances in the nuclear medicine literature. As usual, we are several years behind the general trends in medical research, now dominated by the Human Genome Project to sequence the human genome and a multitude of gene therapy trials. But hopefully we can accelerate our learning processes and catch up quickly. Abstracts 2–43 and 2–44 are worthwhile reading to show you what the next century will bring for nuclear medicine.

R. Neumann, M.D.

Comparative Properties of a Technetium-99m-labeled Single-stranded Natural DNA and a Phosphorothioate Derivative *In Vitro* and in Mice
Hnatowich DJ, Mardirossian G, Fogarasi M, et al (Univ of Massachusetts, Worcester; Boston Univ)
J Pharmacol Exp Ther 276:326–334, 1996   2–45

Background.—DNA and RNA oligonucleotides may be useful as radiopharmaceuticals in nuclear imaging studies. A method of radiolabeling single-stranded DNA with technetium-99m has recently been developed. Technetium-99m will probably be the preferred imaging radionuclide, partly because of its short 6-hour half-life. The natural phosphodiester DNA has been considered for these applications, but the unmodified single-stranded oligonucleotides are very susceptible to degradation by nucleases. Attempts have been made to improve stability by altering the phosphodiester backbone of natural oligonucleotides. Studies have shown that the properties of radiolabeled oligonucleotides can depend on the method of radiolabeling and other factors. A synthetic 22-base single-stranded phosphodiester DNA was compared with its phosphorothioate analogue after both were radiolabeled with ^{99m}Tc using the hydrazino nicotinamide chelator.

Methods.—Two synthetic 22-base single-stranded DNA chains were used for most experiments. These two DNA chains differed in their phosphate backbone only. They were radiolabeled with ^{99m}Tc by transchelation. The evaluation of the labeled oligonucleotides included blood and serum incubation studies, tissue homogenate and urine analyses, urine incubations, and animal biodistribution studies.

Results.—Whole-body clearance of the label decreased when introduced on the phosphorothioate because of accumulation in the liver. In both cases, the label was present in urine chiefly on low–molecular weight catabolites. High-performance liquid chromatography analysis of 37°C serum incubates was performed and revealed serum protein binding of ^{99m}Tc in both cases, but to different proteins. Analysis of liver and kidney homogenates showed different behavior in protein binding: the phosphodiester label was nearly quantitatively converted to lower molecular weight catabolites after 15 minutes, but the phosphorothioate label was mainly on proteins. Quick digestion of the phosphodiester by nucleases was not seen, perhaps because protein binding of labeled oligonucleotides stabilized against degradation.

Conclusions.—The high liver uptake of ^{99m}Tc-labeled phosphorothioate DNA may decrease the value of this modified DNA as an imaging agent. The ^{99m}Tc phosphodiester may be a better choice because the label does not accumulate in the liver to the same degree and it is stable to degradation in serum.

3 Infection and Inflammation

Introduction

Infectious diseases are still a leading cause of death worldwide. There continues to be an increase in treatment-resistant human infections and emergence of more challenging infections caused by formerly friendly bacteria and fungi, particularly in the immunocompromised patient. The 1996 Pharmaceutical Research and Manufacturers of America survey reported that 125 medicines and vaccines are now in development for infectious diseases—an increase of 33% over the number reported during the previous survey 2 years earlier. And yet our nuclear medicine literature did not contain a large number of publications in the field of infection and inflammation this past year.

I have tried to pick some of the best articles for this chapter from an ever-increasing pool. Two excellent review articles lead off: the first reviews the basic mechanisms of inflammation; the second reviews the techniques appropriate for infection scintigraphy in the immunocompromised patient. The middle group of articles are reports on our current radiopharmaceuticals and promising new ones for application in infections and inflammation. The final selection of papers contains those dealing with application of our current techniques to the various diseases.

I hope we can somehow inspire more research in these topics, particularly the development and testing of new radiopharmaceuticals for these diseases. I believe we are still a long way from having optimal tests for such patients. Why do we still have such a tough time diagnosing osteomyelitis, especially in its chronic form, from our scans? Let's get to work!

Ronald Neumann, M.D.

The Uptake Mechanisms of Inflammation- and Infection-localizing Agents

Oyen WJG, Boerman OC, van der Laken CJ, et al (Univ Hosp Nijmegen, The Netherlands)
Eur J Nucl Med 23:459–465, 1996   3–1

Introduction.—Many different radiopharmaceuticals have been suggested for use in the scintigraphic study of inflammatory and infectious diseases (Table 1). All of these agents provide functional imaging of some process in the cascade of inflammation, which can be triggered by various types of tissue injury. The biodistribution, kinetics, and mechanisms of the different radiopharmaceuticals studied for use in scintigraphic study of focal inflammation and infection were reviewed.

Agents.—Gallium-67–citrate scanning is a well-established technique, particularly for studying pulmonary and musculoskeletal inflammation. This tracer has been shown to bind to transferrin in the blood. In vitro–labeled white blood cells were introduced in an attempt to find a more specific technique for imaging of inflammation. After initial entrapment in the lungs, the labeled cells migrate to the extravascular space in inflammatory foci. Labeling with indium-111 is more stable than labeling with technetium-99m. Although ^{99m}Tc-labeled nanocolloid has been investigated, it shows poor accumulation in inflammatory foci. Labeled liposomes seem unlikely to be useful in the detection of inflammation, although it may be possible to "fine-tune" liposomes by altering their composition.

Other studies use labeled large proteins, such as nonspecific and specific immunoglobulins. The pathophysiologic principle of this approach is increased vascular permeability and extravasation of large protein. In the case of nonspecific immunoglobulins, labeled antibodies are retained by the specific interaction between the antibody and the antigen expressed on

TABLE 1.—Mechanism of Uptake of Radiopharmaceuticals Used for Imaging Infection and Inflammation

	Influx of Leukocytes	Binding to Activated Leukocytes	Increased Vascular Permeability	Binding to Proteins	Binding to Bacteria
Ga-67 citrate		■		■	■
Leukocytes	■				
Nanocolloid			■		
Liposomes			■		
Non-specific IgG			■		■(?)
Antigranulocyte antibodies		■	■		
Chemotactic peptides		■			
Interleukins		■			
Ciprofloxacin				■(?)	■(?)

activated granulocytes. A monoclonal antibody against E-selectin has been investigated as well. Other studies have investigated labeled receptor-specific small proteins and peptides, such as chemotactic peptides and interleukins. Finally, ^{99m}Tc-labeled ciprofloxacin has been proposed for scintigraphic imaging of infection.

Summary.—Labeled leukocytes may be used to visualize specific processes in the inflammatory cascade, whereas polyclonal immunoglobulin scintigraphy can be used to depict the nonspecific effects of inflammation. None of the approaches described is clearly superior to the others; any claims made will have to be confirmed in clinical studies.

Radionuclide Imaging of Infection in the Immunocompromised Host
Rubin RH, Fischman AJ (Harvard Med School, Boston; Harvard-Massachusetts Inst of Techhnology, Cambridge)
Clin Infect Dis 22:414–422, 1996   3–2

Objective.—The inflammatory response to microbial invasion is impaired in patients with AIDS and other forms of immunocompromise, which makes it difficult to make an early diagnosis of infection. Radionuclide scintigraphy has the potential for overcoming these problems. The use of radionuclide imaging of infection in immunocompromised patients was reviewed, focusing on the chest and abdomen.

Discussion.—Radioscintigraphy permits early diagnosis of infection—even in patients with surgically altered anatomy—in that it depicts leukocyte delivery to the infection site or capillary leakiness to radiolabeled proteins. In addition, whole-body imaging can detect focal sites of infection that otherwise would be unsuspected, and serial studies can be performed to assess the response to therapy. Gallium-67–citrate and radiolabeled leukocytes are available for use in thoracic and abdominal imaging of infection in immunocompromised patients, and indium-111–labeled nonspecific polyclonal IgG will be available soon.

Gallium-67–citrate can permit a specific diagnosis in patients with thoracic disease, although its accumulation in healthy bowel makes abdominal evaluation difficult (Fig 1)). Although ^{111}In-labeled white blood cells can also detect infections, the need for blood-handling procedures is problematic in HIV-infected patients. Radiolabeled autologous leukocytes cannot be used in patients with granulocytopenia. Indium-111–labeled IgG combines many of the advantages of the other techniques; however, all require a delay of 18–24 hours between injection and imaging. This difficulty may be overcome by experimental agents such as technetium-99m–labeled chemotactic peptides, which require delays of less than 3 hours.

Summary.—Radionuclide imaging has the potential to overcome the difficulty of early diagnosis of infection in immunocompromised patients. With further study, ^{111}In-IgG could become the radiopharmaceutical of choice for this purpose.

PULMONARY ACCUMULATION OF GALLIUM

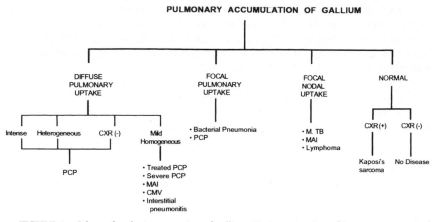

FIGURE 1.—Scheme for the interpretation of gallium-67–citrate imaging of immunocompromised patients. (Courtesy of Rubin RH, Fischman AJ: Radionuclide imaging of infection in the immunocompromised host. *Clin Infect Dis* 22:414–422, 1996. Published by the University of Chicago.)

▶ We are fortunate that these 2 excellent review articles examining nuclear medicine techniques for detecting and evaluating infections appeared. In the first one by Oyen and associates (Abstract 3–1), there is an accurate assessment of the state-of-the-art in radiopharmaceutical development for infection/inflammation scintigraphy. The second (Abstract 3–2), by Rubin and Fischman, provides insight in applying these techniques to detect infections of the immunocompromised host. With the increase in the numbers of immunocompromised patients from all causes, most nuclear medicine practitioners will benefit from a careful reading of these 2 papers in their entirety.

R. Neumann, M.D.

Functional Upregulation of Granulocytes Labeled With Technetium-99m-HMPAO and Indium-111-Oxinate

Bertrand-Caix J, Freyburger G, Bordenave L, et al (Univ of Bordeaux II, France; Hôpital Pellegrin, Bordeaux, France)
J Nucl Med 37:863–868, 1996   3–3

Background.—Recent diagnostic imaging developments in the detection of inflammatory and septic lesions have involved a number of scintigraphic methods of labeling leukocytes and granulocytes. One method uses indium-111–oxinate and another uses technetium-99m–hexamethylpropyleneamine oxime. Both of these labels are trapped in cellular cytoplasm after diffusing through the cell membrane and binding intracellularly. The influence of these radiotracers on the following neutrophil functions was examined: the expression of adhesion molecules after chemoattraction stimulation, adhesion to endothelium, and activation in response to reactive oxygen metabolites.

Methods.—Blood was obtained from 10 healthy volunteers, and the neutrophils (PMN) were isolated. Each PMN suspension was divided into

3 parts, which were labeled with ^{111}In-oxinate, with ^{99m}Tc-HMPAO, and kept unlabeled as a control. Surface expression of CD11b in the neutrophil suspensions was measured after exposure to formylmethionyleucyl-phenylalanine using immunofluorescence flow cytometry. Polymorphonuclear cell adherence to cultured human endothelial cells was determined after incubation for 7, 15, 30, and 60 minutes. Polymorphonuclear cell migration toward formyl-methionyleucyl-phenylalanine chemoattractant was determined to assess chemotaxis. Phagocytosis and hydrogen peroxide production was assessed using staphylococci labeled with propidium iodide

Results.—The CD11b expression on quiescent PMN was increased with both radiotracers, compared with control PMN, with greater increases with ^{111}In-oxinate. Polymorphonuclear cell adhesion to endothelial cells was greater with ^{111}In-oxinate labeling than with ^{99m}Tc-HMPAO labeling. Polymorphonuclear cell migration toward the chemoattractant was decreased with both radiolabels, but the decrease was more pronounced with ^{111}In-oxinate. There were no differences between the control granulocytes and either of the labeled granulocytes in phagocytosis. Hydrogen peroxide production was slightly increased with ^{99m}Tc-HMPAO labeling and significantly increased with ^{111}In-oxinate labeling.

Conclusions.—Neutrophil functions are significantly affected by radiotracers. Therefore, quality control of PMN functions after radiolabeling needs to be reappraised to improve detection of inflammation or infection.

▶ There have always been concerns about the effects of the radiolabeling process on the postlabeling functions of blood cells and platelets. Have we interfered somehow with the normal cell's ability to carry out its role(s) by the very processes necessary to attach a radionuclide label? This paper presents an evaluation of the in vitro functional abilities of leukocytes labeled by the 2 most common methods: ^{111}In-oxinate and ^{99m}Tc-HMPAO. The results indicate that both methods can produce labeled leukocytes sufficient for scintigraphy, but these are not the same old leukocytes anymore; most leukocyte functions assayed were stimulated, but chemotaxis was decreased by the presence of the radiotracers.

R. Neumann, M.D.

Contribution of Phagocytic Cells and Bacteria to the Accumulation of Technetium-99m Labelled Polyclonal Human Immunoglobulin at Sites of Inflammation

Calame W, Welling M, Feitsma HIJ, et al (Univ Hosp, Leiden, The Netherlands; Hercules European Research Ctr, Barneveld, The Netherlands; Mallinckrodt Med, Petten, The Netherlands)
Eur J Nucl Med 22:638–644, 1995   3–4

Background.—Radiolabeled polyclonal human immunoglobulin (Ig) has proven effectiveness in the detection of sites of inflammation. However, the mode of action of IgG accumulation at sites of inflammation is unclear. Although it is generally agreed that vascular leakage plays a role in this accumulation, the role of cellular binding is controversial. The contribution of cells and bacteria to IgG accumulation was examined using an experimental peritoneal inflammation model in mice.

Methods.—Pathogen-free mice were divided into 3 groups and injected intraperitoneally with either *Staphylococcus aureus* (SA), newborn calf serum (NBCS) (to induce a nonbacterial inflammation), or physiologic saline (control group). One hour later, all animals were given IV injections of technetium-99m–labeled polyclonal human immunoglobulin. Animals in each group were killed at various intervals to examine the number of peritoneal cells and bacteria and the activity of each cell fraction at the inflammation site.

Results.—The activity in the peritoneal cavity compared with activity in the total organism never exceeded a 6% increase in any animals. The peak activity occurred at 4 hours after injection of either inducing material and was greatest in the SA group, with significant differences from the other groups at 4, 18, and 24 hours. The SA group also had the greatest total number of cells and of neutrophils, followed by the NBCS group and then the control group. Only the SA group also had a greater number of macrophages than the other 2 groups. In multiple regression analysis, the neutrophils contributed significantly more than the macrophages to the increase in the total number of cells in both the SA and the NBCS groups, but not in the control group.

Cell-bound labeled activity was significantly lower in the control animals than in the other 2 groups and was significantly greater at 18 and 24 hours in the SA group than in the NBCS group. Cell-bound activity showed a time-dependent increase in the SA group and was relatively constant in the NBCS and control groups. Free bacteria decreased and cell-associated bacteria increased in a time-dependent pattern. Cell-bound activity was positively correlated with the total number of cells in all groups. In the 2 inflammation groups, cell-bound activity was positively correlated with the number of neutrophils. In addition, there was correlation between cell-bound activity and the number of cell-associated bacteria.

Conclusions.—Both phagocytic cells and cell-associated bacteria are significant contributors to the labeled IgG accumulation at the site of inflammation. Neutrophils play a particularly important role in the binding of labeled IgG.

Specific Targeting of Infectious Foci With Radioiodinated Human Recombinant Interleukin-1 in an Experimental Model
van der Laken CJ, Boerman OC, Oyen WJG, et al (Univ Hosp Nijmegen, The Netherlands)
Eur J Nucl Med 22:1249–1255, 1995   3–5

Background.—Interleukin-1 (IL-1) is a 17-kd protein produced mainly by mononuclear phagocytes after an inflammatory stimulus. It occurs in 2 forms—IL-1α and IL-1β. An influx of leukocytes, primarily IL-1R positive, characterizes infection and inflammation. Interleukin-1 may be able to target these inflammatory cells specifically because of its high affinity for its receptors. The potential of radioiodinated human recombinant IL-1 to image infectious foci in vivo was investigated in an animal model of infection.

Methods and Findings.—Mice were injected intravenously with iodine-125–labeled IL-1 and iodine-131–labeled myoglobin, a size-matched control agent, 24 hours after a *Staphylococcus aureus* abscess was induced in the left calf muscle. Biodistribution studies showed that radioiodinated IL-1 cleared rapidly from the body. After 12 hours the abscess had the highest activity. Compared with ^{131}I-myoglobin, the absolute abscess uptake of ^{125}I–IL-1 remained high. Thus, abscess-to-muscle ratios of ^{125}I–IL-1 were significantly higher than ^{131}I-myoglobin. The ratios of ^{125}I–IL-1 peaked at a mean 44.4 at 48 hours after inoculation. The ratios of ^{131}I-myoglobin did not exceed a mean of 5.9.

Conclusions.—Radioiodinated IL-1 is retained specifically in the abscess, presumably by IL-1 interaction with its receptor on the inflammatory cells. The high target-to-background ratios obtained over time suggest that the IL-1 receptor is a useful target for imaging infectious foci.

▶ The search goes on for the "Holy Grail" of radiopharmaceuticals to be applied in scintigraphy of infection and inflammation. The "grandfather," gallium-67–citrate, stands alongside labeled leukocytes, labeled polyclonal antibodies, and the latest experimental generation of labeled peptides to give the nuclear medicine physician a family of radiopharmaceuticals from which to select as needed in scintigraphy of inflammation and infection. Abstracts 3–4 and 3–5 present interesting data; one concerning the mechanisms by which ^{99m}Tc-labeled polyclonal human immunoglobulins accumulate at such disease sites and the second presenting a novel new agent based on the recombinant IL-1 molecule.

R. Neumann, M.D.

Quantitative Assessment of Overall Inflammatory Bowel Disease Activity Using Labelled Leucocytes: A Direct Comparison Between Indium-111 and Technetium-99m HMPAO Methods
Mansfield JC, Giaffer MH, Tindale WB, et al (Royal Hallamshire Hosp, Sheffield, England)
Gut 37:679–683, 1995   3–6

Background.—The ideal method for imaging inflammatory bowel disease would reliably show inflammation, intestinal location, and disease severity. Scintigraphic methods of quantifying overall disease activity using indium-111 and technetium-99m–hexamethylpropylenamine oxime (HMPAO)-labeled leukocyte scans were compared.

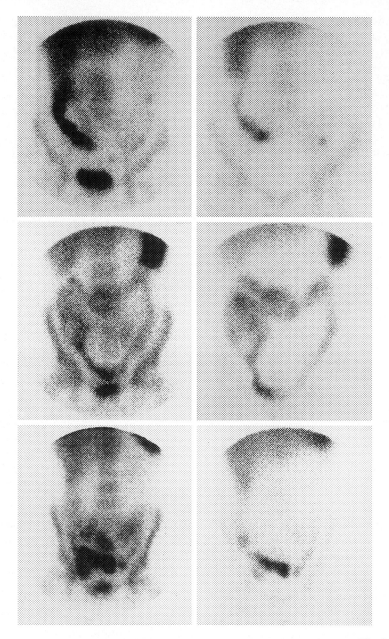

(*Continued*)

FIGURE 2 (cont.)

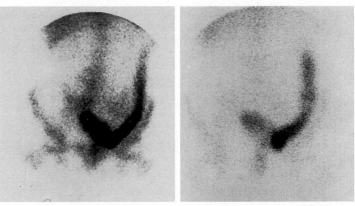

FIGURE 2.—Four pairs of indium-111 and technetium-99m–hexamethylpropylenamine oxine (*HMPAO*) images, showing the superior image quality of that obtained using ^{99m}Tc-HMPAO. All the ^{99m}Tc-HMPAO images were acquired at 120 minutes after injection. (Courtesy of Mansfield JC, Giaffer MH, Tindale WB, et al: Quantitative assessment of overall inflammatory bowel disease activity using labelled leucocytes: A direct comparison between indium-111 and technetium-99m HMPAO methods. *Gut* 37:679–683, 1995.)

Methods.—Twenty-four patients known to have inflammatory bowel disease were included in the study. The 4-day fecal excretion of ^{111}In was measured after ^{111}In scintigraphy. These patients also had ^{99m}Tc-HMPAO scanning within 10 days of initial scanning, with no treatment changes between assessments.

Findings.—Inflammatory activity defined by fecal ^{111}In excretion was closely correlated with the scan score produced by the computer analysis of the ^{99m}Tc-HMPAO image. Accurate information for localizing inflammatory activity could be obtained by a simple visual assessment of both image types, although image quality was better with ^{99m}Tc-HMPAO. Disease activity qualification on ^{99m}Tc-HMPAO images by visual grading showed a wide variability, with the scores of 3 graders being similar in only 69% of the scans. Reproducibility was better in computer-generated analyses (Fig 2).

Conclusions.—The findings of ^{99m}Tc-HMPAO scintigraphy and fecal ^{111}In excretion were well correlated in patients with inflammatory bowel disease. Inflammation can be quantified and localized by either method. Scanning with ^{99m}Tc-HMPAO may be preferred, because it yields faster results, involves a lower radiation dose, and does not require fecal collection.

▶ These authors compared ^{111}In tropolonate– and ^{99m}Tc-HMPAO–labeled leukocytes for their in vivo ability to reliably detect inflammatory bowel disease, correctly identify involved bowel segments, and assess the severity of the inflammation. As noted in Dr. McAfee's review in the 1995 YEAR BOOK OF NUCLEAR MEDICINE,[1] such studies have captured more attention in Europe than the United States, as this very fine paper from England demonstrates.

The authors' conclusions, i.e., that ^{99m}Tc-HMPAO scintigraphy provided accurate assessment quickly and without the need to count the ^{111}In activity in stool samples may expand the role of scintigraphic evaluation of inflammatory bowel disease worldwide.

R. Neumann, M.D.

Reference

1. 1995 YEAR BOOK OF NUCLEAR MEDICINE, pp 93–94.

Sterically Stabilized Liposomes Labeled With Indium-111 to Image Focal Infection

Boerman OC, Storm G, Oyen WJG, et al (Univ Hosp, Nijmegen, The Netherlands; Univ of Utrecht, The Netherlands)
J Nucl Med 36:1639–1644, 1995   3–7

Background.—Several radiopharmaceuticals have been investigated for use in localizing infectious and inflammatory lesions. One recently developed approach is sterically stabilized liposomes. Uptake of these liposomes by the mononuclear phagocyte system is reduced, which prolongs their circulation time and increases their chances of targeting other tissues, possibly including infectious foci. Sterically stabilized liposomes were studied for their ability to image infectious and inflammatory foci in rats.

Methods.—The in vivo study used indium-111–labeled liposomes coated with polyethylene glycol (PEGylated), which were injected IV in rats with *Staphylococcus aureus*–induced calf muscle abscesses. Some animals were killed for biodistribution studies up to 48 hours after injection; others underwent gamma camera imaging before they were killed. Studies with ^{111}In-IgG were performed for comparison.

Results.—Clearance from the blood compartment was similar (half-time about 20 hours) for PEGylated liposomes and ^{111}In-IgG. However, uptake by the abscess was twice as high with ^{111}In liposomes as with ^{111}In-IgG, with values of 2.7% vs. 1.1% ID/g after 48 hours. On gamma counting of dissected tissues, abscess-to-muscle ratios reached 20 at 24 hours and 34 at 48 hours; abscess-to-blood ratios continued to increase for up to 48 hours as well (Fig 1). Scintigraphic imaging of the abscesses was possible as soon as 1 hour after ^{111}In-liposome injection.

Conclusion.—The findings suggest that radiolabeled, sterically stabilized liposomes are a potentially valuable tool for the imaging of infections. Liposomes have some important advantages over radiolabeled leukocytes for this purpose: They are readily available and do not carry blood-derived infectious agents.

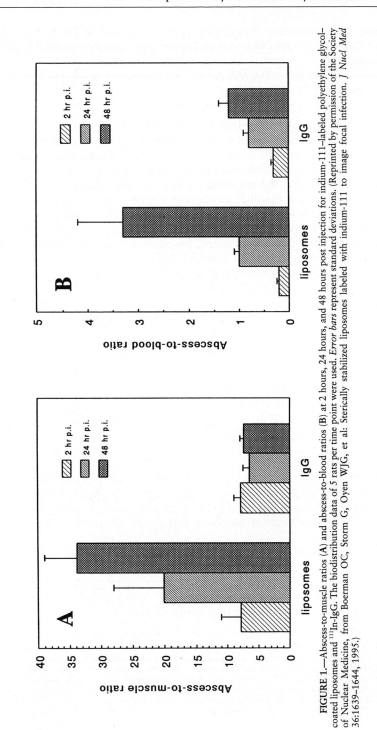

FIGURE 1.—Abscess-to-muscle ratios (A) and abscess-to-blood ratios (B) at 2 hours, 24 hours, and 48 hours post injection for indium-111–labeled polyethylene glycol–coated liposomes and ¹¹¹In-IgG. The biodistribution data of 5 rats per time point were used. *Error bars* represent standard deviations. (Reprinted by permission of the Society of Nuclear Medicine, from Boerman OC, Storm G, Oyen WJG, et al: Sterically stabilized liposomes labeled with indium-111 to image focal infection. *J Nucl Med* 36:1639–1644, 1995.)

Cranial Osteomyelitis: Diagnosis and Follow-up With In-111 White Blood Cell and Tc-99m Methylene Diphosphonate Bone SPECT, CT, and MR Imaging

Seabold JE, Simonson TM, Weber PC, et al (Univ of Iowa, Iowa City)
Radiology 196:779–788, 1995   3–8

Introduction.—Osteomyelitis can be difficult to diagnose on radiographs, especially in patients with concurrent bone destruction and repair resulting from a noninfectious process. Computed tomography and MRI are both useful in the detection of osteomyelitis, although they are not helpful in monitoring the response to therapy. With the new multidetector SPECT systems, it is possible to perform simultaneous acquisition of dual radiotracers, with improved low-photon flux studies. Simultaneous indium-111 white blood cell and technetium-99m methylene diphosphonate (MPD) bone SPECT were evaluated, together with CT and MRI, for use in imaging patients with cranial osteomyelitis.

Methods.—The retrospective study included 26 cases of suspected cranial osteomyelitis in 25 patients during a 5-year period. The patients were 13 males and 12 females (mean age, 55 years); there were 16 postoperative cases. Twenty-four cases were investigated by ^{111}In white blood cell and ^{99m}Tc MDP bone SPECT using a 3-detector system with medium-energy collimators. All patients underwent CT, and 11 patients with suspected infection at the skull base underwent MRI. The imaging findings were compared with the final diagnosis, which was established by bone culture in 18 cases and by clinical follow-up in 8.

Results.—Of the total 35 CT scans obtained, 10 were true positive (TP), 3 were false negative (FN), 13 were true negative (TN), 1 was false positive (FP), and 8 were equivocal. Thirty-six SPECT scans were analyzed, showing 19 TP, 13 TN, 1 FP, 1 FN, and 2 equivocal. The results of 11 MRI scans were TP in 4, TN in 5, and FN in 2. The most effective methods in identifying osteomyelitis in skull areas with little or no bone marrow were CT and bone SPECT scintigraphy. To image osteomyelitis involving the skull base, MRI and bone SPECT were the most sensitive techniques, whereas MRI was best for assessing soft-tissue infection in this area (Fig 4).

Conclusion.—To differentiate between infections of the soft tissue and bone, CT is the best choice. Studies of the calvaria and skull base are best performed using MRI. When the goal is to detect postoperative cranial osteomyelitis or to look for active cranial osteomyelitis after treatment, SPECT appears to be the imaging study of choice.

FIGURE 4.—Images of a 36-year-old woman with persistent pain on the left side of the head for 2 months after a 6-week course of IV antibiotic treatment and a left radical mastoidectomy for recurrent mastoiditis and osteomyelitis. **A,** planar indium-111 white blood cell and technetium-99m methylene diphosphonate (*MDP*) bone SPECT images show faint ^{111}In white blood cell localization (*arrows*) in the left mastoid region that corresponds to focal ^{99m}Tc MDP bone localization (*arrowheads*). It is difficult to determine whether the ^{111}In white blood cell uptake is localized in soft tissue or bone. **B,** [111]In white blood cell and ^{99m}Tc MDP bone SPECT transaxial images show focal ^{111}In white blood cell localization that

(Continued)

FIGURE 4 (cont.)

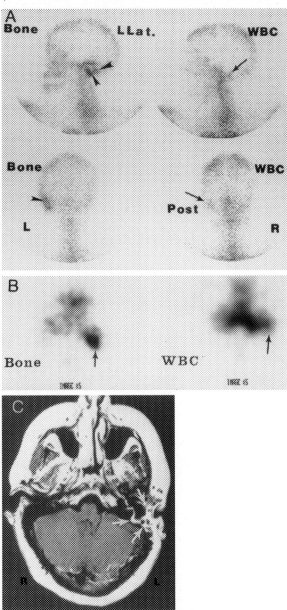

corresponds to areas of focal ^{99m}Tc MDP bone uptake in the left mastoid region (*arrows*; true positive study). **C,** T1-weighted MR image (500/15) reveals a postoperative gadolinium-enhanced scar in the left mastoid region (*arrows*). There are no specific findings to suggest osteomyelitis (false negative). (Courtesy of Seabold JE, Simonson TM, Weber PC, et al: Cranial osteomyelitis: Diagnosis and follow-up with In-111 white blood cell and Tc-99m methylene diphosphonate bone SPECT, CT, and MR Imaging. Radiology 196:779–788, 1995, Radiological Society of North America.)

4 Musculoskeletal

Introduction

Nearly one half of the articles I've chosen for this chapter deal with "quality control" issues. Scintigraphy techniques for bone imaging are in a mature phase now, and proper attention to how we do things is always prudent. With the application of SPECT to bone scintigraphy, we all think we are adding value, but please read the article by Littenberg and colleagues (Abstract 4–4). We do not seem to have published enough of the research now requested by payment providers to document cost-effectiveness or improved patient outcome for SPECT bone scintigraphy.

Positron emission tomography has seldom been used for bone scintigraphy in benign diseases, but the article by Bending et al. (Abstract 4–8) is a particularly exciting application of [18F]fluoride ion PET scans to evaluate bone grafting procedures.

Ronald Neumann, M.D.

Age-related Change of Technetium-99m-HMDP Distribution in the Skeleton

Kigami Y, Yamamoto I, Ohnishi H, et al (Shiga Univ, Japan)
J Nucl Med 37:815–818, 1996
4–1

Background.—Bone scintigraphy can survey the bone metabolism of the entire body, with radiopharmaceutical uptake reflecting local bone turnover, whereas biochemical markers generally reflect total-body bone metabolic activity. Age-related changes in whole-body bone scintigraphy patterns have been reported. To study these changes, regional and total-body skeletal uptake changes in bone scintigraphic patterns associated with age were quantified and correlated with biochemical metabolic bone markers.

Methods.—Bone scintigraphy was done with technetium-99m hydroxy-methane-diphosphonate in 144 women and 130 men. None of the selected patients had focal abnormalities of skeletal uptake. Whole-body skeletal uptake (WBSU) was calculated as the simple mathematical mean of the anterior and posterior views. Bone uptake in the head, the thoracic region, and the lower legs also was quantified as the ratio of uptake in these regions to the WBSU. When the bone scan was done, blood samples also were obtained and were analyzed for C-terminal propeptide of type 1 procollagen (P1CP) and alkaline phosphatase, as markers of bone formation, and C-terminal telopeptide of type 1 collagen, as a marker of bone resorption.

Results.—Both men and women had increasing WBSUs with increasing age. The differences in WBSUs between patients younger and older than age 50 years were statistically significant. In men, the skeletal uptakes increased proportionally in the 3 studied regions, whereas in women, there were significantly greater relative uptakes in the head and legs with aging. Whole-body skeletal uptake was significantly correlated with P1CP in men and with P1CP and alkaline phosphatase in women. Head uptake was correlated with all 3 serum biochemical markers: positively in women and negatively in men.

Conclusions.—Skeletal turnover increases generally with aging in both men and women. Regional skeletal turnover patterns are sex-dependent. These age-related changes in local bone metabolism may indicate progressive bone loss.

The Aetiology and Distinguishing Features of Solitary Spinal Hot Spots on Planar Bone Scans

Coakley FV, Jones AR, Finlay DB, et al (Leicester Royal Infirmary, England)
Clin Radiol 50:327–330, 1995   4–2

Background.—Solitary spinal hot spots are common findings on bone scintigraphy. Management then becomes a clinical challenge, because the cause could be either a benign degenerative change or malignant disease. The cause of solitary spinal hot spots on planar bone scans was determined in patients with and without known malignancy, and radiographic and scintigraphic features distinguishing benign from malignant causes were sought.

Methods.—Whole-body scans with solitary spinal hot spots from 81 patients were reviewed, including 41 identified prospectively and 40 identified retrospectively. Of the 81 patients, 42 had a known malignancy. The cause was determined, using imaging and long-term clinical findings, in 73 patients. The hot spot's location was classified as paravertebral (at the lateral spinal margin), panvertebral (diffusely increased uptake confined within a vertebra), hemivertebral (between the midline and lateral spinal margin), or complex (all other patterns or irregularly outlined uptake).

Results.—Clinical findings (including follow-up) and other imaging findings showed the cause of the spinal hot spot to be benign in 55 patients and malignant in 18. All 18 patients with a spinal metastasis had a known malignancy. There were suggestive findings on the plain radiographs in only 8 of the 18 patients with spinal metastasis. Age and etiology were not associated. The spinal hot spot was located in the cervical area in 3 patients (all with a benign cause), in the thoracic area in 16 patients (of whom 8 had a benign cause), and in the lumbar area in 54 patients (of whom 44 had a benign cause). The location was paravertebral in 21 patients (all with a benign cause), panvertebral in 24 patients (of whom 20 had a benign cause), hemivertebral in 13 patients (of whom 10 had a benign cause), and complex in 15 patients (of whom 4 had a benign cause).

Conclusions.—The solitary spinal hot spots were benign in 75% of the patients overall and in 57% of the patients with a known malignancy. Almost half of the malignant spinal lesions could not be detected radiographically. Abnormal uptake in the thoracic spine or a complex uptake pattern should raise suspicion, whereas a paravertebral uptake pattern can be a reassuring finding.

Observer Variation in the Interpretation of Bone Scintigraphy
Ore L, Hardoff R, Gips S, et al (Lady Davis Carmel Hosp, Haifa, Israel; Israel Inst of Technology, Haifa)
J Clin Epidemiol 49:67–71, 1996   4–3

Background.—Although bone scintigraphy is widely used as a diagnostic test, its validity has not been examined in the medical literature. The validity of a diagnostic test is examined by comparing it with another test considered the "gold standard." If there is no gold standard test, interobserver and intraobserver variability are used to evaluate the test's reliability. The reliability of bone scintigraphy was examined by determining the κ coefficients of the description of findings, diagnostic interpretation, and recommendations for additional radiographic studies.

Methods.—One hundred randomly selected bone scintigraphic studies performed on patients with oncologic and nononcologic conditions were interpreted in groups of 15 studies per session by 2 independent readers. Each observer read each set of studies twice, separated by 3 weeks. They were asked to produce 3 interpretative elements: a description of the findings, a diagnostic interpretation, and recommendations for further radiographic studies. Intraobserver and interobserver agreement was calculated for each of the 3 elements.

Results.—Overall, high agreement was found among and between observers for normal descriptive findings, but the κ values for the various descriptive categories varied from 0.53 to 0.72. Among the anatomical locations of increased activity, intraobserver agreement was high for the skull, the lower limbs, the ribs, and the pelvis and was less reliable for the cervical spine and the upper limbs. Interobserver agreement was high for multifocal skeletal involvement, the lower limbs, the hip joints, the skull, the ribs, and the pelvis. Diagnostic interpretation had high κ coefficients for both intraobserver and interobserver variation for bone metastasis, but there was only moderate reliability for degenerative changes. Regarding recommendations for further radiographic studies, the κ values for intraobserver agreement were 0.20–0.54, with lower κ values for interobserver agreement (0.32).

Conclusions.—The interpretation of bone metastases or normal scintigrams were reliable in the research setting. However, interpretations of bone scintigraphy were less reliable with degenerative changes, and this diagnosis requires radiographic evaluation.

▶ Lest we become complacent in our abilities to practice nuclear medicine, it is always wise to "return to the fundamentals," as successful football coaches repeat at every opportunity. These 3 papers (Abstracts 4–1 to 4–3) deal with the fundamentals of bone scintigraphy.

In the first, a Japanese group took the time to study sex- and age-related changes in bone metabolism by quantifying whole-body bone scans and attempting a correlation with biochemical bone markers. They found that whole-body skeletal uptake actually showed an increase with age in both sexes, but in women the head and leg uptake increased more relative to the thorax; in men, there was no such relative increase in any area. They conclude that their results confirm an age-related increase in skeletal turnover and sex-dependent regional differences in skeletal metabolism.

Coakley and associates took on the difficult task of determining the cause of solitary spinal hot spots in the spine. Eighty-one scans with this feature were collected, the location of the lesion was classified, and the cause was determined as well as possible from all available information. The authors found that most solitary hot spots were benign; even in patients with a known malignancy, 57% were benign. Once again, although most malignant lesions were positive on bone scintigraphy, they were occult radiographically.

Finally, the third of these papers by Ore et al. examines how reliably physicians interpret bone scintigrams. A random sample of 100 bone scans was reviewed twice by each of 2 experienced nuclear medicine physicians. Good to excellent agreement was found both intraobserver and interobserver when reporting normal scans and metastatic disease. However, for degenerative bone disease lesions and other pathologies, not metastatic disease, only moderate correlations were found. The authors conclude that we must improve our reliability as interpreters of many bone studies.

R. Neumann, M.D.

Clinical Efficacy of SPECT Bone Imaging for Low Back Pain
Littenberg B, Siegel A, Tosteson ANA, et al (Dartmouth-Hitchcock Med Ctr, Lebanon, NH)
J Nucl Med 36:1707–1713, 1995   4–4

Objective.—The use of SPECT has been proposed as an accurate method of diagnosing low back pain. A careful literature search was performed to find evidence documenting the diagnostic accuracy, clinical usefulness, and cost-effectiveness of SPECT in patients with low back pain.

Methods.—The review sought to summarize any valid clinical trials estimating the accuracy of SPECT in patients with low back pain; to identify any literature demonstrating the clinical usefulness of SPECT in this situation, i.e., its effect on patient management; and to locate any studies of the cost-effectiveness or other societal benefits of SPECT. The study protocol was carefully designed to avoid bias or error.

Findings.—Of 13 reports that met the inclusion criteria, none included information on the clinical usefulness or cost-effectiveness of SPECT in low back pain. The most recent study provided data on 233 patients undergoing SPECT of the lumbar spine, including 75 patients with known malignancy but no known spinal metastases. Some SPECT abnormality was found in almost all patients, including the 28 with metastases and the 43 with benign conditions. There was a 1.01 likelihood ratio for a positive test. The results suggested that lesions in the pedicle were more likely to be positive and those in the vertebral body to be benign; however, there were insufficient data to determine the value of SPECT in differentiating between patients with and without metastatic spread.

In a study of athletes with back pain, SPECT abnormalities were common, but only 45% of them were also detected by planar bone scan. No external validation of the scintigraphic diagnoses and no clinical outcome data were provided. Another report suggested that SPECT results are positive in patients with painful pars fractures and negative in those with asymptomatic fractures; again, no clinical outcome data were provided.

There were very few data on the accuracy of SPECT in low back pain. One small study concluded that SPECT is highly accurate in detecting pseudarthroses in patients with failed back surgery. A study of cancer patients found that SPECT was of little help in detecting spinal metastases because results were almost always positive. A small, retrospective study suggested that SPECT correctly classified 14 of 15 young patients with low back pain.

Discussion.—There are few research data to support the accuracy, clinical effectiveness, or cost-effectiveness of SPECT imaging for patients with low back pain. Truly useful studies of SPECT would require a large cohort, perhaps up to thousands of subjects; systematic enrolling of all subjects with back pain for whom SPECT might reasonably be helpful; and blinded use of SPECT as the index test and some reference test. Although SPECT could be useful in certain specific situations, there are no data to justify its use in most patients with low back pain.

Metastases Seen on SPECT Imaging Despite a Normal Planar Bone Scan
Roland J, van den Weyngaert D, Krug B, et al (Middelheim Gen Hosp, Antwerp, Belgium)
Clin Nucl Med 20:1052–1054, 1995   4–5

Background.—Bone scintigraphy is highly sensitive but nonspecific in the detection of bone lesions. However, some small lesions embedded in large metabolically normal bone structures may be missed by bone scintigraphy. The use of SPECT in the evaluation of such lesions was examined in a patient with carcinoma of the breast who had occult bone metastasis 1 year later.

> *Case Report.*—Woman, 45, who was premenopausal, was re-evaluated 1 year after treatment of a small adenocarcinoma of the breast with surgery, regional radiotherapy, and chemotherapy. Her serum CA 15-3 level was elevated, although no metastases were detected on planar whole-body bone imaging. Single-photon emission CT imaging with a triple-headed high-resolution system revealed several focal areas of increased activity in the following vertebral bodies: L2–L5, T6, and T8–T12. The activity extended toward the posterior arch in some sites. An area of hypointensity in the T8 vertebral body was detected with T1-weighted MR images in the sagittal plane. The patient was treated with hormonal therapy. However, the serum CA 15-3 level continued to increase. Six weeks later, extensive metastatic involvement was detected with planar bone imaging.

Discussion.—Single-photon emission CT imaging provides cross-section details with greater contrast and anatomical clarity, which can enable both greater sensitivity and some degree of specificity in the evaluation of the metabolic activity of bone. Small focal lesions can be identified more easily because of the ability to separate the metabolic activity of the lesion from that of the underlying and overlying normal bone.

▶ Studies using SPECT are a way of life for most of us now, but not always for bone scintigraphy. Proponents of SPECT suggest that the increased resolution and contrast will improve the clinical practice of bone scintigraphy, but they apparently aren't publishing enough proper studies to prove it, or so say Littenberg and associates (Abstract 4–4). These authors reviewed 940 literature citations from 1966 through September 1993 in a search for the accuracy of SPECT for evaluating low back pain. Only 13 reported on accuracy; of these, only 3 provided a reasonable standard for reference and thus permitted calculation of sensitivity and specificity. They concluded that there is only weak evidence for SPECT's usefulness in 3 settings: detecting pseudoarthroses after failed spinal, evaluating young patients with back pain, and distinguishing benign from malignant lesions in patients with cancer. There were no reports of clinical outcome or cost-effectiveness.

Wake up, colleagues! This is what technology assessment is all about. How can we expect to be paid for tests we haven't properly evaluated? We write and read too many case reports like the one by Roland et al. (Abstract 4–5). This is surely a fine case report, but unfortunately such papers do not convince the HMOs, insurance providers, and health care decision makers. Let's be kind to the forests and not use so much paper on case reports.

R. Neumann, M.D.

Multimodality Imaging of Osteomyelitis

Elgazzar AH, Abdel-Dayem HM, Clark JD, et al (Univ of Cincinnati, Ohio; New York Med College, Valhalla, NY)
Eur J Nucl Med 22:1043–1063, 1995   4–6

Objective.—Even with advances in diagnosis and treatment, osteomyelitis remains a common clinical condition that is difficult to diagnose early. Of the many imaging techniques used in diagnosing osteomyelitis, none is optimal for all cases. The choice of imaging technique depends on an understanding of the different pathophysiologic forms of the disease. Imaging considerations in the diagnosis of osteomyelitis were reviewed.

Imaging of Osteomyelitis.—The choice of imaging modalities to investigate osteomyelitis must take into consideration whether the bone has been previously violated as well as the site of disease. Although conventional radiographs can demonstrate the classic bone destruction and periosteal reaction of osteomyelitis, they may not become abnormal for weeks after the start of the infection. Radiography is nonspecific in patients with violated bone. The initial study of choice for patients suspected of having osteomyelitis is multiphase bone scanning. Study results become positive within 24–48 hours after the start of symptoms, with classical findings of increased regional perfusion as seen in flow and blood pool images and increased uptake on delayed images. Bone scintigraphy is highly sensitive in early diagnosis of osteomyelitis and is highly specific when the bone has not been previously violated. Gallium-67–citrate scanning results also become positive shortly after the onset of symptoms; in addition, unlike multiphase bone scanning, it is useful for monitoring the response to treatment. Labeled leukocyte studies using indium-111 oxime and technetium-99m–hexamethylpropyleneamine oxime are recognized as specific agents for the diagnosis of infection. Recent studies have explored the use of ^{99m}Tc nanocolloid scintigraphy and immunoscintigraphy to diagnose osteomyelitis. Also, because of its ability to distinguish between soft tissue and bone infection, MRI is replacing CT for use in diagnosing osteomyelitis.

Distinctive Forms.—Imaging considerations may vary for patients with distinctive forms of osteomyelitis. For example, bone scanning cannot confirm the presence of active or chronic osteomyelitis, although a negative scan excludes active disease. For diabetic foot osteomyelitis, ^{111}In leukocyte imaging constitutes a sensitive and specific test, particularly when combined with 3-phase bone scanning (Fig 8). Indium-111 leukocyte scanning is also useful in the assessment of osteomyelitis associated with orthopedic prostheses and can be made even more specific with the addition of ^{99m}Tc sulfur colloid bone marrow (Fig 12). The imaging considerations for vertebral osteomyelitis, osteomyelitis associated with sickle cell disease or pressure sores, and chronic recurrent osteomyelitis are discussed as well.

Summary.—No single imaging technique is best for all cases of osteomyelitis. To choose the best study, the diagnostician must understand the

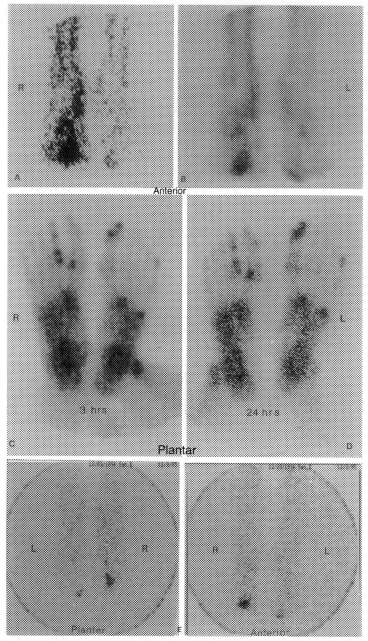

Anterior

Plantar

3 hrs

24 hrs

FIGURE 8.—A 47-year-old male diabetic with a history of pain in the right second and left first toes was referred for a bone scan to rule out osteomyelitis. There is increased flow (**A**), blood pool activity (**B**), and delayed uptake (**C**) in the areas of suspected infection. Twenty-four–hour image (**D**) revealed persistently increased uptake in these areas. An indium-111 white blood cell study (**E**) obtained 2 days later demonstrated foci of increased uptake in the regions of the left first toe and the mid portion of the right second toe, indicating osteomyelitis. The bone scan was essential for proper localization of leukocyte scan abnormalities. (Courtesy of Elgazzar AH, Abdel-Dayem HM, Clark JD, et al: Multimodality imaging of osteomyelitis. *Eur J Nucl Med* 22:1043–1063, 1995. Copyright Springer-Verlag.)

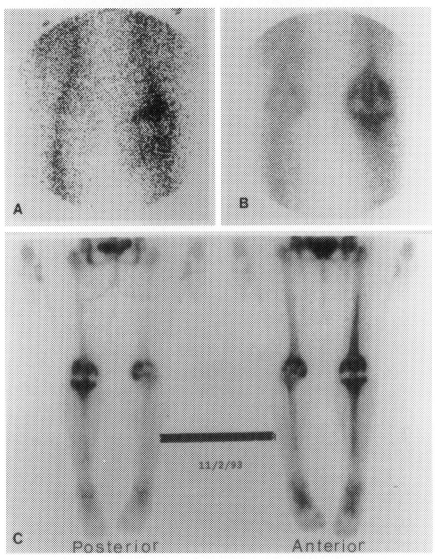

FIGURE 12.—Multiple images of a 62-year-old woman who had had a left knee replacement 7 months earlier. The patient was referred to the Nuclear Medicine Service to rule out postarthroplastic infection because of pain in both knees (worse on the left side) of 2 weeks' duration. Flow (**A**) and blood pool (**B**) images revealed increased perfusion around the left knee prosthesis. Increased uptake was also noted on the delayed images (**C**) around the prosthesis and extending to the shafts of the left femur and tibia.

(*Continued*)

FIGURE 12 (cont.)

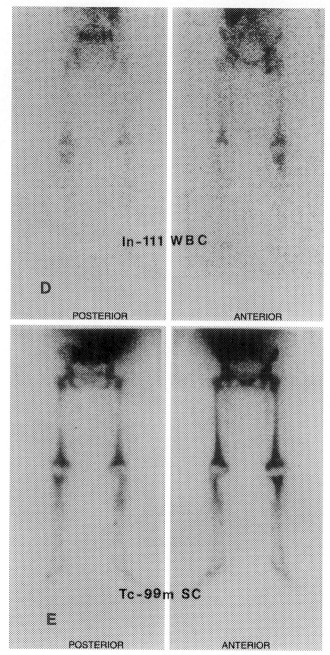

Increased uptake in the right knee suggested arthritis. An indium-111 white blood cell study (D) obtained the next morning revealed increased uptake in the distal femora and proximal left tibia, corresponding to the uptake seen on the subsequently obtained technetium-99m sulfur colloid bone marrow scan (E). These findings indicate that the ^{111}In uptake pattern was caused by active bone marrow uptake with no evidence of osteomyelitis. (Courtesy of Elgazzar AH, Abdel-Dayem HM, Clark JD, et al: Multimodality imaging of osteomyelitis. *Eur J Nucl Med* 22:1043–1063, 1995. Copyright Springer-Verlag.)

pathophysiology of osteomyelitis and the individual patient's medical history. The article includes a simplified algorithm summarizing the recommended approach to imaging studies in patients with osteomyelitis; the vertebral vs. nonvertebral site of the infection is a key consideration

▶ Osteomyelitis continues to provide a diagnostic problem for all of us in the imaging specialties. Despite years of attention, we still do not have a simple definitive test for use in all suspected cases of osteomyelitis. This paper goes a long way in providing a summary of the current methods available and provides excellent summaries of the literature-reported sensitivities and specificities for each. The authors also give a brief review of the pathophysiology of acute, subacute, and chronic forms of this disease. The appropriate use of the different imaging tests, their advantages and disadvantages, and their application in the different types of osteomyelitis are discussed. All in all, this paper is well worth reading.

R. Neumann, M.D.

Scintigraphic and Radiographic Patterns of Skeletal Metastases in Breast Cancer: Value of Sequential Imaging in Predicting Outcome
Janicek MJ, Shaffer K (Harvard Med School, Boston)
Skeletal Radiol 24:597–600, 1995   4–7

Background.—Scintigraphic and radiographic imaging is used to detect skeletal metastases in patients with breast cancer. In roughly 70% of patients with metastatic breast cancer, skeletal lesions develop. In 62% to 78% of patients, the skeleton is the first site of distant recurrence. Findings in a previous study of a healing flare and its predictive value, indicated that in patients with breast cancer and skeletal metastases, scintigraphic healing flare was not associated with a survival benefit. Also, scintigraphic stabilization of bony metastatic disease was found to be favorable. To evaluate the predictive value of temporal changes in findings from scintigraphy and bone radiography, records from patients with breast cancer skeletal metastases were reviewed.

Methods.—Bone scan readings and radiographs of 101 randomly selected patients with skeletal metastases from breast cancer were reviewed retrospectively. Images were correlated with survival rates after metastases were detected.

Results.—There was a correlation between survival and the time to detection of skeletal metastases and the length of time patients were radiologically stable after skeletal metastases developed. There was an association between significantly lower survival and failure to develop a radiographically and scintigraphically stable posttreatment pattern. Compared with all other patterns, scintigraphic regression of metastases correlated with a significant survival benefit and longer stabilization of disease.

Conclusions.—Sequential scintigraphic and radiographic imaging is helpful in managing patients with breast cancer because it can be used to detect metastases, monitor treatment, and provide prognostic information.

▶ After the 10th or 12th metastatic disease bone scan of the day, some of us, I'm sure, find it all too easy to let the mind ask "Am I really providing an essential service to this patient?" Read this paper. The authors provide a retrospective study of bone scans and radiographs from 101 randomly selected patients with skeletal metastases. Their goal was to determine whether temporal changes in the scintigraphic and bone radiograph findings have any prognostic significance for patients with skeletal metastases from breast cancer.

The good news is that these tests are useful for patients with breast cancer. The test results are not only good at finding metastatic disease and monitoring treatment effects, but they also can provide valuable prognostic information. Please read this paper and be of good cheer!

R. Neumann, M.D.

Evaluation of the Incorporation of Bone Grafts Used in Maxillofacial Surgery With [¹⁸F] Fluoride Ion and Dynamic Positron Emission Tomography

Berding G, Burchert W, van den Hoff J, et al (Medizinische Hochschule Hannover, Germany)

Eur J Nucl Med 22:1133–1140, 1995   4–8

Background.—Successful bone grafting is dependent on complex biological processes, including blood supply and osteoblastic vitality. Fluoride is extracted from the blood by bone during bone formation only. Therefore, dynamic PET with [¹⁸F]fluoride ion may provide useful information on bone blood flow (K_1) and fluoride influx to bone (K_{mlf}) to characterize graft incorporation with different kinds of grafts at different times postoperatively.

Methods.—Nine patients were studied, including 5 patients receiving autologous bone grafts for mandibular reconstruction (4 with a vascular pedicle and 1 without) and 4 patients receiving onlay grafts for alveolar atrophy (all transferred without a vascular pedicle). All grafts healed without complications. Positron emission tomography studies with [¹⁸F]fluoride tracer were done, with 8 studies done within 5–42 days and 3 performed within 144–248 days. Multilinear least squares fitting was used to calculate K_1 and K_{mlf}. Patlak plot analysis also was used to calculate fluoride influx (K_{pat}). These parameters were calculated using cervical vertebral bodies as a comparison reference.

Results.—The cervical vertebral bodies had a mean K_1 value of 0.1162 mL/min/mL, a mean K_{mlf} value of 0.0508 mL/min/mL, and a mean K_{pat} value of 0.0385 mL/min/mL. The early PET studies showed that the osteosyntheses and onlay grafts had significantly elevated blood flow and fluoride influx, whereas blood flow, but not fluoride influx, was significantly elevated in pedicle grafts. Onlay grafts had a significantly greater fluoride influx than pedicle grafts. Between the early and late postoperative PET studies, there was a significant decrease in blood flow in the onlay grafts and pedicle grafts and a significant decrease in blood flow and fluoride influx in osteosyntheses.

Conclusions.—During the early postoperative period, bone repair in the graft and host bone is indicated by increased blood flow and osteoblastic activity in onlay grafts and areas of osteosynthesis. Both parameters decrease in the areas of osteosynthesis over time during uncomplicated healing. Increased blood flow in conjunction with no increase in influx suggests some necrosis in pedicle grafts.

▶ This paper represents an exciting application of the dynamic PET technique to bone healing assessment after maxillofacial surgery. Kinetic modeling and quantitative methodology permitted the investigators to provide insight into the biology of bone graft incorporation. With PET, [^{18}F]fluoride ion bone scans may become an example of the expression "what goes around comes around," with a return to radiofluoride bone scintigraphy.

R. Neumann, M.D.

Pattern Recognition in Five-phase Bone Scintigraphy: Diagnostic Patterns of Reflex Sympathetic Dystrophy in Adults
Leitha T, Staudenherz A, Korpan M, et al (Univ Clinic of Nuclear Medicine, Vienna)
Eur J Nucl Med 23:256–262, 1996   4–9

Background.—Reflex sympathetic dystrophy (RSD), a pain syndrome of unknown causes, usually develops after minor or major trauma. Bone scintigraphy often is performed to aid inexperienced clinicians in the differential diagnosis of RSD. However, the best acquisition protocol, diagnostic patterns, and usefulness of quantification are still debated. To increase the diagnostic value of bone scintigraphy in RSD, the qualitative and quantitative patterns of tracer accumulation were studied.

Methods and Findings.—One hundred twenty patients with a high clinical suspicion of RSD were included. In 96 patients, RSD was confirmed during follow-up. The other 24 patients served as controls. In a discriminant analysis, the combination of 3 signs had the greatest diagnostic accuracy, independent of localization, sex, age, and precipitating factors. These signs were diffuse uptake in the carpus or tarsus, diffuse uptake in all small joints, and increased activity ratio in the late blood pool phase. If the osseous structures can be delineated clearly on the early bone phase image, the late bone phase image can be omitted (Tables 3 and 4).

Conclusions.—The diagnosis of RSD is based on the combination of a diffuse periarticular uptake in the carpus or tarsus and in all small joints

TABLE 3.—Scintigraphic Data of the Initial 5-Phase Bone Scintigraphy in 96 Patients With Reflex Sympathetic Dystrophy

		Statistics
Scintigraphic data		
Ratio I (arterial phase)	2.3±1.9	vs II: $P<0.05$; vs V: $P <0.01$
Ratio II (early blood pool phase)	2.0±0.9	vs III: $P<0.01$; vs IV: $P <0.01$; vs V: $P <0.01$
Ratio III (late blood pool phase)	2.1±0.9	vs IV: $P<0.01$; vs V: $P<0.01$
Ratio IV (early bone phase)	2.4±1.0	vs V: $P<0.01$
Ratio V (delayed bone phase)	2.8±1.9	
Scintigraphic signs (present:absent)		
1: Diffuse periarticular uptake	84:12	
2: Diffuse uptake in all small joints	76:20	
3: Diffuse diaphyseal uptake	20:76	
4: Diffuse uptake in large joint	27:69	
5: Visible uptake of fracture	34:62	

(Courtesy of Leitha T, Staudenherz A, Korpan M, et al: Pattern recognition in five-phase bone scintigraphy: Diagnostic patterns of reflex sympathetic dystrophy in adults. *Eur J Nucl Med* 23:256–262, 1996, Copyright Springer-Verlag.)

of the affected extremity plus an increased uptake in the late blood pool phase. This combination of signs is useful for diagnosing RSD in the upper and lower extremities.

▶ This article by Leitha and colleagues is worth reviewing. Using discriminant analysis, the authors found that the combination of 3 signs (diffuse uptake in carpus/tarsus, diffuse uptake in all small joints, and an increased activity ratio in the late blood pool phase) was the pattern with the highest diagnostic accuracy.

R. Neumann, M.D.

TABLE 4.—Comparison of the Initial and the Follow-up Study in 41 Patients With Reflex Sympathetic Dystrophy

	Initial	Follow-up	Statistics
Scintigraphic ratios			
Ratio I (arterial phase)	2.5±2.3	2.1±1.9	NS
Ratio II (early blood pool phase)	2.0±0.8	1.7±0.8	<0.05
Ratio III (late blood pool phase)	2.2±0.8	1.9±0.9	<0.01
Ratio IV (early bone phase)	2.7±1.0	2.1±0.8	<0.01
Ratio V (late bone phase)	3.2±1.1	2.5±1.0	<0.01
Scintigraphic signs (present:absent)			
1: Diffuse periarticular uptake	39:8	30:17	<0.01
2: Diffuse uptake in all small joints	37:10	28:19	<0.01
3: Diffuse diaphyseal uptake	15:32	9:38	<0.05
4: Diffuse uptake in large joint	15:32	11:36	NS
5: Visible uptake of fracture	18:29	13:34	NS

(Courtesy of Leitha T, Staudenherz A, Korpan M, et al: Pattern recognition in five-phase bone scintigraphy: Diagnostic patterns of reflex sympathetic dystrophy in adults. *Eur J Nucl Med* 23:256–262, 1996, Copyright Springer-Verlag.)

Clinical Pathological Correlation: Wrist Pain
Kwan W, Strauss HW (Stanford Univ, Calif)
J Nucl Med 37:534–535, 1996   4–10

Background.—Repetitive movements of certain types can damage the microvascular supply of bone, ligament, or tendon, resulting in pain and functional limitations. These musculoskeletal injuries may be difficult to diagnose objectively. Three patients underwent 3-phase bone scanning during the evaluation of wrist pain.

Case 1.—Woman, 39, had a 3-month history of diffuse right wrist pain when typing at her computer keyboard at work. The physical examination revealed normal sensation, range of motion, and strength in the wrist, and an absence of Tinel's sign. The patient was managed with rest, nonsteroidal anti-inflammatory drugs, and job modification, but she had no improvement. Plain radiographs revealed no abnormalities. A 3-phase bone scan with dynamic images of the forearms, wrists, and hands in the palmar views showed a subtle increase in activity in the lunate region on static images and increased uptake in the triquetral and lunate bones at the area of pain on delayed images. An area of increased uptake in the lunate of her other wrist suggested a metabolic response to a wrist injury.

Case 2.—Man, 28, an airplane mechanic, had a softball injury involving hyperextension of his left wrist 1 year earlier. He reported increasing pain in his left wrist that was exacerbated by specific movements, such as using a wrench. Treatment with a wrist brace brought no improvement. He had focal tenderness in the triquetrum region. There were no abnormalities on plain radiographs, but MRI results indicated possible edema in the area of pain. A 3-phase bone scan showed a marked increase in activity at the ulnar aspect of the proximal carpal row. This activity and the focal tenderness suggested fracture with nonunion.

Case 3.—Woman, 20, a triple jumper and weight lifter, reported a 4-month history of right midulnar pain radiating to the wrist with no trauma. She had tenderness along the midshaft of the right distal ulnar. On a 3-phase bone scan, the perfusion and immediate static images showed increased perfusion and blood-pool activity in the mid-ulnar. The delayed images showed increased uptake in the middle third of the right ulnar diaphysis. This area also showed increased T2 signal within the bone marrow on an MRI.

Discussion.—Musculoskeletal injury caused by repetitive joint movements may not be discerned on plain radiographs. Three-phase bone scanning is more sensitive to subtle fracture and metabolic abnormalities and may therefore be important in the evaluation of patients with otherwise undiagnosed wrist pain.

Additional Reading

Devillers A, Moisan A, Jean S, et al: Technetium-99m hexamethylpropylene amine
oxime leucocyte scintigraphy for the diagnosis of bone and joint infections: A
retrospective study in 116 patients. *Eur J Nucl Med* 22:302–307, 1995.
▶ Although a number of nuclear medicine scintigraphy tests are now available
to us for confirming bone or joint infections in patients, few of the tests have
been extensively evaluated in a truly large number of patients. This paper adds
a retrospective review of 116 patients to determine the diagnostic value of
technetium-99m–hexamethylpropyleneamine oxime leukocyte scintigraphy for
detecting bone and joint infections. The patients were divided into 3 groups:
those with an infection suspected to involve orthopedic implants, those with
acute or chronic osteomyelitis, and those with suspected septic arthritis. The
corresponding values for sensitivity and specificity were: 97% and 87%, respectively, for group I; 100% and 100%, respectively, for group II; and 80% and
83%, respectively, for group III. The authors conclude that ^{99m}Tc-HMPAO-LS is
an effective tool for diagnosis of bone infection involving implants and even
chronic osteomyelitis.

R. Neumann, M.D.

5 Endocrinology

Introduction

The basic applications of nuclear medicine in endocrinology continue to be directed mainly at somatostatin imaging of neuroendocrine tumors, imaging and evaluation of thyroid disease, and the detection of parathyroid adenomas and hyperplasia. Nothing dramatic has occurred since the 1996 YEAR BOOK OF NUCLEAR MEDICINE. What we are looking at is a continuing refinement of the techniques and applications in these areas. Octreotide remains the only FDA-approved receptor-based imaging agent in the United States. It certainly has lived up to its promise and proven to be an extremely useful agent. The only limitation of this agent is that it addresses a relatively uncommon condition. If the expression of specific receptors in other types of tumors that are more common could be identified and imaging agents developed, they could have an extraordinary impact on nuclear medicine diagnosis.

It is an advantage of PET imaging that FDG is not only taken up by a large number of malignant tumors but that the tumors in which it does appear to be useful are relatively common among neoplasms so that the impact of the technique can be very profound. Similar agents that can be used with planar or SPECT imaging would certainly be of great value in oncology and in staging of lymphomas and surgical disease, but they have not yet appeared on the clinical scene.

The great progress that has occurred in in vitro thyroid diagnosis has greatly reduced the role of nuclear medicine. However, the role of radioiodine therapy in both hyperthyroidism and thyroid cancer continues to be of great importance. The articles reviewed in this issue help to put medical treatment of hyperthyroidism, radioiodine treatment of hyperthyroidism, and the role of nuclear medicine in the diagnosis and therapy of hyperthyroidism into perspective.

Finally, a great deal of interest continues to be directed at parathyroid diagnosis. The recent development of handheld probes holds promise of being of great value in this field. Some authors have looked at double-phase imaging of the parathyroid, including flow studies, to see whether this could enhance diagnosis. I am not particularly an advocate of perfusion imaging, and I believe that there are very few conditions for which perfusion imaging substantially contributes to nuclear medicine diagnosis.

The remarkable relationship between cardiac imaging agents and parathyroid scintigraphy continues unabated. Sestamibi, thallium, and now tetrofosmin all can be used to image the parathyroid. Perhaps next year we will be able to determine which appears to be the best agent.

M. Donald Blaufox, M.D., Ph.D.

Dynamic Octreotide Scintigraphy in Neuroendocrine Tumours
Bajc M, Ingvar C, Persson B, et al (Univ Hosp, Lund, Sweden)
Acta Radiol 36:474–477, 1995   5–1

Background.—Scintigraphy with the radiolabeled somatostatin analogue octreotide is a promising modality. Octreotide enables visualization of primary tumors and metastases that are undetectable by CT. Octreotide scintigraphy also has been found to be useful in localizing neuroendocrine tumors. The optimal timing of scintigraphy after octreotide injection was investigated. The role of SPECT was also assessed.

Methods.—Twenty-two patients with known or suspected neuroendocrine tumors were included in the study. One SPECT examination and as many as 4 whole-body scans were performed in each patient at 0.5, 5, 24, and 48 hours after 110 MBq of indium-DTPA–octreotide was injected. Altogether, 98 scintigrams were obtained.

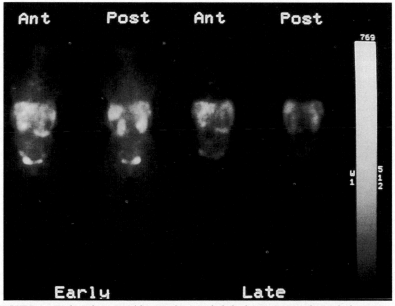

FIGURE 1.—Early (5 hours) and late (24 hours) whole-body scintigrams obtained after injection of octreotide in a patient with midgut carcinoid tumor. Pathologic uptake is visible in the mediastinum, liver, bowel, peritoneum, and ovaries. The late image has a higher signal-to-noise ratio, but pathologic uptake is already present in the early image. (Courtesy of Bajc M, Ingvar C, Persson B, et al: Dynamic octreotide scintigraphy in neuroendocrine tumours. *Acta Radiol* 36:474–477, 1995.)

Findings.—Nineteen patients had a pathologic uptake of octreotide. Early scintigrams, obtained at 0.5 and 5 hours after injection, were most useful in 3 patients. In 4 patients, scintigrams obtained at 24 and 48 hours were best (Fig 1). In 13 patients, SPECT was of value. Abnormal uptake not detected in the whole-body scintigrams was visualized on SPECT images in 2 of these patients. In another 5 patients, SPECT images clearly demonstrated abnormal uptake that was seen only as possible abnormal uptake on the whole-body scintigrams. In another 6 patients, SPECT images were useful for localizing tumors. SPECT did not add to the whole-body scintigrams in the remaining 8 patients.

Conclusion.—To correctly interpret octreotide scintigraphy, clinicians must obtain both early and late planar studies and perform SPECT. The SPECT study is needed to localize small tumors and resolve the problems of superposition.

▶ The introduction of octreotide imaging has been a welcome addition to nuclear medicine. Unfortunately, its very great cost has limited its utilization. However, there remains the need to define how the procedure should be done. As the procedure is increasingly refined and its sensitivity and specificity are improved, hopefully it will achieve greater utilization. Greater utilization is an end in itself, because this will ultimately lead to a reduction in the price and make the technique more suitable on an economic basis for general applications in nuclear medicine. Unfortunately, the conclusions of this study—that octreotide scintigraphy should be carried out with early and late planar scintigrams as well as SPECT—if proven correct, will tend to have a negative impact on the overall cost of the procedure, even if the radiopharmaceutical cost is reduced.

M.D. Blaufox, M.D., Ph.D.

Value of Somatostatin Receptor Scintigraphy for Preoperative Localization of Carcinoids
Kisker O, Weinel RJ, Geks J, et al (Philipps-Univ Marburg, Germany)
World J Surg 20:162–167, 1996   5–2

Background.—Carcinoid tumors are rare and can occur in the intestines, lungs, thymus, pancreas, and ovary. Most go undetected for years, until they cause complications or until they are detected by chance during other procedures. They are rarely suspected before surgery. Preoperative detection of the primary tumor can be achieved by CT, MRI, ultrasonography (US), or iodine-131–metaiodobenzylguanidine scintigraphy with varying degrees of success. Because somatostatin receptors are expressed by 87% of carcinoid tumors, scintigraphy using radiolableled somatostatin analogues may aid detection. The value of somatostatin receptor scintigraphy in detecting carcinoid tumors was determined.

Methods.—In 22 patients with carcinoid tumors who had not undergone surgery for removal of the primary tumor, somatostatin receptor scintigraphy, CT, and US were performed and results compared.

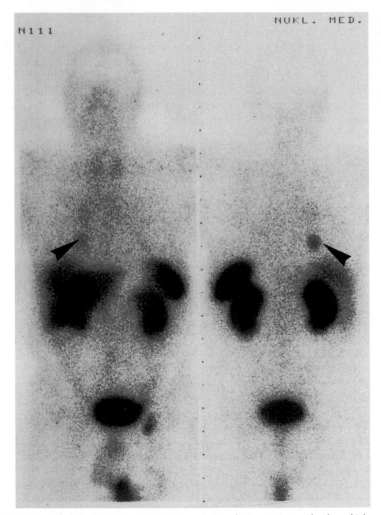

FIGURE 1.—Whole-body somatostatin receptor scintigraphy in a patient with a bronchial carcinoid tumor (*arrowheads*). This tumor was correctly localized by CT and somatostatin receptor scintigraphy. **Left,** frontal view **right,** posterior view. (Courtesy of Kisker O, Weinel RJ, Geks J, et al: Value of somatostatin receptor scintigraphy for preoperative localization of carcinoids. *World J Surg* 20: 162–167, 1996. Copyright Springer-Verlag.)

Results.—Of 10 patients with no evidence of diffuse metastases by CT and US, 2 had bronchial carcinoid tumors localized by CT and somatostatin receptor scintigraphy (Fig 1), and 8 had gut carcinoids. Six of the 8 were correctly diagnosed by somatostatin receptor scintigraphy. For detecting primary lesions, there was no advantage of somatostatin receptor scintigraphy over CT or US. All techniques detected tumors larger than 2 cm. For detecting liver metastases, somatostatin receptor scintigraphy was not superior to CT or US. Computed tomography and US detected liver metastases in all patients; somatostatin receptor scintigraphy detected liver metastases in 16 of 18 patients. Whole-body somatostatin receptor scintigraphy was superior to CT and US for localization of extrahepatic abdominal and extra-abdominal metastases.

Conclusion.—For localization of small, primary carcinoid tumors, somatostatin receptor scintigraphy is not superior to CT or US. Results of somatostatin receptor scintigraphy were similar to those of other imaging techniques for localization of liver metastases. Somatostatin receptor scintigraphy successfully detected extra-abdominal and extrahepatic abdominal carcinoid metastases. Somatostatin receptor scintigraphy identified receptor-positive tumors and should always be used in patients with known carcinoid tumors.

▶ Correlative studies are appearing increasingly in the literature as medical providers are being pressed to demonstrate the effectiveness of a treatment or diagnostic modality. In this study, as in many others, no single modality clearly fulfilled all needs. For instance, although the authors conclude that somatostatin receptor imaging is not superior to CT or US for localization of primary carcinoids or liver metastases, they do report its value in visualizing extrahepatic and extra-abdominal tumor spread. They also suggest that it is useful in identifying those tumors that may respond to treatment with somatostatin analogues. This nicely demonstrates the great problem the physician is faced with in being increasingly told to chose 1 modality to test the hypothesis of the patient's disease because the insurer will not pay for 2.

Often there is no single modality that will provide all the answers needed. Therefore, if a single modality is chosen, some vital information may be lost. Although it is nice to try to develop a cost-efficacious approach to medicine, it remains a problem in a field that is more an art than a science. From an individual patient's point of view, the justification that 80% of all individuals will benefit from a single diagnostic modality is of little comfort if that person falls within the 20% who continue to be undiagnosed or untreated.

Perhaps someday society will come to grips with the reality that good medical care is very expensive. I personally find it difficult to be concerned about the fact that medical care represents a significant fraction of the gross national product as long as "defense" still represents a considerably greater fraction. I would rather see more money spent in preserving my health than in destroying that of other persons.

M.D. Blaufox, M.D., Ph.D.

Somatostatin Receptor Scintigraphy in Patients With Carcinoid Tumors
Kwekkeboom DJ, Krenning EP (Univ Hosp Dijkzigt, Rotterdam, The Netherlands)
World J Surg 20:157–161, 1996   5–3

Background.—Carcinoid tumors are sometimes detected because of symptoms of hormone overproduction, local expanding growth, or by chance. It can be difficult to detect tumor sites with conventional imaging, but choice of treatment sometimes depends on information regarding these sites. Tumor sites can be detected with [indium-111–DTPA-D-Phe[1]]-octreotide scintigraphy in 80% to 90% of patients with carcinoid tumors. The effectiveness of combinations of octreotide scintigraphy and conventional imaging in localizing carcinoid tumors were compared.

Methods.—In 52 patients with carcinoid tumors, suspected carcinoids, or at risk for these tumors, scintigraphy was performed with [iodine-123–Tyr[3]]-octreotide or [^{111}In-DTPA-D-Phe[1]]-octreotide. Results were analyzed and compared.

Results.—More tumor sites were detected with octreotide scintigraphy alone or combined with other imaging techniques than with any combination of conventional imaging modalities. In all patients with lesions detectable by any means, the combination of octreotide scintigraphy, chest radiography, and ultrasonography of the upper abdomen detected lesions with a sensitivity of 87%. This imaging regimen was more expensive than combined conventional imaging, but the benefit was at least 1 lesion detected in 11% of patients in whom no abnormalities were detected with conventional imaging. This means an extra 65 lesions would be detected per 100 patients if these results were extrapolated to a group of 100 patients.

Discussion.—The decision to perform surgery can depend on detecting more tumor sites in patients in whom 1 tumor site is detected with conventional imaging. Octreotide scintigraphy can localize tumors, aid in choice of treatment, and, in the near future, select patients for radiotherapy.

▶ Here is yet another study supporting the great potential value of somatostatin receptor imaging in this highly selective group of patients.

M.D. Blaufox, M.D., Ph.D.

An Update on Diagnostic Methods in the Investigation of Diseases of the Thyroid
Reinhardt MJ, Moser E (Albert-Ludwigs-Univ, Freiburg, Germany)
Eur J Nucl Med 23:587–594, 1996   5–4

Introduction.—Thyroid disease remains a significant problem in the countries of central, eastern, and southern Europe. The insufficient iodine supply in these regions causes goiter in 15% to 80% of the population. This needs to be considered when comparing data from countries in which thyroid deficiency is not pandemic. There are several recent and important developments in the detection of thyroid disease. Current diagnostic procedures in patients with various thyroid diseases were reviewed.

In Vitro Thyroid Function Tests.—The diagnostic accuracy of thyroid-stimulating hormone (TSH) determination has been improved in the detection of borderline thyroid function using second- and third-generation TSH assays. The simultaneous measurement of TSH and free thyroxine provides maximum sensitivity and specificity for detecting hyperthyroidism and hypothyroidism. The differentiation of blocking and stimulating TSH receptor antibodies may be helpful in the presence of discrepant thyroid function results. Glycosaminoglycans have been found to be significantly increased in some patients with endocrine ophthalmopathy.

Ultrasonography and Fine-needle Aspiration Cytology.—The diagnostic method of choice for the detection of morphologic changes of the thyroid is ultrasonography. Scintigraphy should be performed if any focal abnormalities are visible. The prevalence of malignancy in lesions with increased echogenicity is below 1% and is 10% in hypoechoic lesions. In lesions that show a scintigraphically cold nodule, the malignancy rate is 20%. Fine-needle aspiration (FNA) cytology can accurately diagnose 90% to 98% of such nodules. About 50% to 70% of patients with suspected malignancy can avoid diagnostic surgery because of the use of FNA. Only follicular neoplasia cannot be differentiated by FNA.

Scintigraphy.—Quantitative high-resolution gamma camera scintigraphy has significantly enhanced the detectability of hot and cold lesions within the thyroid. New imaging agents have added to the ability of scintigraphy to be useful in thyroid disease: technetium-99m pertechnetate under TSH suppression may be helpful in determining individual dosage for radioiodine therapy; somatostatin receptor imaging has been used in Graves' ophthalmopathy and medullary thyroid carcinoma; positron emission tomography using FDG may be helpful in detecting metastases of differentiated thyroid cancer that does not accumulate radioiodine.

Conclusion.—The accuracy of thyroid diagnostics has markedly improved over recent years. The application of gene technology to thyroid in vitro tests, the use of ultrasonography and FNA cytology, and the development of functional and quantitative imaging techniques in thyroid scintigraphy have all expanded the ability to detect thyroid disease.

▶ As the authors themselves point out, "while there has not been a revolution in thyroid diagnostics, there has been much evolution and improvement." We have seen the steady evolution and change of both in vitro and in vivo diagnostic techniques for thyroid diagnosis. The ubiquitous thyroid scan and uptake, which at one point represented close to a majority of all nuclear medicine procedures, have now given way in large part to in vitro diagnostic tests that do not even require the use of radioactivity. These and many other related changes have greatly improved our ability to diagnose and treat patients with thyroid disease. In spite of this, the treatment of thyroid cancer still remains an almost mystical experience, so there is no question that there is still room for improvement in our thyroid armamentarium.

M.D. Blaufox, M.D., Ph.D.

Prediction of Remission in Graves' Disease Treated With Long-term Carbimazole Therapy: Evaluation of Technetium-99m Thyroid Uptake and TSH Concentrations as Prognostic Indicators

Prakash R (Batra Hosp, New Delhi, India)
Eur J Nucl Med 23:118–122, 1996   5–5

Background.—Graves' disease is characterized by increased levels of thyroid receptor antibodies, which stimulate the thyroid in a manner similar to thyrotropin. This results in enlargement of the thyroid and release of thyroid hormones. This hyperthyroidism can be controlled by thionamide, but many patients have recurrent hyperthyroidism after completing antithyroid drug treatment. The value of technetium-99m pertechnetate thyroid uptake and thyrotropin levels as predictors of remission in patients with Graves' disease treated with carbimazole was assessed.

Methods.—There were 45 patients with Graves' disease between 22 and 70 years of age. Patients were treated with carbimazole for 18 months. Before and after carbimazole therapy, ^{99m}Tc thyroid uptake was estimated. Thyrotropin levels were also estimated with an immunoradiometric assay. Follow-up was for 3 years.

Results.—Before carbimazole therapy, all patients had increased ^{99m}Tc thyroid uptake and subnormal thyrotropin levels. During follow-up, recurrent hyperthyroidism developed in 22 patients. Thyroid uptake was persistently elevated at the end of drug therapy in 20 of these 22 patients

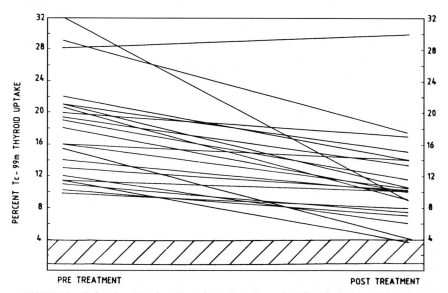

FIGURE 4.—Technetium-99m thyroid uptake in 22 patients who relapsed after completion of carbimazole therapy. Individual patient values before and after treatment are plotted on the left- and right-hand sides of the y-axis, respectively. The *hatched area* represents the normal range of 20-minute ^{99m}Tc thyroid uptake. (Courtesy of Prakash R: Prediction of remission of Graves' disease treated with long-term carbimazole therapy: Evaluation of technetium-99m thyroid uptake and TSH concentrations as prognostic indicators. *Eur J Nucl Med* 23:118–122, 1996. Copyright Springer-Verlag.)

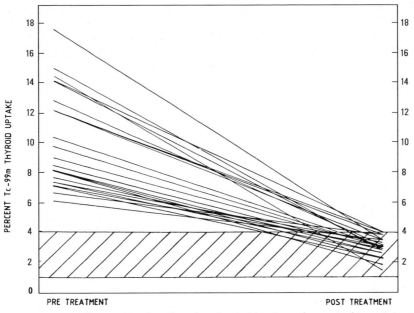

FIGURE 2.—Technetium-99m thyroid uptake values in 23 patients who remained in remission after carbimazole therapy. Individual patient values before and after treatment are plotted on the left- and right-hand sides of the *y*-axis, respectively. The *hatched area* represents the normal range of 20-minute ^{99m}Tc thyroid uptake. (Courtesy of Prakash R: Prediction of remission in Graves' disease treated with long-term carbimazole therapy: Evaluation of technetium-99m thyroid uptake and TSH concentrations as prognostic indicators. *Eur J Nucl Med* 23:118–122, 1996. Copyright Springer-Verlag.)

(Fig 4). Thyrotropin levels were subnormal in 18 of these patients. Thyroid uptake was normal at the end of drug therapy in the 23 patients who remained in remission throughout the follow-up period (Fig 2). Thyrotropin levels were normal at the end of drug therapy in 19 of these 23 patients in remission but were subnormal in 4 patients.

Conclusion.—These findings indicate that there is a high risk of relapse in patients with persistently elevated ^{99m}Tc thyroid uptake and subnormal thyrotropin levels after a full course of antithyroid drug therapy. Patients are likely to stay in remission if ^{99m}Tc thyroid uptake and thyrotropin levels have returned to normal.

▶ The role of thyroid uptake has been diminishing in clinical medicine over the years as we develop increasingly sophisticated in vitro tests. The suggestion here that there is a dissociation between thyrotropin levels and thyroid ^{99m}Tc uptake is an interesting one. The investigator suggests that this information is useful because it would help to chose patients in whom long-term antithyroid drug treatment, or perhaps surgery or radioiodine therapy, should be initiated. However, as the author himself notes, the high accuracy of the ^{99m}Tc uptake in predicting relapse in their study is not in agreement with that of other investigators who found the value to be a poor parameter. The author suggests that differences in methodology and long-term follow-up explain the difference in his results. Further investigations will be needed to determine whether the author's suggestion that this is a reliable and relatively inexpensive method for predicting relapse in Graves' disease is correct.

M.D. Blaufox, M.D., Ph.D.

Transient Hypothyroidism After Iodine-131 Therapy for Grave's Disease
Gómez N, Gómez JM, Orti A, et al (Univ of Bellvitge, Barcelona)
J Nucl Med 36:1539–1542, 1995   5–6

Background.—Because antithyroid drugs do not always induce remission of Graves' disease, most patients require therapy with iodine-131 or subtotal thyroidectomy. Although treatment with ^{131}I is safe and effective, hypothyroidism will occur. Some patients have transient hypothyroidism, but its incidence and characteristics are unknown. This study attempted to characterize transient hypothyroidism and its predictive value after therapy with ^{131}I for Graves' disease and to differentiate transient from permanent hypothyroidism.

Methods.—Participants were 355 patients with Graves' disease. Of these, 333 were treated with ^{131}I lower than 10 mCi, and 22 were treated with ^{131}I higher than 10 mCi. Transient hypothyroidism was diagnosed by

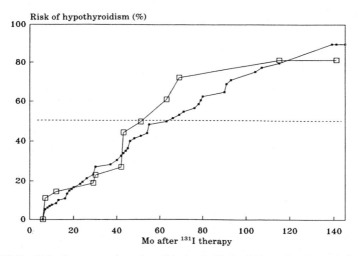

FIGURE 2.—Risk of permanent hypothyroidism by the Kaplan-Meier estimation according to the development of transient hypothyroidism. *Horizontal dashed line* represents the median probability of permanent hypothyroidism. (Reprinted by permission of the Society of Nuclear Medicine, from Gómez N, Gómez JM, Orti A, et al: Transient hypothyroidism after iodine-131 therapy for Grave's disease. *J Nucl Med* 36:1539–1542, 1995.)

low levels of thyroxine, regardless of thyrotropin, within 1 year after therapy with ^{131}I followed by recovery of normal levels of thyroxine and thyrotropin.

Results.—Of patients who received less than 10 mCi of ^{131}I, 40 had transient hypothyroidism within the first year. In 15 of these patients, transient hypothyroidism was symptomatic. No patient who received more than 10 mCi of ^{131}I had transient hypothyroidism. A risk factor for transient hypothyroidism was ^{131}I uptake of more than 70% at 2 hours before treatment. When transient hypothyroidism was diagnosed, basal levels of thyrotropin were high, normal, or low, and, therefore, transient hypothyroidism was not related to pituitary function. No patient with basal thyrotropin levels higher than 45 mU/L developed transient hypothyroidism. There was a risk of 81.4% of permanent hypothyroidism 141 months after therapy with ^{131}I in patients who previously had transient hypothyroidism compared with a risk of 89.9% those who did not (Fig 2).

Conclusion.—Transient hypothyroidism did not affect long-term thyroid function. Before diagnosing definitive hypothyroidism within a few months of therapy with ^{131}I, spontaneous recovery of thyroid function should be considered, especially if levels of thyrotropin are lower than 45 mU/L. Thyroid function should be assessed 6 months after ^{131}I therapy, when thyroid function may be recovered after transient hypothyroidism.

▶ This article reviews some of the factors associated with the development of transient hypothyroidism during the first 6 months after ^{131}I therapy for Graves' disease to try to identify those patients who may need chronic thyroid replacement. The authors make the important point that during this time, evidence of reduced thyroid function may be transient and, therefore, does not necessarily warrant long-term thyroid replacement therapy. In their series, however, there was a very high risk of subsequent development of hypothyroidism. Although the authors indicate that an ^{131}I uptake of greater than 70% at 2 hours is a risk factor for transient hypothyroidism, they give a 95% confidence interval for their odds ratio of 0.9 to 9.4. Because this odds ratio risk crosses 1, even this predictive factor would appear to be relatively unreliable.

M.D. Blaufox, M.D., Ph.D.

A Patient With an Autonomously Functioning Thyroid Nodule With Papillary Adenocarcinoma Associated With Graves' Hyperthyroidism

Tsuboi M, Shigemasa C, Ueta Y, et al (Tottori Univ, Yonago, Japan)
Clin Nucl Med 20:985–988, 1995   5–7

Purpose.—Few Japanese patients have an autonomously functioning thyroid nodule (AFTN). However, it is well known that functioning thyroid-stimulating hormone (TSH) receptors can occur in differentiated thyroid cancer cell membranes. Given that the circulating thyroid-stimulating antibody (TSAb) found in Graves' hyperthyroidism is one of the antibodies against the TSH receptor, it is interesting to note that Graves' hyperthy-

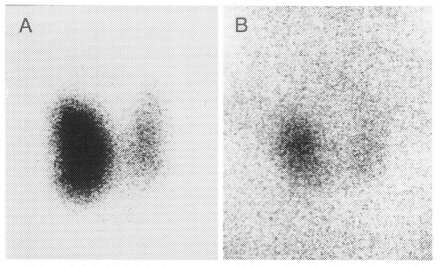

FIGURE 1.—Thyroid iodine-123 scintigram (A) shows high uptake into almost the entire right lobe and partially suppressed uptake into the left lobe. Thallium-201 scintigram (B) shows uptake almost entirely confined to the nodule in the right lobe. (Courtesy of Tsuboi M, Shigemasa C, Ueta Y, et al: A patient with an autonomously functioning thyroid nodule with papillary adenocarcinoma associated with Graves' hyperthyroidism. *Clin Nucl Med* 20:985-988, 1995.)

roidism and thyroid cancer can occur concomitantly. A rare case of autonomously functioning thyroid papillary adenocarcinoma in a patient with Graves' hyperthyroidism was reported.

> *Case Report.*—Man, 69, was seen with palpitation and dyspnea, finger tremor, and weight loss. He was hyperthyroid and had a right lobe thyroid nodule that was hyperfunctional on iodine-123 imaging (Fig 1A). On thallium-201 imaging, tracer uptake was confined almost entirely to the hyperfunctional nodule, which was identified as papillary adenocarcinoma on aspiration (Fig 1B). This diagnosis was confirmed at surgery, which also revealed diffuse hyperplasia around the nodule and some enlargement of the left thyroid lobe. Retrospective measurement of serum TSAb activity showed that it was 920% before the start of treatment for hyperthyroidism and 255% 3 months after surgery, compared with a normal level of less than 134%.

Discussion.—In this case, a carcinomatous nodule in the right lobe showed elevated uptake on ^{123}I scintigraphy, with partial suppression of uptake in the left lobe. The reason for uptake suppression in the left lobe—despite high TSAb activity—is unknown. It may be that the response of cancer tissue to TSAb is different from that of extranodular thyroid tissue.

▶ It is axiomatic that nothing in life is one hundred percent certain. Fortunately, the association of functioning thyroid tissue and adenocarcinoma is an extraordinarily rare occurrence. This case is particularly complex because of the presence of thyroid stimulating antibody as well. This abstract has been included to remind us never to take anything for granted.

M.D. Blaufox, M.D., Ph.D.

Intraoperative Identification of Parathyroid Gland Pathology: A New Approach

Martinez DA, King DR, Romshe C, et al (Ohio State Univ, Columbus; Children's Hosp, Columbus, Ohio)
J Pediatr Surg 30:1306–1309, 1995   5–8

Background.—Technetium-99m–sestamibi (^{99m}Tc-MIBI) scintigraphy accurately detects parathyroid adenoma in adults. Use of this isotope and a handheld gamma-detecting probe to identify abnormal parathyroid tissue intraoperatively in children was studied.

Methods.—For 3 teenage patients with hypercalcemia, ^{99m}Tc-MIBI scanning revealed abnormal isotopic uptake in the thyroid or the mediastinum, suggesting the presence of excessive parathyroid activity. Before surgery, each patient received an IV dose of ^{99m}Tc-MIBI. Intraoperatively, the surgical field was scanned with the handheld gamma-detecting probe and background noise was squelched. A second scan was performed, identifying tissues with increased isotope uptake. These tissues were then removed.

Results.—For 2 patients, significantly increased uptake was found in tissues that subsequently proved adenomatous (Table 1). This included 1 patient who had previously undergone an unsuccessful neck exploration, in whom an adenoma was found beneath the ascending aortic arch. For 1 patient, tissue was visibly enlarged at surgery but did not show increased uptake. Serum calcium and parathormone levels reverted to normal postoperatively in all patients.

Conclusion.—This technique may be useful in localizing abnormal parathyroid tissue in children during surgery.

▶ The use of small handheld probes for localizing radioactivity in areas of disease uptake is very old indeed. However, the incredible advances in

TABLE 1.—Intraoperative Gamma-probe Counts

Case 1		Case 2		Case 3	
Tissue	GPC, $\overline{X} \pm$ SD	Tissue	GPC, $\overline{X} \pm$ SD	Tissue	GPC, $\overline{X} \pm$ SD
Chest wall	238 ± 24	Thyroid, L lobe	38 ± 4	Thyroid, R lobe	55 ± 3
Aorta	256 ± 19	Thyroid, R lobe	40 ± 4	Hyperplasia, R superior	80 ± 1*
Thymus	196 ± 15	Adenoma	45 ± 3	Hyperplasia, R inferior	95 ± 9*
Adenoma	349 ± 6*			Thyroid, L lobe	64 ± 8
				Hyperplasia, L superior	73 ± 4
				Hyperplasia, L inferior	104 ± 8*

* Gamma-probe counts exceeded criterion of "mean plus 3 times the square root of the mean."
Abbreviations: GPC, gamma-probe counts; *L*, left; *R*, right; *SD*, standard deviation.
(Courtesy of Martinez DA, King DR, Romshe C, et al: Intraoperative identification of parathyroid gland pathology: A new approach. *J Pediatr Surg* 30:1306–1309, 1995.)

electronics and instrumentation have now returned these devices to the marketplace in a greatly improved manner and with hope for their more widespread application. In particular, the use of the handheld probe to detect sentinel nodes in the breast or malignant melanoma has proven very promising, especially in malignant melanoma. This is one more potential application of a handheld probe that seems quite interesting and exciting.

M.D. Blaufox, M.D., Ph.D.

Hyperparathyroidism in High-risk Surgical Patients: Evaluation With Double-phase Technetium-99m Sestamibi Imaging
Lee VS, Wilkinson RH Jr, Leight GS Jr, et al (Duke Univ, Durham, NC)
Radiology 197:627–633, 1995   5–9

Background.—Thallium-201 scintigraphy of parathyroid glands with technetium-99m pertechnetate subtraction of thyroid is a effective scintigraphic technique for evaluation of hyperparathyroidism. Recent studies, however, report a low sensitivity for technetium-thallium imaging in this setting. Technetium-99m–sestamibi was examined for its accuracy in detecting and localizing hyperfunctioning parathyroid tissue in high-risk surgical patients.

Patients and Methods.—Fifty-one patients with suspected hyperparathyroidism underwent 52 preoperative ^{99m}Tc-sestamibi imaging studies between November 1992 and February 1995. Imaging was indicated because of previous neck surgery in 23 patients, severe renal osteodystrophy in 5, and a history of radioactive iodine therapy in 3; 11 patients had a medical condition that placed them at high risk. Thirty-eight patients had a total of 39 operations, and 1 patient, who died of hypercalcemic crisis, underwent autopsy. Thus, 40 double-phase ^{99m}Tc-sestamibi studies with histopathologic correlation were available for analysis.

Results.—Surgical findings were solitary adenomas in 29 patients and hyperplastic glands in 9. The patient who died and was examined at autopsy had a parathyroid adenoma that was correctly localized with sestamibi imaging. All but 2 of the 38 surgical patients became normocalcemic after surgery. Localization was achieved with double-phase sesta-

TABLE 1.—Results of 40 Double-phase Technetium-99m–Sestamibi Studies in 39 Patients

Finding	True-Positive	False-Positive	True-Negative	False-Negative
Adenomas ($n = 30$)	28	1	42	2
Hyperplasia ($n = 30$)	18	0	1	12
Negative study ($n = 0$)	—	—	1	0
Total	46	1	44	14

(Courtesy of Lee VS, Wilkinson RH Jr, Leight GS Jr, et al: Hyperparathyroidism in high-risk surgical patients: Evaluation with double-phase technetium-99m sestamibi imaging. *Radiology* 197:627–633, 1995, Radiological Society of North America.)

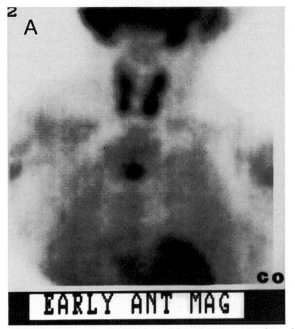

FIGURE 1A.—Immediate image of a double-phase technetium-99m–sestamibi study in a man, 18, with severe secondary hyperparathyroidism. Five hyperplastic glands were resected during neck and limited mediastinal exploration. (Courtesy of Lee VS, Wilkinson RJ Jr, Leight GS Jr, et al: Hyperparathyroidism in high-risk surgical patients: Evaluation with double-phase technetium-99m sestamibi imaging. *Radiology* 197:627–633, 1995, Radiological Society of North America.)

mibi imaging in 77% of abnormal glands (Table 1). The rate of accurate localization was higher for adenomas (93%) than for hyperplastic glands (60%). There was 1 false positive study, for a specificity of 98%. Multiple gland disease was present in 7 patients (Fig 1A). Bilateral abnormalities could be seen in all patients. Gland weight and vascularity were statistically significant predictors of uptake of sestamibi. Neither a history of neck surgery nor preoperative serum levels of intact parathyroid hormone or of calcium were related to the rate of correct preoperative localization.

Conclusion.—Double-phase ^{99m}Tc-sestamibi imaging offers promise as a means of localizing parathyroid adenomas in high-risk surgical patients. The imaging technique was less accurate in localizing multiple hyperplastic glands. Preoperative sestamibi imaging can reduce operating time and the need for reoperation.

▶ The literature has been literally flooded with the application of nuclear imaging in hyperparathyroidism, perhaps totally out of proportion to the frequency of the disease. However, its role in this disease is becoming increasingly firm. As this occurs, it is necessary to define more clearly the exact clinical characteristics of patients in whom sestamibi imaging will potentially be valuable.

The authors suggest that routine parathyroid imaging may not be of very great clinical value but that, in patients defined as high risk because of a history of prior neck surgery, prior radioactive iodine therapy, renal osteodystrophy, or other medical conditions (including advanced age, severe obesity, and severe hypercalcemia), the use of sestamibi imaging can be helpful in reducing the operative risk through preoperative localization. Whether the restrictions should be narrowed to this degree, as the authors themselves point out, is controversial, but certainly in the patients as defined by the authors there can be little doubt of the potential value of parathyroid imaging.

M.D. Blaufox, M.D., Ph.D.

Early and Delayed Thallium-201 Scintigraphy in Thyroid Nodules: The Relationship Between Early Thallium-201 Uptake and Perfusion

Derebek E, Biberoglu S, Kut O, et al (Dokuz Eylul Univ, Izmir, Turkey)
Eur J Nucl Med 23:504–510, 1996   5–10

Introduction.—Preoperative differential diagnosis is important in patients with cold thyroid nodules. The tumor-seeking properties of thallium-201 have been observed, but its role in early and delayed ^{201}Tl imaging has not been determined. The role of early and delayed ^{201}Tl scintigraphy in differentiating malignant and benign thyroid nodules and the relationship between perfusion and ^{201}Tl uptake were analyzed.

Methods.—Seventy-six patients with thyroid nodules and normal thyroid function were evaluated. Sixty-three patients underwent technetium-99m–pertechnetate perfusion and ^{201}Tl testing. The remaining 13 patients underwent ^{201}Tl testing only. Twenty-four patients underwent surgery because of fine-needle aspiration (FNA) and other clinical findings. The remaining patients were followed for 1 year with FNA and ultrasonography. The thyroid was imaged 15 minutes and 3 hours after injecting 74 MBq of [201]Tl. Then 185 Mbq of ^{99m}Tc-pertechnetate was injected and 1-minute and 20-minute perfusion images were taken.

Results.—There was an increased ^{201}Tl uptake consistent with malignant criteria on early and delayed images in 18 nodules. Benign findings were present in 43 nodules. The sensitivity, specificity, and negative predictive values were 85%, 64%, and 78%, respectively, in patients who underwent surgery. When findings of patients who underwent repetitive FNA were included, the respective overall sensitivity, specificity, and negative predictive values were 86%, 87%, and 95%. Poor correlation was observed in a comparison of the relationship between perfusion and early ^{201}Tl uptake in thyroid nodules. The correlation was very poor in hyperactive nodules. Hyperperfusion and normal ^{201}Tl uptake were observed in most of the hyperactive nodules. Perfusion and [210]Tl uptake were variable in hypoactive nodules and the correlation between them was poor. All 3 perfusion patterns were observed in malignant nodules and there was increased ^{201}Tl uptake in all malignant nodules.

Conclusion.—Findings suggest that early and delayed ^{201}Tl imaging should not be used in the differential diagnosis of cold thyroid nodules. The role of perfusion of thyroid nodules is limited in ^{201}Tl localization. Early ^{201}Tl uptake may be more closely related to factors other than perfusion.

▶ Although the primary thrust of this article is toward the differentiation of benign and malignant thyroid nodules, I have included it in the YEAR BOOK for another reason. As thallium and ^{99m}Tc-sestamibi are increasingly being used to localize parathyroid adenomas and parathyroid hyperplasia, we are frequently encountering problems in differentiating between normal thyroid uptake and parathyroid uptake. This article provides considerable information about the pharmacodynamics of ^{201}Tl uptake in thyroid nodules. An understanding of the kinetics of thallium uptake in the thyroid should be of value in helping to localize parathyroid adenomas with greater accuracy. Unfortunately, thallium uptake does not appear to be of any great value in the differential diagnosis of thyroid nodules.

M.D. Blaufox, M.D., Ph.D.

Rapid Washout of Technetium-99m-MIBI From a Large Parathyroid Adenoma
Bénard F, Lefebvre B, Beuvon F, et al (Université de Sherbrooke, Québec, Canada)
J Nucl Med 36:241–243, 1995   5–11

Introduction.—The use of technetium-99m–methoxyisobutylisonitrile (MIBI) for imaging of the parathyroid using a subtraction method with iodine-123–iodide is suggested for evaluation of primary hyperparathyroidism. In 1992, a double-phase method was proposed to take advantage of the faster clearance of ^{99m}Tc-MIBI from normal thyroid tissue. This method does not use ^{123}I and eliminates the need for subtraction images. A case of rapid clearance of ^{99m}Tc-MIBI from a large parathyroid adenoma was presented.

> *Case Report.*—Woman, 62, was evaluated for primary hyperparathyroidism. Double-phase ^{99m}Tc-MIBI parathyroid scintigraphy was performed, and a large parathyroid adenoma was observed caudal to the left lobe of the thyroid gland. The scintigrams showed rapid washout of the tracer. The parathyroid adenoma was surgically removed, and histologic examination confirmed the absence of oxyphil cells.

Conclusion.—Technetium-99m–MIBI parathyroid scintigraphy is the best imaging technique for locating abnormal parathyroid tissue in hyperparathyroidism, but slow washout of the radiotracer is not invariable, and rapid release can occur in some adenomas when the double-phase method is used.

▶ The authors point out a potential cause of false negative ^{99m}Tc-MIBI imaging in parathyroid disease. Although the sensitivity of this technique is high, suggesting that this is a relatively uncommon problem, an awareness of this potential source of error can make the test even more useful.

M.D. Blaufox, M.D., Ph.D.

Technetium-99m-Sestamibi Imaging Before Reoperation for Primary Hyperparathyroidism
Chen CC, Skarulis MC, Fraker DL, et al (Natl Inst of Diabetes, Digestive and Kidney Diseases, Bethesda, Md; Natl Cancer Inst, Bethesda, Md)
J Nucl Med 36:2186–2191, 1995   5–12

Background.—High sensitivities have been reported for parathyroid localization with technetium-99m–sestamibi. Previous research has used either iodine-123/^{99m}Tc-sestamibi or a double-phase sestamibi scanning method, focusing mainly on patients undergoing initial surgery. One experience with ^{123}I/^{99m}Tc-sestamibi subtraction combined with delayed ^{99m}Tc-sestamibi imaging in patients referred for reoperative surgery was reviewed.

Methods.—Thirty-five patients underwent early and delayed double-phase sestamibi scanning. Twenty-five patients also underwent evaluable ^{123}I/^{99m}Tc-sestamibi subtraction studies. Findings were correlated with surgical results in 32 patients and with clinical outcomes in 3 patients undergoing radiologic ablation for mediastinal lesions.

Findings.—Double-phase sestamibi imaging detected 59% of 39 abnormal parathyroid glands. Seventy percent of 27 abnormal parathyroid glands were detected on ^{123}I/^{99m}Tc-sestamibi imaging. Oblique imaging, delayed imaging, and ^{123}I subtraction were all contributors to sensitivity. In patients with partial thyroid suppression, ^{123}I subtraction proved useful. In 2 patients, lesions visible on the early sestamibi images were not visualized at all on the delayed scans. Four diagnoses were false positive.

Conclusion.—The evaluation of all patients scheduled for reoperation for primary hyperparathyroidism should include ^{123}I/^{99m}Tc-sestamibi subtraction scanning, even when the patients are thyroid suppressed. The number of thyroid-suppressed patients should be minimized by scheduling CT scans after the radionuclide study and, when possible, reducing or discontinuing levothyroxine treatment before study. All patients should have early and delayed double-phase imaging as well as right and left anterior oblique ^{99m}Tc-sestamibi images. Imaging with SPECT is done as needed. It is important to keep in mind that differences in washout rates between thyroid and parathyroid tissues are not always obvious with the double-phase technique. Also, because of rapid tracer washout, some parathyroid abnormalities may be seen only on early images. Thus, delayed imaging alone is unreliable, and early ^{99m}Tc-sestamibi images are indicated for ^{123}I/^{99m}Tc-sestamibi subtraction.

▶ It would be nice if we could do parathyroid studies using only double-phase sestamibi scanning, obviating the need for 2 radionuclides. This study suggests that this simplification may result in a loss of sensitivity. Therefore, the axiom that simplification leads to a loss in accuracy appears to continue to be true. Of course, this group of patients was a particularly difficult one because they were referred after having undergone previous surgeries. Perhaps we should reserve dual-isotope imaging for patients in this category and use the double-phase sestamibi technique for patients with less-complicated disease.

M.D. Blaufox, M.D., Ph.D.

Utility of ^{99m}Tc-Sestamibi Scintigraphy as a First-line Imaging Procedure in the Preoperative Evaluation of Hyperparathyroidism
Caixàs A, Bernà L, Piera J, et al (Universitat Autònoma de Barcelona)
Clin Endocrinol 43:525–530, 1995   5–13

Background.—Many of the imaging techniques currently used for preoperative assessment of patients with hyperparathyroidism are not sensitive and specific enough to justify routine use. The sensitivity and specificity of technetium-99m–sestamibi scintigraphy used in the management of patients with different types of hyperparathyroidism was evaluated

Patients and Methods.—Twenty-one patients with primary and 4 with secondary hyperparathyroidism underwent preoperative imaging with ^{99m}Tc-sestamibi scintigraphy. Planar images of the neck and upper chest were obtained in the anterior view 15 and 120 minutes after injection of 740 MBq of ^{99m}Tc-sestamibi (Fig 2). At least one other imaging modality, including CT, ultrasound, MRI, or thallium-201/^{99m}Tc subtraction scintigraphy, also was performed. Imaging results were correlated with those obtained at surgery.

Results.—Correct localization of 20 of 21 adenomas was obtained with ^{99m}Tc-sestamibi scintigraphy, yielding a sensitivity of 95.2%. This was considerably higher than that obtained with the other imaging techniques: CT, 41.7%; ultrasound, 75%; MRI, 33%; and ^{201}Tl/^{99m}Tc subtraction scintigraphy, 57.1%. Of all 17 glands identified as hyperplastic at surgery and verified by pathologic studies, positive images were obtained with ^{99m}Tc-sestamibi scintigraphy in 10, for a sensitivity of 58.8%. This was again higher than that noted with the other imagining techniques. There were no false positive results with ^{99m}Tc-sestamibi. All ectopic adenomas were detected before surgery; this had a significant effect on surgical approach.

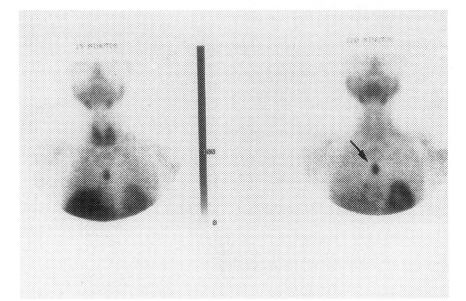

FIGURE 2.—Technetium-99m–sestamibi scintigraphy of a female, 59, who was evaluated preoperatively for hyperparathyroidism (**left,** 15 minutes; **right,** 120 minutes). The 120-minute scan showed increased tracer uptake located in the mediastinum, which was identified surgically as an ectopic parathyroid adenoma weighing 2.47 g; postoperative calcium and parathyroid hormone levels were normal. (Courtesy of Caixàs A, Bernà L, Piera J, et al: Utility of ^{99m}Tc-sestamibi scintigraphy as a first-line imaging procedure in the preoperative evaluation of hyperparathyroidism. *Clin Endocrinol* 43:525–530, 1995, Blackwell Science Ltd.)

Conclusions.—Use of ^{99m}Tc-sestamibi scintigraphy for preoperative localization of pathologic parathyroid glands is associated with a high sensitivity and specificity and may be considered a first-line imaging procedure.

▶ Strong evidence is being accumulated of the value of sestamibi imaging in patients with hyperparathyroidism who require a second surgery or in patients with more complex forms of the disease. This article is of note because the authors are suggesting a very high sensitivity and specificity for sestamibi imaging in primary diagnosis. It is also of note that the investigators report that in their experience, sestamibi imaging provided a better sensitivity than did ultrasonography, thallium imaging, CT, and MRI. There can be little doubt that sestamibi imaging of the parathyroid is here to stay.

M.D. Blaufox, M.D., Ph.D.

Parathyroid Scintigraphy: Comparison of Technetium-99m Methoxy-isobutylisonitrile and Technetium-99m Tetrofosmin Studies

Aigner RM, Fueger GF, Nicoletti R (Univ Hosp Graz, Austria)
Eur J Nucl Med 23:693–696, 1996   5–14

Background.—The myocardial perfusion scanning agents technetium-99m tetrofosmin and ⁹⁹ᵐTc-methoxyisobutylisonitrile (MIBI) are currently used in scintigraphic studies of various oncologic entities. Tetrofosmin, unlike MIBI, has not yet been used in parathyroid scintigraphy. The diagnostic value of parathyroid scintigraphy using this tracer in patients with increased serum levels of parathyroid hormone was investigated prospectively.

Methods and Findings.—Ten patients, aged 49–66 years, with primary chronic hyperparathyroidism underwent parathyroid imaging using MIBI and tetrofosmin within 3–5 days. Both tracers identified the parathyroid adenomas correctly by focal prolonged tracer retention. On visual examination, MIBI generally yielded higher image contrast than did tetrofosmin. In 6 patients, tetrofosmin was eliminated more slowly from the parathyroid adenomas than MIBI (Fig 3.)

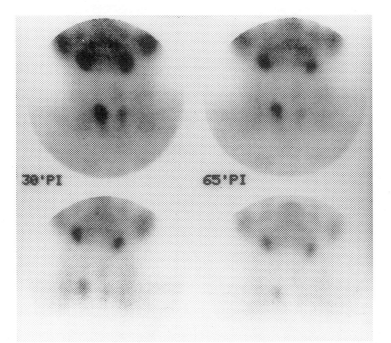

FIGURE 3.—Static technetium-99m tetrofosmin images up to 180 minutes after injection. Right superior parathyroid adenoma. (Courtesy of Aigner RM, Fueger GF, Nicoletti R: Parathyroid scintigraphy: Comparison of technetium-99m methoxyisobutylisonitrile and technetium-99m tetrofosmin studies. *Eur J Nucl Med* 23:693–696, 1996. Copyright Springer-Verlag.)

Conclusions.—Tetrofosmin appears to be a feasible, sensitive tracer in parathyroid scintigraphy. This tracer may be an alternative to MIBI for routine use because of its rapid kit preparation without heating and lower radiation dose. Additional research is needed to determine which tracer is more sensitive for detecting parathyroid adenomas and which properties better indicate the extent of endocrine activity.

▶ I suppose it should not be surprising in view of the great success that ^{99m}Tc-MIBI imaging has had in parathyroid disease that somebody would try using tetrofosmin. Nor should it be surprising that tetrofosmin also should prove to be a useful agent in this disease. It would appear that, within the next year or 2, we should be able to clearly identify the best imaging agent for evaluation of parathyroid disease and to delineate the clinical conditions in which such imaging is indicated. Hopefully there will be a good review article that serves this purpose soon. In the meantime, the place of nuclear medicine in the evaluation of patients with parathyroid disease appears to be secure.

M.D. Blaufox, M.D., Ph.D.

6 Renal

Introduction

Although the dramatic innovations that have occurred in recent years in renal nuclear medicine, such as captopril renography and the introduction of mercaptoacetyltriglycine (MAG_3), have slowed down, there continues to be a considerable amount of solid work in this area. I have chosen to start this chapter of the YEAR BOOK with citations of some articles relating to the use of technetium-99m–dimercaptosuccinic acid (DMSA) in urinary tract infection. This continues to be an underutilized area that should be the gold standard for pediatric urinary tract infection. The application of SPECT imaging to patients undergoing ^{99m}Tc-DMSA scintigraphy promises to further refine the technique.

Diuretic renography continues to be a major application in renal nuclear medicine and, although many of us have been cautious in using this in newborns, it is encouraging that MAG_3 may not suffer from a limitation in this age group.

I have taken the liberty of including an article from my group (Abstract 6–8), because I believe that it is important and presents a model for the evaluation of cost efficacy. There is no question we are increasingly being called on to demonstrate the cost-effectiveness of our procedures, and although this article represents a certain amount of nepotism, I believe that it provides some very interesting and useful data.

Articles on captopril renography have fallen off somewhat and are more addressed toward fine-tuning the use of this technique than toward general support of its application. Other articles in this section are directed at measurement of renal function, evaluation of kinetics of various radiopharmaceuticals, and again basically refinements in our understanding and use of prior knowledge. Most encouraging is the report by Behr and associates (Abstract 6–17) that the use of amino acid infusion can reduce monoclonal antibody uptake by the kidney, which can have a dual role of both improving our evaluation of abdominal monoclonal imaging and of potentially facilitating monoclonal imaging of the kidney and eliminating the interference of nonspecific uptake. Ethylenedicysteine continues to be a focus of interest and we are learning more about the handling of this agent and the specifics of its potential role in renal disease. The ubiquitous gallium continues to find a role in renal nuclear medicine, as it does in all other areas.

Overall, the contributions from nuclear medicine to the study of the kidney continue to demonstrate that this field is very much alive and well.

M. Donald Blaufox, M.D., Ph.D.

Technetium-99m-DMSA Studies in Pediatric Urinary Tract Infection
Clarke SEM, Smellie JM, Prescod N, et al (Guy's Hosp, London)
J Nucl Med 37:823–828, 1996   6–1

Introduction.—The major risk of urinary tract infection (UTI) in children is renal scarring of reflux nephropathy with subsequent hypertension

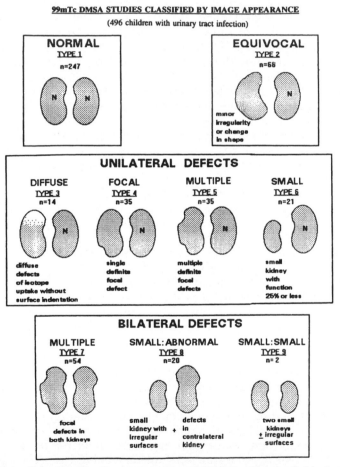

FIGURE 1.—Technetium-99m–dimercaptosuccinic acid (*DMSA*) studies classified by image appearance in 496 children with urinary tract infection. (Reprinted by permission of the Society of Nuclear Medicine, from Clarke SEM, Smellie JM, Prescod N, et al: Technetium-99m-DMSA studies in pediatric urinary tract infection. *J Nucl Med* 37:823–828, 1996.)

TABLE 1.—Relationship Between Image Appearance and Percentage Contribution of One Kidney to Total Function

DMSA image appearance	Image type	Percent function in one kidney					Total children
		45–50%	40–44%	30–39%	20–29%	10–19%	
Normal	1	247	—	—	—	—	247
Equivocal	2	36	31	1	—	—	68
Abnormal unilateral	3	10	4	—	—	—	14
	4	17	13	3	2	—	35
	5	12	6	11	6	—	35
	6	—	—	3	10	8	21
Abnormal bilateral	7	13	13	22	6	—	54
	8	—	—	4	11	5	20
	9	1	—	1	—	—	2
Total		336	67	45	35	13	496

(Reprinted by permission of the Society of Nuclear Medicine, from Clarke SEM, Smellie JM, Prescod N, et al: Technetium-99m-DMSA studies in pediatric urinary tract infection. *J Nucl Med* 37:823–828, 1996.)

and renal failure. Renal scarring has been observed in 12% of children with UTI undergoing IV urography and 25% of patients with recurrent infection. In the pediatric population, this is almost always associated with vesicoureteral reflux (VUR). Renal scars may be prevented with effective early treatment of UTI. An imaging technique is needed that can identify infants and children with or at risk of having renal damage. A cross-sectional analysis of technetium-99m–dimercaptosuccinic acid (DMSA) findings in 496 consecutive children with bacteriologically proven UTI was done.

Methods.—A standard ^{99m}Tc-DMSA protocol was used for imaging of 157 male and 339 female patients with an age range of birth to 14 years. Findings were analyzed in relation to age and sex, history of UTI, timing of the most recent infection, and presence or absence of VUR on contrast micturating cystourethrography (MCU). The appearance and extent of any functional defect was used to categorize renal images (Fig 1).

Results.—Of 496 children, 222 were evaluated after the first proven UTI. One hundred sixty-one had proven and 113 had suspected recurrent symptomatic infections. The images were normal in appearance and the differential function was within normal limits in about half of the children. One kidney contributed 47% to 50% of total function in 212 children (86%) (Table 1). The differential function was within normal limits in 53% of 68 children with equivocal image changes. In 181 children with abnormal images, function was within normal limits in 37% of those with unilateral defects and in 18% of the 76 children with bilateral abnormalities. The highest proportions of abnormal findings were seen in infant boys and girls age 5 years and older. Girls comprised 75% of the children with a history of recurrent infection, compared with an overall recurrence rate of 67%. A finding of VUR was present in 84% of children with abnormal images. This was seen in 72% of children with unilateral abnormalities and 98% of children with bilateral changes.

Conclusion.—After a UTI, a wide range of ^{99m}Tc-DMSA images can be seen throughout childhood, with fairly equal incidence in boys and girls. Boys younger than 1 year of age and girls older than age 5 years with recurrent infections had the most abnormal images. The finding of VUR was present in almost all children with bilateral abnormalities. Investigation is important at all ages to prevent potential complications of UTI.

▶ I have said it before and I will say it again and again, the use of ^{99m}Tc-DMSA or glucoheptonate studies in urinary tract infection is an extraordinarily valuable and greatly underutilized procedure. This very extensive review of findings in 496 patients certainly provides a great deal of information about this technique. It demonstrates the large amount of useful clinical information that can be derived from DMSA scanning in patients with urinary tract infection. It also makes it clear that the scan may show a wide variety of changes, and the paper tries to categorize these to make interpretation and understanding of these changes easier. It is noteworthy that the authors report that in patients with bilateral abnormalities, VUR was almost invariably present.

M.D. Blaufox, M.D., Ph.D.

Tc-99m DMSA SPECT Imaging in Patients With Acute Symptoms or History of UTI: Comparison With Ultrasonography
Mastin ST, Drane WE, Iravani A (Univ of Florida, Gainesville)
Clin Nucl Med 20:407–412, 1995   6–2

Introduction.—Acute pyelonephritis is difficult to diagnose in pediatric patients and can result in a significant loss of renal function. Planar cortical scintigraphy has been found to be a sensitive test for the detection of renal infection and scarring; however, the dose of Technetium-99m–dimercaptosuccinic acid (DMSA) needed is high. It has been suggested that SPECT is a sensitive method for detecting renal scarring and infection while using a lower dose of ^{99m}Tc-DMSA. Reduced-dose ^{99m}Tc-DMSA SPECT was compared with ultrasonography in the identification of acute pyelonephritis and renal scarring.

Methods.—Thirty-six patients (67 kidneys) with recurrent (11 patients) or recent symptoms of (25 patients) urinary tract infection were evaluated using SPECT imaging. Patient ages ranged from 1 month to 55 years. A SPECT scan was performed 2 hours after the administration of a weight-adjusted IV dose of ^{99m}Tc-DMSA. The SPECT images were evaluated for functional mass size, areas of decreased activity within the cortex, and cortical defects. An ultrasonogram was also performed. The SPECT and ultrasonogram results were obtained within 1 week of each other.

Results.—Cortical defects consistent with pyelonephritis were found on SPECT scans in 19 of 25 patients with symptoms; scans were considered

TABLE 1.—Dimercaptosuccinic Acid and Ultrasonography Findings in Symptomatic and Asymptomatic Patients—Predominant Findings by Patient

	DMSA					US					
	Round or Central Defect	Diffuse Decrease/ NL Size	Equivocal Appearance	Peripheral Defect/ Small Size	Normal	Hydro- nephrosis	Large	Small	Focal Defect	Not Seen	Normal
Symptomatic patients (N = 25)											
Urine culture (+) (N = 16)	5	1		5	5	4		1			11
Urine culture (−) (N = 7)			3	3	1						7
Culture deferred (N = 2)				2				1			1
Asymptomatic patients (N = 11)	1		1	5	4		1	1	1		8
Totals (N = 36)	6	1	4	15	10	4	1	3	1		27

Abbreviations: DMSA, dimercaptosuccinic acid; *US,* ultrasonography.
(Courtesy of Mastin ST, Drane WE, Iravani A: Tc-99m DMSA SPECT imaging in patients with acute symptoms or history of UTI: Comparison with ultrasonography. *Clin Nucl Med* 20:407–412, 1995.)

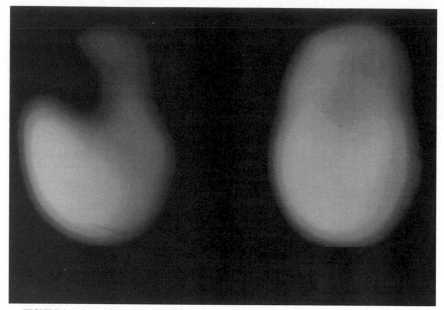

FIGURE 3.—Coronal images of the right kidney at the time of acute presentation and 10 months after therapy. The first image demonstrates a wedge-shaped defect with some central extension suspicious for pyelonephritis, and the second demonstrates no defect after treatment. (Courtesy of Mastin ST, Drane WE, Iravani A: Tc-99m DMSA SPECT imaging in patients with acute symptoms or history of UTI: Comparison with ultrasonography. *Clin Nucl Med* 20:407–412, 1995.)

normal in the remaining 6 patients (Table 1). Single-photon emission CT scans were repeated in 4 patients in whom pyelonephritis was suspected (Fig 3). Abnormalities persisted in 3 patients at 10 months. Results from ultrasonography found evidence of pyelonephritis (hydronephrosis) in only 4 of 25 symptomatic patients. Two patients had small kidneys, suggesting scarring, and ultrasonography was normal in the remaining 19 patients. Cortical defects were found by SPECT in 7 of 11 asymptomatic patients; the results for the remaining 4 patients were normal. Ultrasonography found scarring in 2 of the 11 patients, enlarged kidneys in 1 patient, and no abnormalities in the remaining 8 patients. Overall, SPECT found statistically more abnormalities than did ultrasonography. In patients with symptoms, SPECT found abnormalities in 24 of 46 kidneys as compared with 9 of 46 found by ultrasonography. In asymptomatic patients, abnormalities were found in 11 of 21 kidneys by SPECT, as compared with 4 of 21 by ultrasonography.

   Conclusion.—In this series of patients, ^{99m}Tc-DMSA SPECT was found to be a more sensitive method of determining kidney abnormalities than was ultrasonography. The use of SPECT imaging may be a more appropriate means of following patients with recurrent kidney infections and for identifying cortical infections and scarring.

▶ Perhaps our initial reaction that the role of SPECT in renal nuclear medicine was limited was erroneous. We are beginning to see mounting evidence of a variety of situations in which SPECT imaging can improve our diagnostic accuracy. Urinary tract infection would appear to be a natural use for SPECT imaging because it often can be difficult to differentiate between the abnormality that may be induced in the kidney by local infection and changes in renal appearance that are related to position and other extraneous factors.

This is a very encouraging article in terms of the role of SPECT and of the role of nuclear medicine in renal infection. Furthermore, the authors have been sensitive to the issue of a high radiation dose associated with the administration of ⁹⁹ᵐTc-DMSA and have reduced the dose proportionately. Also noteworthy in this study is that significantly more abnormalities were found in their population using DMSA SPECT than using ultrasound. It would be nice to know how many of the patients with ultrasound abnormalities also had abnormalities on DMSA SPECT scanning. These data do not appear to be contained in the article.

M.D. Blaufox, M.D., Ph.D.

Renal Dysplasia in Infants: Appearance on ⁹⁹ᵐTc DMSA Scintigraphy
Roach PJ, Paltiel HJ, Perez-Atayde A, et al (Harvard Med School, Boston)
Pediatr Radiol 25:472–475, 1995   6–3

Objective.—Abdominal masses frequently are caused by multicystic dysplastic kidney (MCDK) in the neonate. The radiopharmaceutical technetium-99m–dimercaptosuccinic acid (DMSA) is a highly sensitive tracer for renal cortical abnormalities and renal uptake is seen in urinary tract obstruction but not in MCDK. Findings of ⁹⁹ᵐTc-DMSA scintigraphy in infants with renal dysplasia, including MCDK, were evaluated.

Patients and Methods.—Forty-two infants aged 1–12 months with known or suspected MCDK were included in the study. Ultrasound studies were performed within 3 months of scintigraphic evaluations. All ultrasound studies were reviewed by an experienced pediatric radiologist without knowledge of the clinical history or results of other investigations. The ⁹⁹ᵐTc-DMSA scintigrams were reviewed by 2 nuclear medicine physicians blinded to clinical history and ultrasound results. Uptake in the region of each kidney was evaluated using a 4-point system (Fig 1).

Results.—Uptake on ⁹⁹ᵐTc-DMSA scintigraphy was noted in 6 of 41 dysplastic kidneys. In all these scintigrams, the degree of uptake was low grade, and the area of uptake was less than 25% the size of the contralateral kidney. In 7 patients, ultrasonography identified abnormalities in the contralateral kidney, including increased parenchymal echogenicity in 3, pelviceal dilatation in 1, mild ureteral dilatation in 1, and minimal pelvic ectasia in 1. Uptake in the affected kidney was not observed on scintigraphy in any of these patients. The remaining patient demonstrated grade 2 uptake in the affected kidney. In this patient, ultrasonography showed

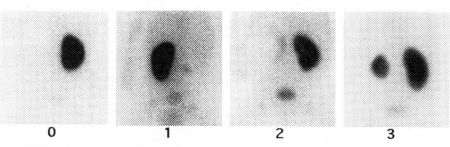

FIGURE 1.—Technetium-99m–dimercaptosuccinic acid classification of infantile renal dysplasia: **grade 0**, no uptake; **grade 1**, uptake seen only with background enhancement; **grade 2**, minimal visualization without computer enhancement; **grade 3**, easily visualized/normal. (Courtesy of Roach PJ, Paltiel HJ, Perez-Atayde A, et al: Renal dysplasia in infants: Appearance of ^{99m}Tc DMSA scintigraphy. *Pediatr Radiol* 25:472–475, 1995. Copyright Springer-Verlag.)

mild hydronephrosis and increased parenchymal echogenicity in the contralateral kidney. Eighteen patients also underwent nephrectomy. On histologic examination, uptake was found to be closely associated with the presence of mature renal cortical tissue in the affected kidney.

Conclusion.—Low-grade uptake on DMSA scintigraphy is found in a small but significant number of MCDKs. The presence of scintigraphic uptake does not definitely exclude MCDK as the cause of renal cystic disease shown by ultrasound in the infant.

▶ Multicystic dysplastic kidneys can be a devastating illness in infants. The diagnosis of this condition is being made infrequently in utero as prenatal ultrasound use increases. These authors suggest that patients with MCDK may have some mature renal cortical tissue, which can take up ^{99m}Tc-DMSA. Although this tends to argue against the use of the combination of ultrasound and ^{99m}Tc-DMSA to definitively diagnose renal dysplasia, it still leaves a useful role. Patients with no DMSA uptake and ultrasound findings can potentially avoid unnecessary surgery or more invasive diagnostic testing through the use of these 2 modalities in conjunction. False positive diagnoses of urinary tract obstruction would not appear to be a major problem because it seems likely that most physicians would prefer to use possible therapeutic intervention if even a small possibility of success exists, rather than risk ignoring, the risk for urinary tract obstruction.

M.D. Blaufox, M.D., Ph.D.

Correlation of Renal Biopsy and Radionuclide Renal Scan Differential Function in Patients With Unilateral Ureteropelvic Junction Obstruction
Stock JA, Krous HF, Heffernan J, et al (Univ of California, San Diego)
J Urol 154:716–718, 1995   6–4

Background.—Urinary tract obstruction is clinically defined as any restriction to urinary outflow that will result in progressive renal deteriora-

TABLE 1.—Characteristics of Patients With Abnormal Biopsies

Pt.–Age at Repair (mos.)	% Differential Function		% Change	Biopsy			
	Preop.	Postop.		Glomeruli	Tubules	Interstitium	Summary
BT-4	15	3	-0.8	Immature, focal podocyte effacement	Focal rupture by Tamm-Horsfall casts	Focal fibrosis and mild chronic inflammation	Focal tubular and interstitial scarring with glomerular sparing
TJ-48	28	23	-0.17	10 of 30 obsolescent	Mild focal atrophy	Focal fibrosis and chronic inflammation	Focal renal cortical scarring
CJ-2	12	3	-0.41	Focal and global sclerosis, focal Bowman's space dilatation	Multifocal atrophy and dropout, numerous proteinaceous casts	Severe chronic inflammation, lymphoid follicles and fibrosis	Focal cortical "end stage" changes
HS-5	31	30	-0.03	Bowman's space dilatation in 4 of 29, focal segmental glomerulosclerosis in 1 of 29	Mild focal atrophy	Normal	Mild glomerular changes
FS-3	30	13	-0.56	Segmental and global sclerosis	Focal distension and rupture by proteinaceous casts	Mild focal fibrosis	Glomerular sclerosis, mild tubulointerstitial changes
BJ-12	50	40	-0.2	1 of 40 obsolescent	Focal atrophy, dropout or dilatation and neutrophilic infiltration	Diffuse fibrosis and chronic inflammation with lymphoid aggregates	Multifocal chronic tubulointerstitial disease

(Courtesy of Stock JA, Krous HF, Heffernan J, et al: Correlation of renal biopsy and radionuclide renal scan differential function in patients with unilateral ureteropelvic junction obstruction. J Urol 154:716–718, 1995.)

TABLE 2.—Characteristics of Patients With Normal Biopsies

Pt.–Age at Surgery (mos.)	% Differential Function		% Change
	Preop.	Postop.	
RC–15	52	48	−0.07
MO–46	48	48	—
CA–1	Symmetrical*	58/42	—
WJ–3	45	50	−0.11
BC–56	48	47	−0.02
BM–2	44	46	+0.04
RJ–7	44	50	+0.13
CL–60	50	48	−0.04
BK–84	44	44	—

*Preoperative study was performed elsewhere and reported as symmetrical function. Percent differential function was not calculated.

(Courtesy of Stock JA, Krous HF, Heffernan J, et al: Correlation of renal biopsy and radionuclide renal scan differential function in patients with unilateral ureteropelvic junction obstruction. J Urol 154:716–718, 1995.)

tion if left untreated. Renal biopsy was performed in a group of children undergoing primary pyeloplasty in an effort to clarify the relationship between renal function measured by diuretic radionuclide renography and the outcome of pyeloplasty.

Patients and Methods.—Seventeen patients (mean age, 20 months) with unilateral ureteropelvic junction obstruction were included in the study. All patients underwent renal biopsy at pyeloplasty. A systematic evaluation of biopsy specimens was performed. One pathologist reviewed the biopsy sections, and findings were correlated with preoperative and postoperative radionuclide renal scan differential function.

Results.—Six of the 17 patients had abnormal renal biopsy specimens (Table 1). A preoperative differential function of less than 33% was noted in 5 of these 6 kidneys, none of which showed postoperative improvement in renal function on follow-up scans, despite technically successful results. In the remaining patient with an abnormal biopsy specimen, the preoperative differential function was 50%. A postoperative differential function of 40% was noted on follow-up scan.

In the remaining 11 kidneys with normal renal biopsy specimens, the preoperative differential function was greater than 44%. Nine of these 11 patients underwent a follow-up scan at 6 months. Changes in preoperative to postoperative differential function were not significant (Table 2).

Conclusion.—The probability of significant histologic changes on biopsy is high and the likelihood of postoperative improvement in differential function is low among patients with ureteropelvic junction obstruction and a differential function of less than 35%. Renal biopsy at pyeloplasty appears to be useful in predicting postoperative functional outcome. The relationship between differential function, renal biopsy results, and functional outcome after pyeloplasty may be clarified further with longer follow-up of these patients.

▶ Although renal imaging generally has been accepted in patients with urinary tract obstruction, there is a paucity of clear objective data to relate the findings on radionuclide scintigraphy of the kidney and the subsequent likelihood of failure of surgical intervention in these patients. Functional correlates are extremely important, but so are direct correlative anatomical studies. Because of the great variability in the way in which various renal radionuclide studies are performed, one must be cautious in directly applying the numbers reported in this study to a general nuclear medicine practice.

Further confirmation is required if we are to conclude that a kidney having less than 35% of the total renal function has a low probability of improvement after surgical intervention. This editor is particularly concerned because 35% would be a relatively mild impairment in renal function. At our institution, we use a range of 50% ± 10% to include the normal. Some institutions use a range of 50% ± 5%, but we believe that this is much too narrow under usual circumstances. Also, it should be noted that there are not sufficient data concerning the methodology in this manuscript. However, the fact still remains that this type of study is greatly needed in this area.

M.D. Blaufox, M.D., Ph.D.

Utility of Technetium-99m-MAG3 Diuretic Renography in the Neonatal Period
Wong JCH, Rossleigh MA, Farnsworth RH (Prince of Wales Hosp, Sydney, Australia)
J Nucl Med 36:2214–2219, 1995   6–5

Objective.—Perinatal ultrasound can detect hydronephrosis and hydroureteronephrosis, raising the need to distinguish between obstructive and nonobstructive causes. The immature renal function of newborns is thought to make diuretic renography an unreliable study for diagnosing obstruction. Technetium-99m–mercaptoacetyltriglycine (MAG_3) diuretic renography was evaluated for use in diagnosing obstruction at the pelviureteric junction (PUJ) or vesicoureteric junction (VUJ) in newborns.

Methods.—The study included 27 newborns (mean age, 17 days) referred for further evaluation of hydronephrosis or hydroureteronephrosis detected on perinatal ultrasound. All infants underwent standard diuretic renography using ^{99m}Tc-MAG_3 with a frusemide dose of 1 mg/kg, followed by another image after gravity-assisted drainage. The analysis included a total of 53 renal units, defined as a kidney and its ureter.

Results.—Excellent diuretic responses with clearance half-times of 0.6 to 7.7 minutes were observed in 17 normal, undilated renal units. Another 18 units were found to have PUJ obstruction, as confirmed at surgery (Fig 1). Of 8 units that were diagnosed as unobstructed, 7 were confirmed as such by serial ultrasound and ^{99m}Tc-MAG_3 imaging. In the remaining unit, pyeloplasty was eventually performed for PUJ obstruction. The renographic findings for PUJ obstruction were indeterminate in 1 unit; how-

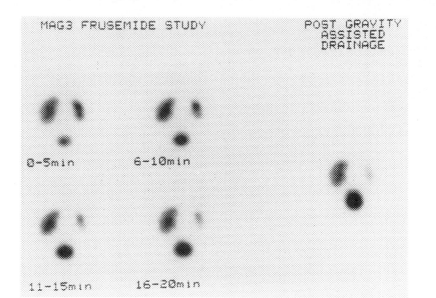

FIGURE 1.—Left pelviureteric junction. Posterior views show a dilated left pelvi-calyceal system that drains poorly during the diuretic phase and that remains essentially unchanged after gravity-assisted drainage. Good drainage is seen from the normal right kidney. The pelvic clearance half-time was infinity for the left and 7.7 minutes for the right. (Reprinted by permission of the Society of Nuclear Medicine, from Wong JCH, Rossleigh MA, Farnsworth RH: Utility of technetium-99m-MAG3 diuretic renography in the neonatal period. *J Nucl Med* 36:2214–2219, 1995.)

ever, it showed good clearance on gravity-assisted drainage, and repeat studies confirmed that it was unobstructed. In eight of 9 renal units, a diagnosis of VUJ was surgically confirmed as such, the final diagnosis remained uncertain in the remaining unit. Two units with PUJ obstruction also had VUJ obstruction. In these cases, insufficient radiotracer drainage through the tight stenosis into the ureter precluded recognition of the VUJ obstruction.

Conclusion.—The use of ^{99m}Tc-MAG$_3$ for diuretic renography produces an adequate diuretic response and thus permits a reliable diagnosis of obstruction in newborns with hydronephrosis and hydroureteronephrosis. Patients in whom this study produces an unobstructed or indeterminate result need follow-up imaging to ensure that obstruction does not develop later. Also, in patients with coexisting VUJ and PUJ obstruction, the VUJ obstruction may be missed. The ^{99m}Tc-MAG$_3$ technique may also be useful in postoperative follow-up to demonstrate improved clearance.

▶ This article is noteworthy in reporting experience with a particularly young cohort of children suspected of having urinary tract obstruction. On a theoretical basis, the handling of both the diuretic and of MAG$_3$ are thought to be somewhat unpredictable in children in the age range studied here, and general practice is to try to delay the radioisotope study as long as feasible in the expectation of obtaining a more accurate result later. This article is encouraging in its suggestion that accurate results can, in fact, be obtained in very young infants, facilitating an early diagnosis and clinical management plan. Hopefully, it will stimulate further studies at this age, which will lead to confirmation. It is particularly important to note, however, that the agent used was MAG$_3$, which does not depend on glomerular filtration, and that early use of DTPA imaging may well be very unreliable, as generally thought. Chung et al.[1] have also reported similar findings, as noted by the authors.

M.D. Blaufox, M.D., Ph.D.

Reference

1. Chung S, Majd M, Rushton HG, et al: Diuretic renography in the evaluation of neonatal hydronephrosis: Is it reliable? *J Urol* 150:765–768, 1993.

Detection of a Poorly Functioning Malpositioned Kidney With Single Ectopic Ureter in Girls With Urinary Dribbling: Imaging Evaluation in Five Patients
Gharagozloo AM, Lebowitz RL (Harvard Med School, Boston)
AJR 164:957–961, 1995   6–6

Background.—In girls with lifelong dribbling of urine despite normal voiding habits, urography or sonography may show evidence of only 1 kidney. It is likely that these patients exhibit a poorly functioning, nonvisualized kidney with a nonduplicated collecting system that has a ureter with an ectopic orifice. Experience with such a group of patients was analyzed to identify the best way to verify the presence and show the location of a possible abnormal kidney.

Materials and Methods.—The medical records and imaging studies of patients who were first seen for evaluation of continuous urinary dribbling between 1975 and 1993 were reviewed. The patients ranged in age from 3.5 to 16 years. Their final diagnosis was a kidney drained by a ureter with an ectopic orifice. Sonography, excretory urography, retrograde and intraoperative antegrade ureterography, vaginography, CT, MRI, and renal cortical scintigraphy with technetium-99m–dimercaptosuccinic acid (DSMA) were among the imaging studies performed.

Results.—In all of the patients, the abnormal kidneys were on the left side. In only 1 of 5 patients did excretory urography or sonography show the abnormal kidney. In 3 girls undergoing renal cortical scintigraphy with DSMA, the malpositioned, abnormal kidney was identified. A CT scan, with special attention given to the area of radionuclide uptake observed on the scintigram, was also performed in 2 of these 3 patients and showed the location of the dysplastic kidney more precisely. In one of 2 patients undergoing both CT and DSMA scintigraphy, the CT was done with and without IV contrast material and showed enhancement of the abnormal kidney (Fig 5).

Conclusion.—It is recommended that girls with incessant dribbling of urine who have been shown to have only 1 kidney have a DSMA scinti-

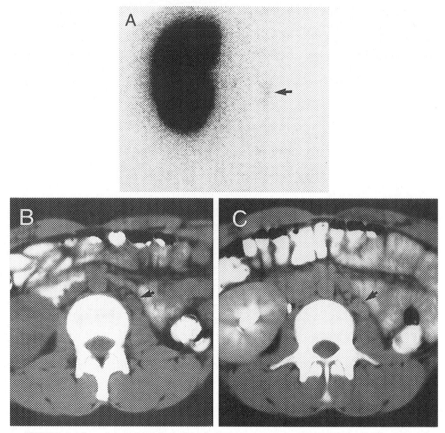

FIGURE 5.—In a patient, 16, who had both dimercaptosuccinic acid (*DMSA*) and CT scintigraphy, DMSA scintigram (**A**) reveals tiny kidney on left side at level of lower margin of hilum of right kidney (*arrow*). **B** and **C**, CT scans without (**B**) and with (**C**) IV contrast material, with special attention to level at which increased radionuclide uptake was seen on DMSA scintigram. On unenhanced CT scan (**B**), dysplastic left kidney (*arrow*) had attenuation value comparable to that of psoas muscle. On contrast-enhanced CT scan (**C**), dysplastic kidney enhanced (*arrow*). Note anatomical splenic flexure of colon in left renal fossa. (Courtesy of Gharagozloo AM, Lebowitz RL: Detection of a poorly functioning malpositioned kidney with single ectopic ureter in girls with urinary dribbling: Imaging evaluation in five patients. *AJR* 164:957–961, 1995.)

gram as their next imaging evaluation. A CT scan directed at the area indicated by the scintigram will more precisely delineate the often ectopic kidney, thereby facilitating removal.

▶ Although the lesson seems to be one that just won't take, the message keeps recurring that nuclear imaging has an important role to play in both adults and children with renal disease. In spite of the exquisite resolution of CT imaging, the data obtained in this series of patients were greatly improved by localizing the dysplastic malpositioned kidneys using DMSA scintigrams. Given these data, the authors still advocate doing an excretory urogram and a sonogram before going on to nuclear imaging. It would seem to this reviewer that the combination of a sonogram and a nuclear scan would provide the optimum information with minimal radiation to the patient.

M.D. Blaufox, M.D., Ph.D.

Detection of Permanent Damage in Kidneys With Vesicoureteral Reflux by Quantitative Single Photon Emission Computerized Tomography (SPECT) Uptake of [99m]Technetium Labeled Dimercaptosuccinic Acid
Groshar D, Gorenberg V, Weissman I, et al (Technion-Israel Inst of Technology, Haifa)
J Urol 155:664–667, 1996   6–7

Introduction.—Nearly one half of children with urinary tract infections have vesicoureteral reflux, and it is present in 1% to 2% of the pediatric population. Although management is controversial, surgical correction and antibiotic prophylaxis have been successful. Quantitative SPECT of dimercaptosuccinic acid (DMSA) uptake has been used to assess renal damage and function in children with vesicoureteral reflux. In this study, SPECT imaging was used to determine the level of permanent renal damage from vesicoureteral reflux that could not be corrected by surgery.

Methods.—Sequential quantitative SPECT imaging was performed at a mean interval of 3.2 years on 19 children (mean age, 5.5 years) with bilateral vesicoureteral reflux. Reflux was grade I to II in 9 patients, grade III in 13 patients, and grade IV or V in 12 patients. Ten patients with reflux greater than grade III had antireflux surgery. Technetium-99m–DMSA was injected (0.75 to 2 mCi) in each patient, and SPECT imaging was performed in 4–6 hours. Renal functional volume and percent uptake of ^{99m}Tc-DMSA were determined.

Results.—For patients who had undergone antireflux surgery, the initial kidney volume was 79 ± 40 cc. Percent of injected dose per cc of renal tissue was 0.33 ± 0.18, with 25.2 ± 14.4% uptake of DMSA (Figure). On the second SPECT image, kidney volume was found to significantly increase (100.5 ± 53.8 cc), with a mean change of 26.5 ± 32.4%. There were no significant changes in percent of injected dose per cc of renal tissue or in percent uptake. Patients who had not undergone surgery for reflux were found to have a significant increase in renal volume from the first to the second scan (84.7 ± 44.7 cc vs. 106.6 ± 49.7 cc). The percent of injected dose per cc of renal tissue was found to significantly decrease from 0.38 ± 0.21 to 0.28 ± 0.16. No significant difference in uptake was found between the 2 scans. In all 34 kidneys evaluated, a 27.2% ± 28.4% change in renal volume was found between the first and second scans. A 15.6% kidney uptake was found to be the threshold for differentiating between kidneys with a greater than 7% change in volume and kidneys with a change in volume of less than 7%. Values less than 15.6% had a 100% positive predictive value for predicting a change in volume of less than 7%; values

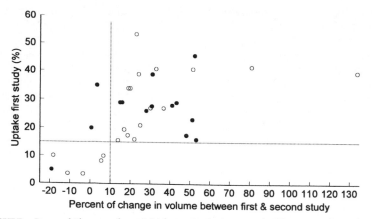

FIGURE.—Percent kidney uptake at initial examination compared with percent change in volume between initial and repeat examinations in kidneys with (*open circles*) and without (*solid circles*) surgical intervention. (Courtesy of Groshar D, Gorenberg V, Weissman I, et al: Detection of permanent damage in kidneys with vesicoureteral reflux by quantitative single photon emission computerized tomography (SPECT) uptake of ⁹⁹ᵐtechnetium labeled dimercaptosuccinic acid. *J Urol* 155:664–667, 1996.)

over 15.6% had a 93% negative predictive value for predicting a greater than 7% change in kidney volume.

Conclusion.—In patients with vesicoureteral reflux, ⁹⁹ᵐTc-DMSA uptake of less than 15.6% during SPECT imaging is indicative of permanent functional damage to the kidney. All patients with vesicoureteral reflux should undergo quantitative SPECT imaging to evaluate the extent of renal function damage.

▶ This study is particularly interesting, as it is an application of SPECT imaging to renal nuclear medicine. In general, the use of SPECT in renal nuclear medicine has been useful but relatively limited. The concept of quantitation using DMSA SPECT is an attractive one. However, the authors suggest that this technique may be easier to perform than measurement of relative glomerular filtration rate with ⁹⁹ᵐTc DTPA or relative tubular uptake with ⁹⁹ᵐTc-mercaptoacetyltriglycine (MAG₃). I do not think that relative renal function using a gamma camera is really more difficult than the quantitative SPECT technique described here. It would be most useful if the investigators or some other group would compare the proposed DMSA method with relative MAG₃ or DTPA to identify exactly what their relative roles and accuracy are.

M.D. Blaufox, M.D., Ph.D.

Cost Efficacy of the Diagnosis and Therapy of Renovascular Hypertension

Blaufox MD, Middleton ML, Bongiovanni J, et al (Albert Einstein College of Medicine, Bronx, NY; Montefiore Med Ctr, Bronx, NY; Univ of Texas Health Science Ctr, Houston)

J Nucl Med 37:171–177, 1996   6–8

Background.—The role of renovascular disease in diagnosing and treating hypertension is controversial. The incidence of renovascular hypertension is estimated at less than 1% in the general population and up to 40% in selected populations. There is little information on the value and relative cost of screening procedures and on long-term benefits of anatomical

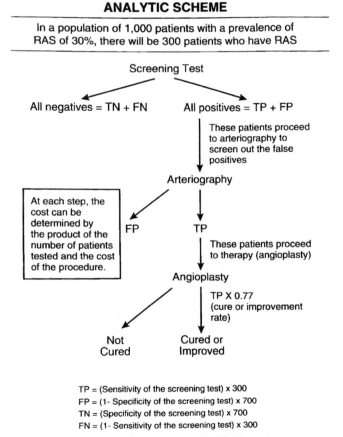

ANALYTIC SCHEME

In a population of 1,000 patients with a prevalence of RAS of 30%, there will be 300 patients who have RAS

Screening Test

All negatives = TN + FN   All positives = TP + FP

These patients proceed to arteriography to screen out the false positives

Arteriography

At each step, the cost can be determined by the product of the number of patients tested and the cost of the procedure.

FP   TP

These patients proceed to therapy (angioplasty)

Angioplasty

TP X 0.77 (cure or improvement rate)

Not Cured   Cured or Improved

TP = (Sensitivity of the screening test) x 300
FP = (1- Specificity of the screening test) x 700
TN = (Specificity of the screening test) x 700
FN = (1- Sensitivity of the screening test) x 300

FIGURE 1.—Schematic illustrates the basic approach to calculating the relative cost of diagnostic and therapeutic procedures available for renovascular hypertension. "Successfully treated patients" include those whose blood pressure reverts to normal and those who have a reduction in medication requirements. The absolute cost efficacy of the procedure depends on the total reduction in medication requirements achieved by the therapy. (Reprinted by permission of the Society of Nuclear Medicine, from Blaufox MD, Middleton ML, Bongiovanni J, et al: Cost efficacy of the diagnosis and therapy of renovascular hypertension. *J Nucl Med* 37: 171–177, 1996.)

TABLE 2.—Meta-analysis Values

Test	Sensitivity	Specificity	(30% RAS) PPV	(RVH) PPV
Captopril renogram (RAS)	89 (86,92)	92 (89,95)	83 (78,88)‡	64 (60,68)
Captopril renogram (RVH)	90 (88,92)	86 (79,93)	NC	66 (56,76)
Captopril test	61 (54,68)	86 (83,89)	65 (60,70)	50 (46,54)
Doppler*	90 (86,94)	98 (97,99)	95 (88,100)	73 (68,78)
Arteriography (RVH)†	NC	NC	100	77 (74,80)

*Only 83% success rate.
†Based on angioplasty data.
‡Numbers in parentheses are 95% confidence intervals.
Abbreviations: PPV, positive predictive value; *RAS*, renal artery stenosis; *RVH*, renovascular hypertension; *NC*, not calculable.
(Reprinted by permission of the Society of Nuclear Medicine, from Blaufox MD, Middleton ML, Bongiovanni J, et al: Cost efficacy of the diagnosis and therapy of renovascular hypertension. *J Nucl Med* 37:171–177, 1996.)

correction of renovascular hypertension. In the past 10 years, there have been dramatic improvements in medical and pharmacologic treatment of hypertension. The cost, sensitivity, and specificity of various screening tests for renovascular hypertension were evaluated, and the cost-effectiveness of correcting renal artery stenosis was compared with other medical treatments.

Methods.—A meta-analysis was conducted of studies of screening procedures for renovascular hypertension and renal artery stenosis. The sensitivity, specificity, and predictive values were calculated for arteriography, Doppler, the captopril test, and captopril renography. The cost per patient improved or cured was compared with the lifetime cost of medical therapy. A hypothetical population was used to estimate cost-effectiveness (Fig 1).

Results.—All modalities, except the captopril test, had similar sensitivity, specificity, and positive predictive value (Table 2); the sensitivity of the captopril test was significantly lower. The specificity of Doppler was the highest, but it had a 17% technical failure rate. Arteriography had the highest cost per patient improved or cured, and the captopril test had the lowest cost per patient improved or cured. The relative values of arteriography and renography were similar; Doppler and the captopril test had the lowest relative value (Table 3). There was an estimated savings of $5,800 to $8,000 per patient if angioplasty reduced medication use by 3 drugs. Surgical treatment was not cost effective, except in highly selected patients.

TABLE 3.—Relative Quality Values
[(1/Cost) × Patients × 1000]

Captopril renography (RVH)	1/13,554 × 208	=	15.35
Captopril renography (RAS)	1/14,875 × 206	=	13.85
Arteriography*	1/15,793 × 231	=	14.63
Doppler	1/15,041 × 172	=	11.44
Captopril test	1/13,881 × 141	=	10.16

*Arteriography will result in 5% complications that are not factored into the quality score.
Abbreviations: RVH, renovascular hypertension; *RAS*, renal artery stenosis.
(Reprinted by permission of the Society of Nuclear Medicine, from Blaufox MD, Middleton ML, Bongiovanni J, et al: Cost efficacy of the diagnosis and therapy of renovascular hypertension. *J Nucl Med* 37:171–177, 1996.)

Conclusion.—The cost effectiveness of arteriography and captopril renography are similar. Captopril renography often eliminates the need for an arteriogram. Most screening tests are less effective in patients with azotemia. Arteriography is the most effective if there is concern about restoring renal function. Any of the screening tests are effective in patients with well-preserved renal function, but captopril renography is the most cost-effective.

▶ It is very difficult to review, in an objective fashion, an article for which the reviewer served as the primary author. Therefore, those of you who may distrust my remarks for this reason are advised to skip over these comments. However, I believe that this is an extremely important article that presents a model of how we in nuclear medicine should be dealing with the procedures we offer. There is clearly a need for very careful, scientific comparisons of the results of various modalities in seeking a solution to a diagnostic problem. I believe that this article presents a very valuable and useful model.

The reader is particularly referred to the many places in this article where it is stated that insufficient information exists for dealing with the resolution of certain very relevant questions. No matter how simplistically we try to approach the problem of cost efficacy, the fact remains that this is not a simple problem; it is extraordinarily expensive, and we simply do not have enough information in most areas to provide the correct answers. I believe this article does the best that can be done under the circumstances, and for those of you who are considering providing captopril renography or who already provide it in the differential diagnosis of renovascular hypertension, I think it provides some very useful information.

M.D. Blaufox, M.D., Ph.D.

Diagnosis of Renovascular Hypertension: Feasibility of Captopril-sensitized Dynamic MR Imaging and Comparison With Captopril Scintigraphy
Grenier N, Trillaud H, Combe C, et al (Groupe Hospitalier Pellegrin, Bordeaux, France; Hôpital Saint-André Bordeaux, France)
AJR 166:835–843, 1996   6–9

Introduction.—To evaluate the feasibility of captopril-sensitized dynamic MRI, imaging studies were performed in 15 patients in whom there was a high suspicion of renovascular hypertension. In experimental models, blockage of glomerular filtration by an angiotensin-converting enzyme inhibitor (ACEI) was detectable with MRI. Renal scintigraphy was also performed to compare captopril-induced changes in the 2 techniques.

Patients and Methods.—Seven men and 8 women with a mean age of 50 years and a duration of hypertension ranging from 2 months to 10 years were studied. All had at least 2 criteria suggestive of renovascular hypertension and had renal artery stenosis demonstrated before MRI. Patients were studied with sequential gadolinium-enhanced MRI after oral admin-

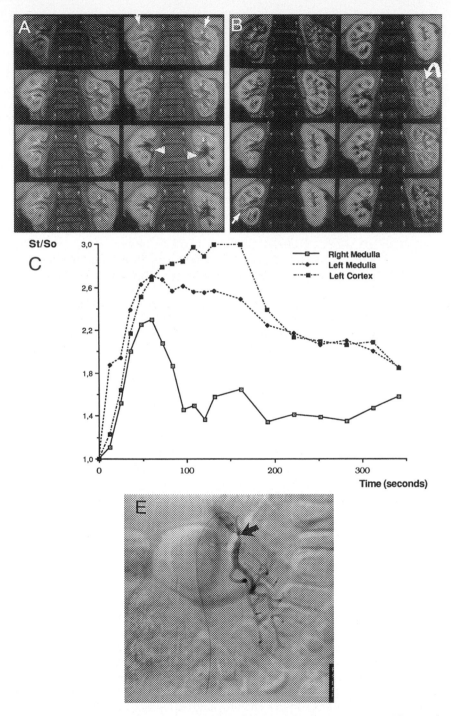

(*Continued*)

istration of 50 mg of the ACEI captopril. Data recorded included symmetry of onset and evolution of tubular phases between the 2 kidneys and medullary signal intensity time curves for each kidney. Patients in whom asymmetry between kidneys was noted underwent the same study 24 hours later without captopril. Renal scintigraphy was performed with captopril, and all patients underwent 3-dimensional time-of-flight angiography.

Results.—Eleven patients showed a symmetric tubular phase after administration of captopril and had negative renal scintigraphic results. Asymmetry of tubular and excretory phases was present after captopril in the remaining 4 patients; 2 had shown slight asymmetry in tubular phases and 2 had normal and symmetric baseline studies (Fig 3). This functional change was segmental in 1 case and affected the whole kidney in 3. Scintigraphy also showed a captopril-induced functional impairment in these 4 patients. In 1 case, however, scintigraphy did not reveal the segmental distribution of filtration impairment seen at MRI. Renal artery stenosis was apparent at MR angiography in 10 patients, 9 in single renal arteries and 1 in the main branch of a double renal artery. The 4 patients with functional renal impairment underwent percutaneous transluminal angioplasty; 2 were cured, 1 experienced improvement, and the procedure was a technical failure in 1 case.

Conclusion.—Captopril-sensitized dynamic MRI of the kidney can be performed in patients with high suspicion of renovascular disease, but tests were not positive in all confirmed cases. Although captopril MRI and captopril scintigraphy yield similar results, the latter study may not demonstrate segmental functional involvement.

▶ I have a great many problems with this article, which is very difficult to read and does not provide the kind of data in which I would be most interested. For instance, the authors indicate that they followed the blood pressures of patients who had intervention for renal artery stenosis, but the relation between blood pressure response and the results of the tests of these individuals is not given in sufficient detail. Furthermore, the discussion of the physiology of renal artery stenosis is rather difficult to follow and confused. Finally, the authors would have been better advised to have used technetium-99m–DTPA for the renograms to compare with the gadolinium-enhanced MR studies, because then they would at least have been comparing 2 agents that had relatively similar renal physiologic characteristics. Regardless of all of these reservations, the investigators have shown that it

---

FIGURE 3 (cont.)

FIGURE 3.—Man 70, with atherosclerosis. **A,** MR images obtained without administration of captopril (from top to bottom, then left to right) show symmetric tubular phase (*arrows*) appearing 60 seconds after beginning of vasculointerstitial phase and symmetric excretory phase (*arrowheads*). **B,** MR images after administration of captopril show tubular phase in right kidney (*straight arrow*) 4 minutes before left side (*curved arrow*), where low signal intensity of medulla migrates centrifugally toward cortex, which appears completely hypointense on late images. **C,** signal-intensity-time curves after administration of captopril show delayed but prolonged decrease in signal intensity within medulla and within cortex of left kidney. **E,** angiogram shows tight stenosis of left renal artery (*arrow*). (Courtesy of Grenier N, Trillaud H, Combe C, et al: Diagnosis of renovascular hypertension: Feasibility of captopril-sensitized dynamic MR imaging and comparison with captopril scintigraphy. *AJR* 166:835–843, 1996.)

is possible to diagnose renovascular hypertension using gadolinium-enhanced dynamic MRI. A full-scale study to show the actual value of this modality and its relative cost compared with captopril renography would appear to be indicated at this time. The authors' data do not appear to suggest any unique advantage or disadvantage of MRI in this setting—they simply show its feasibility.

M.D. Blaufox, M.D., Ph.D.

Interpretation of Captopril Renography by Nuclear Medicine Physicians
Schreij G, van Kroonenburgh MJ, Heidendal GK, et al (Univ Hosp, Maastricht, The Netherlands; Maasland Hosp, Sittard, The Netherlands)
J Nucl Med 36:2192–2195, 1995   6–10

Background.—The interpretation of diagnostic tests may be subject to considerable bias. Intraobserver and interobserver variability is commonly tested to assess the reliability of diagnostic investigations. This strategy was used to determine the diagnostic accuracy of nuclear medicine physicians in their assessment of baseline and captopril renograms.

Methods.—Three experienced nuclear medicine physicians interpreted baseline, captopril, and paired renograms. The renograms of 28 hypertensive patients suspected of having renovascular hypertension on the basis of clinical clues were included in the study. Angiography also was performed in all patients. The interpreters were not aware of the patients' angiographic diagnoses.

❧*Findings.*—Renal artery stenosis was diagnosed in 13 patients on renal angiography. Eight were unilateral and 5 were bilateral. The intraobserver agreement ranged from 64% to 89% and the kappa (observed agreement corrected for chance), from 0.52 to 0.75. Interobserver agreement ranged from 68% to 86%, with a kappa of 0.61 to 0.82. The sensitivity of the physicians' interpretation of paired baseline plus captopril renograms in relation to the angiographic diagnosis was less than 50%. The posttest

TABLE 2.—Observed Agreement (OA) and Kappa of Renographic Diagnosis of Technetium-99m–MAG$_3$ Baseline and Captopril Renograms

Baseline Renogram	OA Intermed.	OA High	Kappa Intermed.	Kappa High
A vs. B	82%	96%	0.78	0.95
A vs. C	68%	100%	0.61	1.0
B vs. C	86%	96%	0.82	0.95
Captopril renogram				
A vs. B	78%	96%	0.74	0.95
A vs. C	64%	96%	0.57	0.95
B vs. C	75%	93%	0.69	0.91

Note: Readers had to determine different levels of probability of renal artery stenosis being present.
Abbreviations: MAG$_3$, mercaptoacetyltriglycine; *intermed.*, intermediate; *high*, high level.
(Reprinted by permission of the Society of Nuclear Medicine, from Schreij G, van Kroonenburgh MJ, Heidendal GK, et al: Interpretation of captopril renography by nuclear medicine physicians. *J Nucl Med* 36:2192–2195, 1995.)

probability of renal artery stenosis in cases of renograms with negative results was similar to the pretest probability of 46%. The readers' accuracy was increased when they were unaware of which renogram was obtained after captopril imaging (Table 2).

Conclusion.—Experienced nuclear medicine physicians had reasonably good intraobserver and interobserver agreement in renographic interpretation. When scan results are positive, blinding interpreters as to which renogram is the precaptopril and which is the postcaptopril image appears to increase diagnostic accuracy.

▶ This article is both encouraging and disappointing. It is encouraging because the authors did find reasonable concordance among 3 different readers. This is particularly important because most captopril renography is evaluated qualitatively, and one would hope that interpretations from center to center would be fairly reproducible. Our experience at my center using blinded interpretations by 2 separate readers has been much more encouraging, with excellent correspondence between the 2 readers.

The disappointing part of the study is the very low sensitivity reported. This may be partially ascribed to the fact that the authors used criteria for renal artery stenosis applied to the DTPA renogram in a study in which the renogram was performed with mercaptoacetyltriglycine (MAG_3). These parameters are really quite different, and one should not apply the same criteria to a DTPA renogram that one would apply to an MAG_3 renogram. Moreover, because of minor variations in technique, any kind of quantitative or semiquantitative parameters have to be carefully validated for the individual center.

The message from this study is a step in the right direction, namely, an effort to determine the interobserver variability in the interpretation of the test. However, the second goal of the study, which was the assessment of the diagnostic accuracy of the nuclear physicians involved, does not appear to be at a level commensurate with general experience.

M.D. Blaufox, M.D., Ph.D.

Techniques for Measuring Renal Transit Time
Russell CD, Japanwalla M, Khan S, et al (Univ of Alabama, Birmingham; VA Med Ctr, Birmingham, Ala)
Eur J Nucl Med 22:1372–1378, 1995   6–11

Introduction.—The prolonged renal transit time resulting from significant renal artery stenosis (RAS) has been used diagnostically since first described in 1963. Alternative methods for measuring transit time were compared in a group of 30 patients undergoing baseline and postcaptopril gamma camera renography, then contrast angiography.

Methods.—All patients were hypertensive, and 3 had previous renal transplants. Low-dose technetium-99m–mercaptoacetyltriglycine (MAG_3) was used for the baseline study. One to 2 hours later, 50 mg of oral

TABLE 3.—Normal Transit Times: Mean and Standard Deviation for 14 Normal Kidneys

	Peak (min)	R20/3 (min)	MTT (min)
Whole	3.91±1.43	0.35±0.33	3.22±0.97
Cortex	3.24±1.25	0.31±0.32	2.62±0.73
Factor	2.76±0.48	(0.18±0.07)	2.04±0.37

Abbreviations: R20/3, ratio of counts at 20 minutes to those at 3 minutes; *MTT,* mean transit time.
(Courtesy of Russell CD, Japanwalla M, Khan S, et al: Techniques for measuring renal transit time. *Eur J Nucl Med* 22:1372–1378, 1995. Copyright Springer-Verlag.)

captopril was given. One hour after captopril administration, a higher dose of ^{99m}Tc-MAG$_3$ was given and the postcaptopril renogram was performed. The peak time, mean transit time, and ratio of background-subtracted counts at 20 minutes to those at 3 minutes (R20/3) were measured. Whole-kidney region of interest (ROI), cortical ROI, and cortical factor were calculated for each index.

Results.—Normal ranges for transit time parameters were estimated using the mean and standard deviation for 14 normal kidneys (Table 3). The greatest correlations between angiographic percent of stenosis and transit time index were seen for the peak time and the R20/3, using the whole-kidney ROI and baseline data without captopril. Administration of captopril shifted the R20/3 curve toward decreased specificity and slightly toward greater sensitivity. This change was not often of diagnostic value because captopril can cause a compensated kidney to decompensate because it interferes with the autoregulatory control mechanism for glomerular filtration rate. A decompensated kidney may show no further change with captopril.

Conclusion.—The simplest measures of transit time (whole-kidney peak time and whole-kidney R20/3) were as accurate as more sophisticated

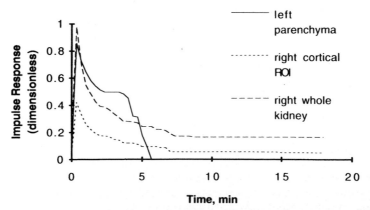

FIGURE 5.—Right-sided renal artery stenosis: deconvoluted parenchymal transit, after captopril. For the stenotic kidney, transit is incomplete at 20 minutes and the cortical ROI and whole-kidney ROI lead to equivalent results. *Abbreviation: ROI,* region of interest. (Courtesy of Russel CD, Japanwalla M, Khan S, et al: Techniques for measuring renal transit time. *Eur J Nucl Med* 22:1372–1378, 1995. Copyright Springer-Verlag.)

methods, such as deconvolution, factor analysis, or use of a cortical ROI (Fig 5). The more sophisticated methods may be preferred in patients with obstruction, a dilated collecting system, or chronic parenchymal disease.

▶ One of the more controversial methodologies in nuclear medicine has been the measurement of renal transit time. This is probably related to the great difficulty in performing this measurement and the many rather poorly constructed commercial programs for its use. Dr. Russell has been one of the pioneers in the use of this methodology and presents here a carefully performed and objective assessment of transit time measurement in a group of 30 patients who also underwent captopril renography.

It is somewhat reassuring that Dr. Russell et al. suggest that the simple measurements of peak time or the ratio of the 20-minute to 3-minute value of activity in the renogram provide results that are just as reliable as the much more complex transit time measurements. Our results have been quite similar. It appears that, although there is a great deal to be learned about renal physiology from the use of mean transit time, in the vast majority of situations more simple qualitative or semiquantitative analyses suffice. It is possible that because of the great complexity of the measurement, the results are highly dependent on user expertise and experience. However, Dr. Russell's credentials in this area can hardly be questioned and lead to the inescapable conclusion that we do not yet know enough about the measurement of renal transit time to use it reliably in renal diagnosis.

M.D. Blaufox, M.D., Ph.D.

Measurement of Renal Function With Technetium-99m-MAG3 in Children and Adults
Russell CD, Taylor AT, Dubovsky EV (Univ of Alabama, Birmingham; Emory Univ, Atlanta, Ga)
J Nucl Med 37:588–593, 1996   6–12

Introduction.—A single-sample technique for determining technetium-99m–mercaptoacetyltriglycine (MAG$_3$) in adults has been described. A single-injection, single-sample technique that is based on a larger and more varied pool and incorporates scaling for patient size so that it is valid for adults and children alike has been developed.

Methods.—An empirical formula was determined by fitting data collected at several centers from 122 adults and 80 children. All measurements in the formula are expressed in dimensionless combinations. The measurements consisted of plasma activity expressed as a percentage of the administered dose per liter of plasma and corresponding sample times that were expressed as time after injection, using at least 6 samples per research subject.

Results.—Findings were scaled to standard adult surface area and were presented in units of mL/min/1.73 m^2. The equation (number 3): Ct/W =

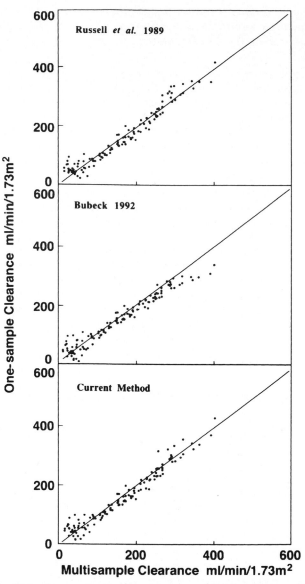

FIGURE 2.—Adult subjects: technetium-99m–mercaptoacetyltriglycine clearance estimated from 1 sample at 45 minutes compared with clearance calculated from multiple samples. The line of identity is shown: (**top**) earlier method of Russell et al.; (**middle**) method of Bubeck; (**bottom**) current method. (Reprinted by permission of the Society of Nuclear Medicine, from Russell CD, Taylor AT, Dubovsky EV: Measurement of renal function with technetium-99m-MAG3 in children and adults. *J Nucl Med* 37:588–593, 1996.)

$222.6 - 168.8X + 52.73X^2 - 11.14X^3$ was used to determine clearance. The agreement between observed and predicted values was shown using equation 3. Increased random error was observed at low clearance values for adults (Fig 2). Higher values were observed in pediatric research

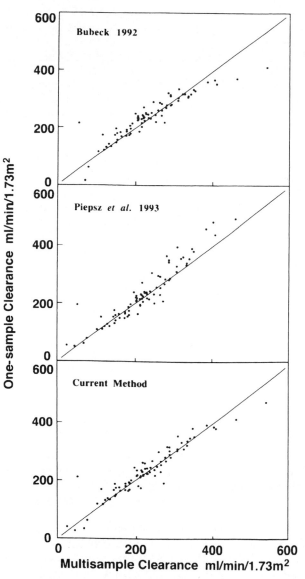

FIGURE 3.—Pediatric subjects: technetium-99m–mercaptoacetyltriglycine clearance estimated from 1 sample at 35 minutes compared with clearance calculated from multiple samples. The line of identity is shown: (**top**) method of Bubeck; (**middle**) method of Piepsz et al.; (**bottom**) current method. (Reprinted by permission of the Society of Nuclear Medicine, from Russell CD, Taylor AT, Dubovsky EV: Measurement of renal function with technetium-99m-MAG3 in children and adults. *J Nucl Med* 37:588–593, 1996.)

subjects after scaling for body surface (Fig 3). For adults, the residual standard deviation (rsd) was 23 and was calculated from a single sample at 45 minutes, using the plasma clearance calculated from a multisample clearance curve as reference. An rsd of 24 was calculated for children (using the new formula from a single sample at 35 minutes). For children, a comparable value of 33 was determined using an already published pediatric formula.

Conclusion.—This new clearance formula is recommended as a replacement for the formula that was previously published. It can be used in the range of sample times from 35 to 50 minutes. It is recommended that sampling be at 35 minutes for children and at 45 minutes for adults to keep the span of time as short as possible without excessive loss of accuracy at low clearance values.

▶ This detailed study of single-injection, single-sample measurement of MAG₃ clearance attempts to provide a basis for use in both children and adults. Like all other single-sample methods, the final result is an empirical formula derived from fitted data. My greatest concern with this article is the concluding statement, "the new clearance formula is recommended as a replacement for the formula we previously published." The problem with all single-sample methods is that as the patient population changes (as it has in this study) and as the number of patients grows, the formula invariably is increasingly refined. Because single-sample clearance techniques are empirical techniques, there will never be a formula that is truly perfect. The validity of the formula will always be affected by the particular patient population being studied, and no single patient population, even if it includes children and adults, can satisfy all the potential variables with which we have to deal. The important thing to keep in mind is that these methods are reproducible, they are an estimate (albeit an accurate estimate), and they must be performed with meticulous technique. In situations in which highly reliable clearance data are needed, the study must be performed under rigidly controlled research conditions with urine collection. For routine clinical applications, however, the single-sample methods suffice, and this paper describes one that is particularly attractive because the authors suggest that this single-sample methodology can be used in both children and adults. Unfortunately, it is a method for MAG₃ clearance, and the information that most nephrologists seek is the glomerular filtration rate.

M.D. Blaufox, M.D., Ph.D.

Renal and Extrarenal Clearance of ^{99m}Tc-MAG₃: A Comparison With ^{125}I-OIH and ^{51}Cr-EDTA in Patients Representing All Levels of Glomerular Filtration Rate
Rehling M, Nielsen BV, Pedersen EB, et al (Skejby Univ Hosp, Aarhus, Denmark)
Eur J Nucl Med 22:1379–1384, 1995   6–13

Introduction. — Technetium-99m–labeled mercaptoacetyltriglycine (MAG₃) is mainly excreted in the urine by tubular secretion. It is excreted by glomerular filtration to a minor degree. Its renal clearance is smaller than the clearance of iodine-125–labeled orthoiodohippurate (OIH) and

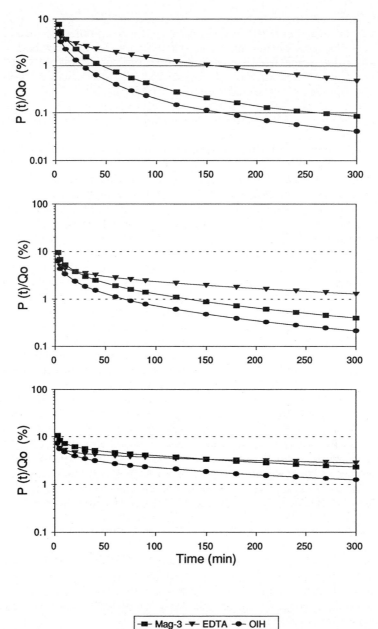

FIGURE 1.—Average arterial concentration per liter of plasma [$P(t)$] in percent of injected dose of technetium-99m-mercaptoacetyltriglycine 3 (*square*), iodine-125 orthoiodohippurate (*circle*), and chromium-51-ethylenediaminetetraacetate (*triangle*) after a simultaneous single IV injection in patients with glomerular filtration rate (*GFR*) > 80 mL/min (**upper part**), GFR between 15 and 80 mL/min (**middle part**), and GFR < 15 mL/min (**lower part**). (Courtesy of Rehling M, Nielsen BV, Pederson EB, et al: Renal and extrarenal clearance of ^{99m}Tc-MAG$_3$: A comparison with ^{125}I-OIH and ^{51}Cr-EDTA in patients representing all levels of glomerular filtration rate. *Eur J Nucl Med* 22:1379–1384, 1995. Copyright Springer-Verlag.)

about 2–3 times the glomerular filtration rate (GFR). Fifty-one patients referred for measurement of GFR underwent a simultaneous injection of MAG_3, OIH, and chromium-51–ethylenediaminetetraacetic acid (^{51}Cr-EDTA) to determine whether the clearance of MAG_3 was more closely correlated to the clearance of OIH than to GFR and whether there is a clinically significant extrarenal clearance of MAG_3.

Methods.—The GFR was between 4 and 132 mL/min in all patients. Plasma clearance was measured from blood samples from 0 to 5 hours after injection. The plasma clearances of MAG_3, OIH, and EDTA were compared. The renal plasma clearance of EDTA was used as a measure of GFR.

Results.—Patients were assigned to 1 of 3 groups: group 1, estimated endogenous creatinine clearance (EECC) greater than 80 mL/min; group 2, EECC between 15 and 80 mL/min; and group 3, EECC less than 15 mL/min. The relative plasma concentration of OIH was less than the concentration of MAG_3 and EDTA in each of the patient groups (Fig 1). Shortly after injection, the EDTA concentration was higher than the concentration of MAG_3 in patients with an EECC greater than 80 mL/min. The intersection of the 2 plasma concentration curves occurred later in groups 2 and 3. The renal plasma clearance of MAG_3 was 2.57 times that of EDTA. The coefficient of variation (CV) was 31.2%. The renal plasma clearance of MAG_3 was 0.57 times that of OIH, with a CV of 13.4%. The corresponding values for the plasma clearance ratios were 2.48, with a CV of 27.0%, and 0.59, with a CV of 14.8%. There was a significantly smaller CV for the MAG_3/OIH ratios, compared with that of the MAG_3/EDTA ratios. Ratios were independent of GFR. A small but significant extrarenal clearance was observed; plasma clearance overestimated renal clearance by 7.0 mL/min for MAG_3 and by 4.1 mL/min for EDTA. This difference was independent of GFR. The difference in plasma and renal plasma OIH of 5.5 mL/min was not significant. The volume of distribution of MAG_3 was significantly lower than the volume of distribution of EDTA and OIH. The percent of body weight was 16.3% for MAG_3, 19.4% for EDTA, and 27.0% for OIH. The percent bound to red blood cells was 2% for MAG_3, 14.6% for OIH, and 0.2% for EDTA. Protein binding was 61.1% for OIH, 86.3% for MAG_3, and 5.9% for EDTA. There was no difference in red blood cell binding or protein binding at 5, 40, or 120 minutes after injection.

Conclusion.—The clearances of MAG_3 and OIH were more closely correlated than was the clearance of MAG_3 with GFR. The extrarenal clearance of MAG_3 was relatively less than the extrarenal clearance of EDTA. Findings suggest that plasma clearance of MAG_3 may be used as a measure of renal tubular function.

▶ Although ^{99m}Tc-MAG_3 has had extensive use in the evaluation of renal function and morphology, it remains a relative newcomer to the area. A wealth of information has been published about the physiologic handling of radioiodine-labeled Hippuran and ^{51}Cr-EDTA. This article is useful in giving us some further insights into the handling of MAG_3 and in particular in its detailed comparison with these 2 other agents about which so much is known. Their finding that extrarenal clearance of MAG_3 is less than the extrarenal clearance of EDTA is an important one, because plasma clearances are very frequently used to estimate renal function and invariably lead to an overestimate because of problems such as extrarenal clearance. This paper serves as an excuse to once again state that it is impossible to perform studies in nuclear medicine properly without a clear understanding of the physiologic handling of the radiopharmaceutical being used.

M.D. Blaufox, M.D., Ph.D.

Determination of the Relative Glomerular Filtration Rate of Each Kidney in Man: Comparison Between Iohexol CT and ^{99m}Tc-DTPA Scintigraphy
Frennby B, Almén T, Lilja B, et al (Univ Hosp, Malmö, Sweden; Univ Hosp, Uppsala, Sweden)
Acta Radiol 36:410–417, 1995   6–14

Objective.—In 43 patients, determinations of the relative glomerular filtration rate (GFR) of each kidney were obtained by 2 methods: first using technetium-99m–DTPA scintigraphy and then using the nonionic contrast medium (CM) iohexol and CT. There are a number of possible advantages associated with CT. One injection of CM would allow both the morphology of the renal region and the GFR to be revealed, and the relative GFR could be obtained at centers with a CT unit but without a gamma camera.

Patients and Methods.—All patients had determinations made of the relative GFR with ^{99m}Tc-DTPA and had no suspicion of a change in GFR in the period between CT and scintigraphy. The patient group included 24 women (mean age, 60 years) and 19 men (mean age, 56 years). The most common clinical diagnoses were renal artery stenosis and hydronephrosis. Scintigraphy and CT were performed 0–7 days apart in 31 of the 43 patients. The amount of any GFR marker accumulating in Bowman's space, tubuli, and the renal pelvis within a few minutes after IV injection, before any marker had left the kidney via the ureter, was defined as proportional to the GFR of that kidney.

Results.—The correlation coefficient between iohexol CT and ^{99m}Tc-DTPA scintigraphy was 0.98. In 30 of 43 patients, the differences between the relative GFR measured with scintigraphy and the relative GFR measured with CT was no more than 5% (Fig 4). The greatest difference, recorded in 3 patients, was 13%. In 1 patient, the relative GFR in the left kidney was 5 percentage points higher with CT than with scintigraphy, whereas in the right kidney, the relative GFR was 5 percentage points lower with CT. No patient experienced an adverse reaction to the CM. The mean absorbed dose to the kidneys was calculated to range from 40 to 55 mGy with CT vs. 0.8 mGy with ^{99m}Tc-DTPA.

Conclusion.—There is a growing interest in using nonlabeled urography CM, especially iohexol, as GFR markers. Results of this study suggest that

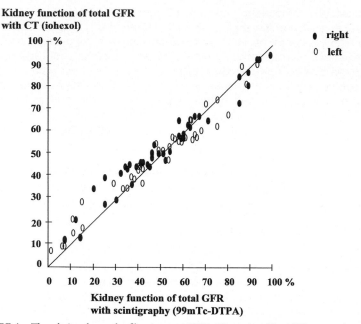

Kidney function of total GFR with CT (iohexol)

FIGURE 4.—The relative glomerular filtration rate (*GFR*) (%) produced by 1 kidney was determined by 2 methods. The *horizontal axis* represents GFR determined by technetium-99m–DTPA scintigraphy. The *vertical axis* represents relative GFR determined by iohexol CT. (Courtesy of Frennby B, Almén T, Lilja B, et al: Determination of the relative glomerular filtration rate of each kidney in man: Comparison between iohexol CT and 99mTc-DTPA scintigraphy. *Acta Radiol* 36:410–417, 1995.)

the relationship between the GFRs of the 2 kidneys can be measured as accurately with CT using iohexol as a GFR marker as with a gamma camera using 99mTc-DTPA. Because there is a higher radiation dose with CT, this method should be used when morphological information is required. Thus, patients with urologic disorders such as hydronephrosis, renal stone disease, and malformations can have relative kidney function and morphological data obtained simultaneously.

▶ The use of CM, iohexol in particular, has become very popular in the Scandinavian countries for the evaluation of renal function. The potential usefulness of this technique has not really been taken advantage of here in the United States, where there is a general lack of application of both radiologic and nuclear techniques for the evaluation of renal function. As the authors point out, however, it is important to keep in mind that with the higher radiation dose from CT than from 99mTc-DTPA injection, relative GFR determinations with CT really are not indicated over nuclear medicine techniques if that is the only information being sought.

M.D. Blaufox, M.D., Ph.D.

Comparison of Single-injection Multisample Renal Clearance Methods With and Without Urine Collection

Russell CD, Dubovsky EV (Univ of Alabama, Birmingham; Dept of Veterans Affairs Med Ctr, Birmingham, Ala)
J Nucl Med 36:603–606, 1995   6–15

Introduction.—Although single-injection methods are much easier than continuous infusion for the measurement of renal clearance, there is concern about their reliability. Total plasma clearance (TPC) and renal plasma clearance (RPC) were compared for accuracy using 2 different radiopharmaceuticals: technetium-99m–mercaptoacetyltriglycine (MAG$_3$) and iodine-131–orthoiodohippurate (OIH).

Methods.—Simultaneous dual-tracer measurements were performed in 20 patients using the 2 radiopharmaceuticals. Nine plasma samples were obtained from an indwelling catheter between 4 and 90 minutes after injection. Urine samples were obtained at 30 and 90 minutes, each with prevoid and postvoid imaging to correct the urine counts for residual bladder activity. Complete data were available for 18 patients.

Results.—Urine samples are required for the RPC method but not for the TPC method. The mean difference between urine-based RPC and urine-free TPC measurements was 1 mL/min for ^{99m}Tc-MAG$_3$ (not significantly different from zero) and 23 mL/min for ^{131}I-OIH. For ^{99m}Tc-MAG$_3$, the regression line did not differ significantly from the line of identity (Fig 1). For both agents, the correlation coefficient was 0.94.

Conclusion.—Single-injection methods for measuring renal clearance have had the reputation of being error-prone, perhaps because of poor results using the terminal slope method. The terminal slope method should not be used with tubular agents. Urine collection is not required to mea-

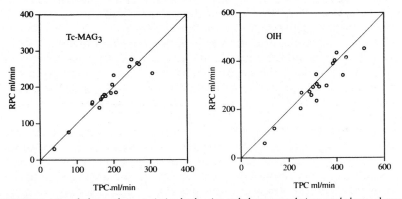

FIGURE 1.—Renal plasma clearance (using both urine and plasma samples) vs. total plasma clearance (using only plasma samples) for technetium 99m–mercaptoacetyltriglycine (*MAG$_3$*) (*left*) and iodine 131–orthoiodohippurate (*OIH*) (*right*). The lines of identity are shown. (Reprinted by permission of the Society of Nuclear Medicine, from Russell CD, Dubovsky EV: Comparison of single-injection multisample renal clearance methods with and without urine collection. *J Nucl Med* 36:603–606, 1995.)

sure renal clearance, except at very low clearance levels, even for tubular agents that are rapidly cleared.

▶ This is another example of the continuing and very important contribution of this group to methods for measurement of renal clearance. The use of plasma clearances without urine collection has been shown time and time again to be accurate and reliable. The authors do offer the caution that at very low levels of renal function, urine collection should be considered because the error of the method, which is very small in terms of the percentage of renal clearance at most levels of renal function, does become a significant percent error at low levels. This recommendation is in keeping with that of the radionuclides in the Nephrology Working Group on Renal Clearances.[1]

M.D. Blaufox, M.D., Ph.D.

Reference

1. Nephrology Working Group on Renal Clearances. *J Nucl Med*, in press.

Tubular Reabsorption of Technetium-99m-DMSA
Müller-Suur R, Gutsche H-U (Karolinska Inst, Stockholm; Inst of Clinical Nephrology, Heide, Germany)
J Nucl Med 36:1654–1658, 1995   6–16

Background.—The mechanism underlying uptake of technetium-99m–dimercaptosuccinic acid (DMSA) in the proximal tubular cells of the kidney is not understood. Study results of renal handling of ^{99m}Tc-DMSA are conflicting, and the debate continues regarding the role of tubular reabsorption of ^{99m}Tc-DMSA from the tubular fluid. The amount of ultrafiltration of ^{99m}Tc-DMSA was measured directly.

Methods.—In fluid collected by micropuncture from Bowman's space of surface glomeruli and from proximal and distal tubules, the concentration of ^{99m}Tc-DMSA along the nephron was measured. Surface proximal tubules were micropunctured and microperfused with ^{99m}Tc-DMSA or ^{99m}Tc pertechnetate for 10 or 20 minutes. Final urine was collected for recovery measurements.

Results.—Only 14% of the ^{99m}Tc activity of arterial plasma was recovered from urine from Bowman's space. This indicates low filtration of ^{99m}Tc-DMSA, probably because of high plasma protein binding. The tubular fluid-to-plasma activity ratios were 0.31 in the proximal tubules and 1.31 in the distal tubules. This indicates that ^{99m}Tc-DMSA is not secreted or reabsorbed along the nephron. Approximately 98% of ^{99m}Tc-DMSA was recovered in the final ipsilateral urine; 0.5% was recovered in the final urine of the contralateral kidney.

Conclusion.—Technetium-99m–DMSA binds to plasma proteins and penetrates the glomerular filter at low rates. The ^{99m}Tc-DMSA in the tubular system is not reabsorbed from the tubular fluid. Peritubular extraction accounts for ^{99m}Tc-DMSA uptake in the proximal tubular cells of the renal cortex.

▶ Müller-Suur's very elegant studies of renal handling of radiopharmaceuticals have greatly supplemented our knowledge of these agents. The authors' findings that DMSA is neither reabsorbed nor secreted from tubular fluid are somewhat at odds with other investigators, including studies carried out at my laboratory with Dr. Yee and Mrs. Lee. It would be interesting to see whether Müller-Suur's group could use their micropuncture technique to try to determine definitively why we noted a very significant defect of acidification on DMSA excretion.

M.D. Blaufox, M.D., Ph.D.

Reduction of Renal Uptake of Monoclonal Antibody Fragments by Amino Acid Infusion
Behr TM, Becker WS, Sharkey RM, et al (Ctr for Molecular Medicine and Immunology, Newark, NJ; Friedrich-Alexander-Univ of Erlangen-Nuremberg, Erlangen, Germany)
J Nucl Med 37:829–833, 1996   6–17

Introduction.—The renal uptake of monoclonal antibody fragments and peptides compromises reliable diagnostic accuracy of radioimmunodetection and therapy. Three previous investigations using semiquantitative analysis have suggested that basic amino acids are effective in decreasing the renal uptake of radiolabeled peptides. It has also been shown that cationic amino acids and amino sugars and their polymers are capable of decreasing the renal uptake of monoclonal antibody fragments (Fab', F(ab')$_2$) with various labels by up to 85%. The clinical results on the reduction of renal uptake of monoclonal antibody Fab' fragments by infusion of a commercially available, low-dose, nutritive amino acid solution were reported.

Methods.—Five patients with recurrent or metastatic carcinoembryonic antigen–expression tumors received 2 L of the amino acid solution intravenously before antibody injection. A volume of saline solution equal to that of the amino acid solution was administered to 75 controls. Whole-body scans were taken at 10 minutes, and 1, 4, and 24 hours after injection. Planar imaging of the pelvis, abdomen, thorax, and head was completed at 4–6 hours and 18–24 hours post injection.

Results.—A significantly lower renal uptake was observed at 4 hours and after 24 hours post injection in the amino acid group, compared with controls. The uptake of all other organs was unaffected. No significant differences were observed at 1 hour post injection. There were no observed effects on the uptake in any other organ or in the blood clearance at any time. There were no fundamental differences in the molecular composition of the activity in the serum between groups. There were significant differ-

TABLE 3.—Molecular Composition of 3-hour Serum Sample and Urine

Total Activity (%)	Serum		Urine	
	Control	Amino acid	Control	Amino acid
F(ab')$_2$	27.3%	29.5%	—	—
Fab'	59.7%	57.5%	7.5%	53.4%
Low-molecular-weight metabolites*	12.2%	8.1%	90.4%	38.2%

Note: Samples from a control subject and an amino-acid–treated patient were collected during a 4-hour period.
* Technetium-99m–cystine and other metabolites.
(Reprinted by permission of the Society of Nuclear Medicine, from Behr TM, Becker WS, Sharkey RM, et al: Reduction of renal uptake of monoclonal antibody fragments by amino acid infusion. *J Nucl Med* 37:829–833, 1996.)

ences between treated patients and controls in molecular species analysis of the urine (Table 3). Gel filtration chromatography of the urine from treated patients indicated that a significantly higher amount of excreted activity was bound to intact Fab', compared with controls (53.4% vs. 7.5%).

Conclusion.—Amino acid infusion can be used to significantly reduce the renal uptake of antibody fragments. This mechanism seems to rely on an inhibition of the tubular reabsorption of glomerularly filtered proteins. Formal toxicologic investigation is needed before application of higher amounts of basic amino acids in human beings.

▶ Interference of abdominal images with monoclonal antibodies caused by renal uptake is a major problem in the clinical application of this technique. The authors suggest that the use of amino acid infusion will significantly reduce monoclonal antibody uptake by the kidney, thereby improving the potential for accurate interpretation of abdominal images. If this study is confirmed both for its efficacy and its safety, this technique will have an important role in abdominal monoclonal antibody imaging.

M.D. Blaufox, M.D., Ph.D.

Technetium-99m-L,L-Ethylenedicysteine Scintigraphy in Patients With Renal Disorders

Gupta NK, Bomanji JB, Waddington W, et al (Middlesex Hosp, London; Katholieke Universiteit Leuven, Belgium)
Eur J Nucl Med 22:617–624, 1995   6–18

Background.—Technetium-99m-L,L-ethylenedicysteine (EC) has been proposed for renal imaging to attempt to overcome the poor image quality and potentially high radiation dose of Hippuran. The applicability of ^{99m}Tc-L,L-EC to renal imaging was studied in healthy volunteers and patients with renal disease.

Methods.—Preparation of the radionuclide was by reconstitution of a labeling kit. Five normal volunteers received ^{99m}Tc-L,L-EC and iodine-131–Hippuran intravenously. The 16 patients received only ^{99m}Tc-L,L-EC. One day later, 5 of these patients were reevaluated using ^{99m}Tc-mercap-

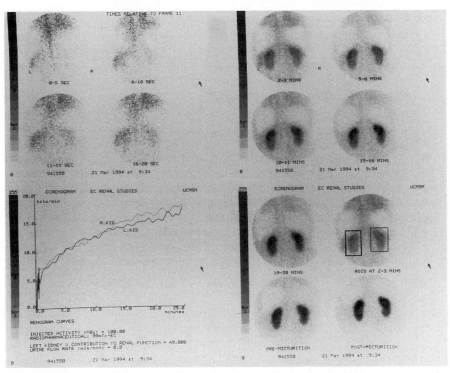

FIGURE 4.—A technetium-99m-L,L-ethylenedicysteine renal study of a patient in renal failure caused by acute tubular necrosis. The patient also had large bilateral pleural effusions that, on the images, appear as photon-deficient areas in the lower part of chest (Courtesy of Gupta NK, Bomanji JB, Waddington W, et al: Technetium-99m-L,L-ethylenedicysteine scintigraphy in patients with renal disorders. *Eur J Nucl Med* 22:617–624, 1995. Copyright Springer-Verlag.)

toacetyltriglycine (MAG₃) for comparison studies. After injection of radionuclide, dynamic imaging was performed, allowing the calculation of parameters of renal function.

Results.—There were no adverse effects reported from any of the participants. In healthy volunteers, the clearance of 99mTc-L,L-EC was an average of 75% of that of 131I-Hippuran. Four of 10 patients suspected of having obstructive uropathy had that diagnosis proven by renogram and parenchymal transit time index. None of the 4 patients referred with possible renovascular hypertension had imaging evidence of angiotensin-II–related disease. The 2 patients with postoperative acute renal failure had progressive tracer accumulation, typical of acute tubular necrosis (Fig 4). Renal time-activity curves, semiquantitative indices, and image quality were not significantly different for 99mTc-L,L-EC, compared with 99mTc-MAG₃ in the 5 patients who received both.

Conclusion.—The 99mTc-L,L-EC provides image quality as good as, and a radiation dose lower than, 131I-Hippuran when used in renal scintigraphy.

▶ This study is surely a step in the right direction. Having done an extensive amount of work with 99mTc-L,L-EC, these investigators are now applying themselves toward its use in patients with renal disease. Unfortunately, the conclusion that ^{99m}Tc-L,L-EC is similar to ^{99m}Tc-MAG$_3$, may not be sufficient to justify its use in the United States. The difference between the clearance of ^{99m}Tc-MAG$_3$ and Hippuran is very significant, and although ^{99m}Tc-L,L-EC has a somewhat higher clearance, it is still only about three quarters of the clearance rate of Hippuran. Although further work should certainly be carried out with ^{99m}Tc-L,L-EC to clearly define its relative advantages or disadvantages when compared with ^{99m}Tc-MAG$_3$ and, especially, its relative price, it seems there still remains room for development of a renal radio-pharmaceutical with more avid uptake.

M.D. Blaufox, M.D., Ph.D.

Evaluation of Technetium-99m-Ethylenedicysteine in Renal Disorders and Determination of Extraction Ratio
Kabasakal L, Atay S, Vural VA, et al (Istanbul Univ, Turkey)
J Nucl Med 36:1398–1403, 1995   6–19

Objective.—The clinical usefulness of technetium-99m–ethylene-dicysteine (EC), a new agent for radionuclide renal function and imaging studies, was evaluated in a group of 20 patients with various renal disorders. Five individuals with normal renal function also were imaged so that extraction ratios of ^{99m}Tc-EC could be determined.

Methods.—The 20 patients, 10 men and 10 women with a mean age of 35.3 years, were referred for renal investigations. Blood samples were withdrawn within 60 minutes of simultaneous IV injection with 200 MBq ^{99m}Tc-EC and 2.5 MBq of iodine-131–orthoiodohippurate (OIH). A 2-compartment model was used to determine plasma clearance. Imaging was performed with the patient in the supine position in the posterior projection. Three groups of images were obtained in each patient. Renal extraction ratios were determined in the 5 volunteers from blood samples obtained from the renal vein and abdominal aorta.

Results.—Use of ^{99m}Tc-EC achieved excellent delineation of the kidneys with high target/background ratios. Renal clearance of this radio-pharmaceutical was significantly lower than that of OIH (Table 1) although the correlation was good (0.53). Protein binding was significantly greater for OIH (nearly twice that of ^{99m}Tc-EC). The volume distribution of EC was slightly greater than that of OIH. Red blood cell binding of ^{99m}Tc-EC was found to be almost negligible. The 2 agents had almost identical mean 60-minute excretion fractions. The extraction ratio of ^{99m}Tc-EC showed no significant change between 5 and 30 minutes, and extraction ratios obtained from plasma samples and blood were similar.

Conclusion.—The new radiopharmaceutical ^{99m}Tc-EC was found to be suitable for routine renal dynamic studies. The quality of images obtained was quite high and its labeling procedure is simple. Although the biological behavior and pharmacokinetics of ^{99m}Tc-EC and OIH differ, clearance of the 2 agents showed a high correlation.

TABLE 1.—Patient Data and Plasma Clearance of Orthoiodohippurate (OIH) and Technetium-99m–Ethylenedicysteine (EC)

Patient No.	Clinical Diagnosis	Creatinine (ml/min/1.73^2)	OIH (ml/min/1.73^2)	^{99m}Tc-EC (ml/min/1.73^2)
1	Hypertension	79	411	325
2	Hypertension	110	541	309
3	Chronic glomerulonephritis	42	257	192
4	Renal amyloidosis	44	211	188
5	Hypertension	81	817	496
6	Chronic renal insufficiency	23	48	39
7	Obstructive renal disease	39	189	190
8	Hypertension	103	670	604
9	Unilateral nephrectomy	75	512	535
10	Obstructive renal disease	52	286	162
11	Unilateral renal hypoplasia	78	400	340
12	Unilateral renal hypoplasia	39	312	249
13	Bilateral hydronephrosis	23	87	60
14	Hypertension	83	556	396
15	Henoch-Shonlein purpura	47	120	69
16	Chronic glomerulonephritis	54	372	224
17	Nephrotic syndrome	27	49	38
18	Nephrotic syndrome	34	89	72
19	Chronic pyelonephritis	89	594	396
20	Hypertension	59	289	196
Mean ± s.e.m.		59 ± 23	341 ± 181	251 ± 136

(Reprinted by permission of the Society of Nuclear Medicine, from Kabasakal L, Atay S, Vural VA, et al: Evaluation of technetium-99m-ethylenedicysteine in renal disorders and determination of extraction ratio. *J Nucl Med* 36:1398–1403, 1995.)

▶ There is no question that ^{99m}Tc-EC is a potentially valuable agent for renal studies. Given the great deal of money that has already been invested in bringing ^{99m}Tc-mercaptoacetyltriglycine (MAG$_3$) to the market and our extensive experience with that agent, the question now to be posed is whether EC offers any real advantage. Unless investigators can either show that EC provides greater diagnostic information or is significantly cheaper than MAG$_3$, it will remain an interesting agent, but it will not become clinically significant. Hopefully, the answer to this question will begin to emerge in the near future. At the present time, however, it is not clear.

M.D. Blaufox, M.D., Ph.D.

Penile Scintigraphy for Priapism in Sickle Cell Disease
Dunn EK, Miller ST, Macchia RJ, et al (State Univ of New York, Brooklyn)
J Nucl Med 36:1404–1407, 1995   6–20

Objective.—Thirteen patients with sickle cell disease and priapism who had undergone penile scintigraphy after IV injection of technetium-99m–pertechnetate were followed to determine the value of this imaging procedure in directing therapy and predicting subsequent sexual potency.

Methods.—The patients, 8 boys and 5 men, ranged in age from 5 to 38 years at the time of penile scintigraphy. All were admitted and treated with a standard protocol that included analgesics, IV hydration, and, as needed, packed-cell exchange transfusion, corporeal irrigation and intracorporeal epinephrine, and glanscavernosa shunt. Scintigraphy was performed after injection of the tracer and with or without prior administration of stannous pyrophosphate for in vivo labeling of red blood cells. Studies were interpreted as high-flow if tracer activity was seen in the corpora cavernosa and corpus spongiosum. During clinical follow-up, the relationship between scintigraphic findings and eventual sexual potency was assessed.

Results.—High-flow scintigraphic findings were present in 5 patients (1 adult and 4 children). Low-flow findings were present in 10 studies obtained in 4 adult and 4 pediatric patients. All 8 patients with low-flow studies had lack of tracer activity in the corpora cavernosa, and 1 demonstrated no activity in the corpus spongiosum as well (Fig 3). Analgesics

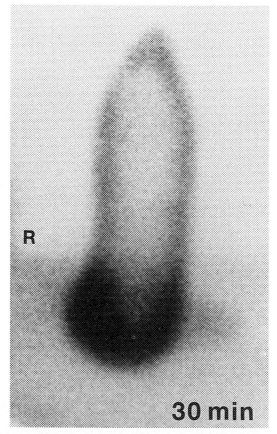

FIGURE 3.—Tricorporal priapism in 1 patient. There is persistent lack of the tracer activity in the corpora cavernosa as well as the corpus spongiosum. (Reprinted by permission of the Society of Nuclear Medicine, from Dunn EK, Miller ST, Macchia RJ, et al: Penile scintigraphy for priapism in sickle cell disease. *J Nucl Med* 36:1404–1407, 1995.)

and hydration were sufficient in 4 of 5 patients with high-flow findings and in 3 of 8 patients with low-flow priapism. Surgical shunting was used in 2 children and 1 adult with low flow, and 2 adults in this group required repeat corporeal irrigation and intracorporeal epinephrine. The 6 pediatric patients available for follow-up were eventually sexually potent, but 4 of 5 adults had persistent impairment of erection.

Conclusion.—Penile scintigraphy reflects the state of vascular circulation through the penis, and a high-flow pattern appears to favor conservative treatment. As seen in half of the patients in this series, however, low flow does not always necessitate aggressive therapy. Scintigraphic findings showed no correlation with subsequent sexual potency, but older patients were less likely to have normal sexual function after an episode of priapism.

▶ I have repeatedly expressed the opinion that penile scintigraphy is a potentially valuable technique in nuclear medicine. Although most previous studies have been directed at problems related to impotence, this study indicates a potential role in patients with sickle cell disease and a new area of study.

M.D. Blaufox, M.D., Ph.D.

Bladder Herniation Detected on a Bone Scan

Vidal-Sicart S, Pons F, Huguet M, et al (Hosp Clinic i Provincial, Barcelona)
Clin Nucl Med 20:949–950, 1995   6–21

Case Study.—Man, 66, known to have prostatic adenocarcinoma underwent technetium-99m–methylene diphosphate bone imaging. In the right inguinal region, a large area of increased activity was noted. Dynamic imaging with ^{99m}Tc pertechnetate demonstrated a photopenic region at the same site. When the patient stood erect, this area filled in. This investigation revealed that the lesion corresponded to a bladder hernia, for which the patient had previously declined treatment (Fig 1).

▶ The potential interference of urinary activity in the bladder with interpretation of the bone scan appears to have limitless possibilities. Here is one more example of the serendipitous discovery of urinary tract abnormalities with bone scanning or, perhaps from the other point of view, the potential interference of urinary tract abnormalities with interpretation of the bone scan.

M.D. Blaufox, M.D., Ph.D.

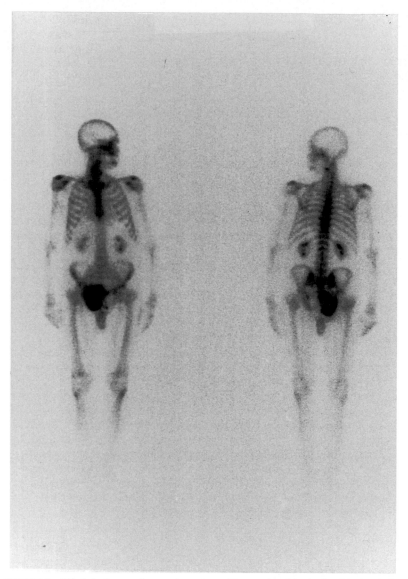

FIGURE 1.—Whole-body scan shows a large area of increased activity in the right inguinal area. Contamination was excluded and the patient was asked to void. (Courtesy of Vidal-Sicard S, Pons F, Huguet M, et al: Bladder herniation detected on a bone scan. *Clin Nucl Med* 20:949–950, 1995.)

Gallium 67 Scintigraphy as a Predictor of Renal Prognosis in Primary Immunoglobulin A Nephropathy

Nomura S, Watanabe Y, Otsuka N, et al (Kawasaki Med School, Kurashiki, Japan)
Am J Kidney Dis 27:204–208, 1996   6–22

Background.—Patients with immunoglobulin A nephropathy (IgAGN) follow a slow but variable course, often ending in chronic renal failure. A number of risk factors have been identified as being potentially helpful in determining the prognosis of end-stage renal disease in these patients. The prognostic value of gallium scintigraphy for renal outcome in IgAGN was studied.

Methods.—Patients with primary IgAGN underwent whole-body scans using gallium-67–citrate and technetium-99–dimercaptosuccinic acid (DMSA), the latter being used to help define the renal region of interest. A ratio of radioisotope uptake in left renal tissue compared with lumbar paravertebral soft tissue (L/S ratio) was calculated. Renal biopsy was performed and appropriate urine and serum tests were obtained from each patient. Patients were followed every 1–2 months with regular tests of the serum creatinine level.

Results.—For 25 patients, the L/S ratio correlated significantly with the 24-hour urinary protein excretion but not with other factors, including serum creatinine, albumin, and immunoglobulin levels. Comparison of those patients with an L/S ratio below the overall mean L/S ratio and those

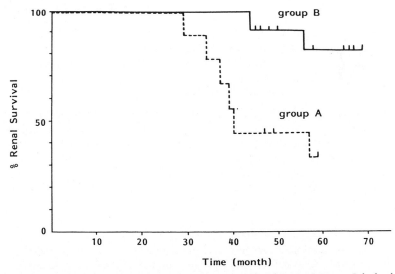

FIGURE 3. Life-table analysis of renal survival. Compared with group A, group B had a better prognosis (*P* < 0.05). *Abbreviation: GA*, gallium. (Courtesy of Nomura S, Watanabe Y, Otsuka N, et al: Gallium 67 scintigraphy as a predictor of renal prognosis in primary immunoglobulin A nephropathy. *Am J Kidney Dis* 27:204–208, 1996.)

whose L/S ratio was above the mean showed a significantly longer renal survival for the group with L/S ratios below the mean (Fig 3).

Conclusion.—Increased renal uptake of gallium correlates with a poorer prognosis for renal survival in patients with IgAGN.

▶ This paper is very interesting in that it suggests the possibility that gallium uptake may play a role in helping to predict the prognosis of patients with IgAGN. I have 2 reservations regarding the report. One is that I would like to have seen a 72-hour uptake, because the relationship between serum creatinine and gallium excretion is well established and a 72-hour uptake may have helped to more clearly separate those patients with significantly reduced renal function from those with little or no impairment.

The other question the paper raises is the fact that 8 of 13 patients in the group with the poorer survival had a serum creatinine level of 1.5 or greater, but only 5 of 12 fell into this serum creatinine range in the group with better survival. Furthermore, the highest serum creatinine value in the group with better survival was only 1.7, whereas 4 patients in the group with poorer survival had higher creatinine levels. Creatinine clearance would perhaps have been even more useful than serum creatinine.

The question remains, if we simply plotted serum creatinine vs. survival, would the same results have been achieved? Although there was no significant difference in the average creatinine values between groups A and B, it would have been helpful to know whether there was a difference in the average creatinine values between those patients who lived and those who died.

M.D. Blaufox, M.D., Ph.D.

Scintigraphic Findings in Renal Malakoplakia
Cox JE, Cowan RJ (Bowman Gray School of Medicine, Winston-Salem, NC)
Clin Nucl Med 20:497–500, 1995   6–23

Introduction.—Malakoplakia is a form of macrophage dysfunction that affects the genitourinary system and is characterized by chronic tubulointerstitial nephritis. It often occurs in patients with recurrent urinary tract infections. Pathologic examination is needed for a definitive diagnosis. Gallium-67 scanning may aid in diagnosis and treatment evaluation. The findings from scintigraphy in a rare case of bilateral renal malakoplakia were reported.

> *Case Report.*—Woman, 50, had acute onset of fever, chills, nausea, vomiting, diarrhea, and myalgia. Past diagnoses included possible scleroderma and chronic pulmonary *Mycobacterium avium* complex infection, for which she had recently completed 27 months of therapy. Ultrasound and CT revealed an enlarged right kidney with bilateral perirenal inflammatory changes. Pyelonephritis was suspected, and although the patient was treated with IV

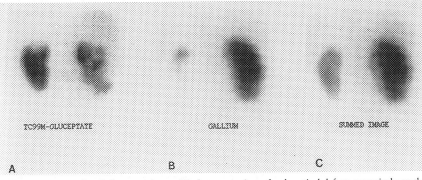

FIGURE 2.—Delayed gluceptate image (**A**) shows prominent focal cortical defects extensively on the right and at the left upper pole. **B**, spot film from gallium-67 scan. **C**, superimposition of the gluceptate renal study and ^{67}Ga images confirm that the abnormal gallium activity is confined to the left upper pole and extensively involves the right kidney. (Courtesy of Cox JE, Cowan RJ: Scintigraphic findings in renal malakoplakia. *Clin Nucl Med* 20:497–500, 1995.)

antibiotics, her fever continued. No abnormal kidney activity was shown by indium-111 leukocyte scanning. Scanning with ^{67}Ga showed intense uptake in the enlarged right kidney and in the upper pole of the left kidney. Scanning with technetium-99m gluceptate showed prominent focal cortical defects on the right and at the upper left pole (Fig 2). This area corresponded to the area of ^{67}Ga abnormality. When the patient's condition had improved little after 2 weeks of antibiotic therapy, treatment was changed and she was discharged without clear improvement. A percutaneous renal biopsy specimen revealed numerous macrophages with abundant periodic acid-Schiff–positive granules and intracytoplasmic calcospherites, which confirmed malakoplakia.

Discussion.—The lack of renal uptake shown by ^{111}In white blood cell scanning may be explained by the fact that most of the indium binds to neutrophils and the infiltrate here was a mixture of macrophages and lymphoplasmacytic elements. In similar cases, renal malignancy or infection initially may be suspected. Renal malakoplakia was considered in this patient after an intensely positive ^{67}Ga scan and a negative ^{111}In white blood cell scan were obtained.

▶ This case report shows, once again, the great potential role of renal imaging for patients with infection and related diseases. It is surprising that whereas the ^{67}Ga study was positive, the ^{111}In leukocyte scan was negative. However, the authors seem to have a valid explanation. It is interesting that with all the problems associated with the use of gallium and gallium imaging, it seems to steadfastly maintain its place in a wide variety of clinical problems subject to nuclear medicine investigation.

M.D. Blaufox, M.D., Ph.D.

7 Gastrointestinal

Introduction

Perhaps the most surprising thing about this section this year is the absence of papers about hepatobiliary imaging. I simply did not come across anything that appealed to me. There were good papers on the use of white blood cells to detect inflammatory disease. I selected a few gastrointestinal bleeding papers. And detection of tumors of various types made a strong comeback this year, including the detection of pancreatic cancer using FDG. I revisit a topic we cover from time to time—the treatment of hepatocellular carcinoma with radioiodinated lipiodol. And we finish with a potpourri of diagnostic tests.

Alexander Gottschalk, M.D.

Validation of ^{99}Tc^m-HMPAO Leucocyte Scintigraphy in Ulcerative Colitis by Comparison With Histology

Middleton SJ, Li D, Wharton S, et al (Addenbrooke's Hosp, Cambridge, England)
Br J Radiol 68:1061–1066, 1995   7–1

Introduction.—When the bowel is severely distended, assessment of the extent and degree of inflammation in patients with inflammatory bowel disease with barium studies and colonoscopy is often poorly tolerated. In these circumstances, a relatively noninvasive study, such as leukocyte

TABLE 2.—Grading Scheme for Abdominal Scintograms With
^{99m}Tc-HMPAO–Labeled Leukocytes

Grade	Abdominal uptake
0	No abdominal uptake
1	Bowel uptake < bone marrow
2	Bowel uptake = bone marrow
3	Bowel uptake > bone marrow
4	Bowel uptake > spleen

Abbreviation: ^{99}Tc^m-HMPAO, technetium-99m–hexamethylpropyleneamine oxime.
(Courtesy of Middleton SJ, Li D, Wharton S, et al: Validation of ^{99}Tc^m-HMPAO leucocyte scintigraphy in ulcerative colitis by comparison with histology. *Br J Radiol* 68:1061–1066, 1995.)

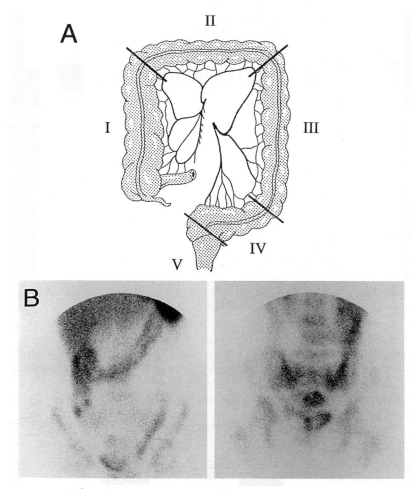

FIGURE 2.—A, the colon was divided in 5 anatomical segments shown. B, each colonic segment was scored for scintigraphic activity according to the system described in Table 2. In this example, the scintigraphic scores are: segment I = 3; segment II = 3, segment III = 1; segment IV = 3; segment V = 3. (Courtesy of Middleton SJ, Li D, Wharton S, et al: Validation of $^{99}Tc^m$-HMPAO leucocyte scintigraphy in ulcerative colitis by comparison with histology. *Br J Radiol* 68:1061–1066, 1995.)

scintigraphy, would be helpful. In detecting gastrointestinal acute inflammation, technetium-99m–hexamethylpropyleneamine oxime leukocyte scintigraphy (TLS) has been compared with biochemical, radiological, and clinical findings and has been found to be highly accurate. An evaluation of the histologic changes associated with positive TLS was conducted.

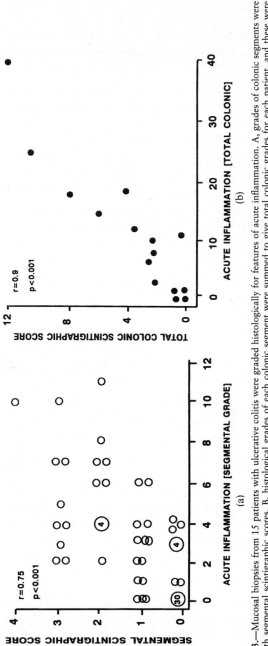

FIGURE 3.—Mucosal biopsies from 15 patients with ulcerative colitis were graded histologically for features of acute inflammation. A, grades of colonic segments were correlated with segmental scintigraphic scores. B, histological grades of each colonic segment were summed to give total colonic grades for each patient, and these were correlated with total colonic scintigraphic activity obtained by summation of segmental scintigraphic scores. (Courtesy of Middleton SJ, Li D, Wharton S, et al: Validation of $^{99}Tc^m$-HMPAO leucocyte scintigraphy in ulcerative colitis by comparison with histology. *Br J Radiol* 68:1061–1066, 1995.)

Methods.—Less than 5 days before colonoscopy, 15 patients with ulcerative colitis, ranging in age from 21 to 70 years, had TLS. Total and segmental colonic TLS scores were compared with histologic features of mucosal biopsies. Grading of scintigraphic activity was conducted by comparing bowel uptake with the normal bone marrow and splenic uptake (Table 2 and Fig 2).

Results.—Histologic grades for acute inflammation and chronic inflammatory cell infiltration in the lamina propria correlated most strongly with segmental and total scintigraphy scores (Fig 3). Patients with ulcerative colitis had acute inflammation of colon detected by TLS, with a negative predictive value of 80% and a sensitivity of 91%. Localized acute inflammation was detected by TLS, with a specificity of 94%, a sensitivity of 82%, a positive predictive value of 94%, an accuracy of 88%, and a negative predictive value of 91%.

Conclusion.—Although negative scintigraphy does not exclude acute inflammation, positive TLS predicts and localizes colonic acute inflammation with a high degree of confidence. It is noninvasive, safe in severely ill patients, has few side effects, and requires no bowel preparation, making it a useful screening test for gastrointestinal inflammation. Histologic changes of chronic ulcerative colitis, such as glandular distortion, were not detected by TLS.

▶ The big problem I have with this type of data is that there is no control group of patients (i.e., those with suspected ulcerative colitis who might or might not have it). As a result, the sensitivity given here is likely to be as good as it gets. In short, there is very little reason to believe that in these patients an area of abnormal uptake is anything other than true ulcerative colitis. Things are likely to go downhill from here; however, I suspect that the hill will not be very large. In general, when inflammation-seeking tracers find something, they do a good job.

Please read on.

A. Gottschalk, M.D.

Comparison of ^{99m}Technetium Hexamethylpropylene-amine Oxime Labelled Leucocyte With ^{111}-Indium Tropolonate Labelled Granulocyte Scanning and Ultrasound in the Diagnosis of Intra-abdominal Abscess
Weldon MJ, Joseph AEA, French A, et al (St George's Hosp, London)
Gut 37:557–564, 1995   7–2

Introduction.—Abscesses should be diagnosed reliably and quickly because they are an important cause of postoperative morbidity and mortality. Ultrasound has been the first line of investigation. White blood cell scanning, such as indium-111 leukocyte scans have had a useful, complementary role. Another method of labeling leukocytes is the use of technetium-99m–hexamethylpropyleneamine oxime (HMPAO), which has

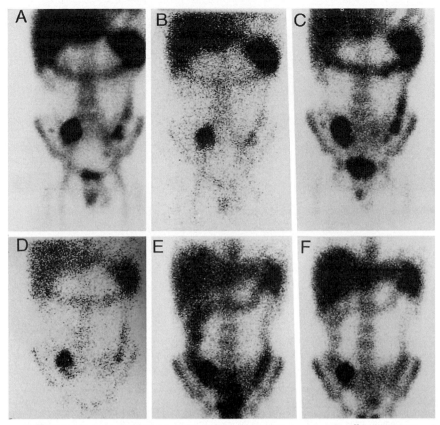

FIGURE 2.—Repeat serial technetium-99m–hexamethylpropyleneamine oxime ($^{99m}Tc\text{-}HMPAO$) and indium-111 (^{111}In) scans performed 19 days later in the patient in figure 1 because of the development of a right iliac fossa mass and tenderness showing the appearances of an abscess. (A) and (B) show the ^{99m}Tc-HMPAO and ^{111}In scans, respectively at 1 hour. (C) and (D) show the ^{99m}Tc-HMPAO and ^{111}In scans, respectively, at 3 hours. (E) and (F) show the ^{99m}Tc-HMPAO and ^{111}In scans, respectively, at 24 hours. (Courtesy of Weldon MJ, Joseph AEA, French A, et al: Comparison of ^{99m}Technetium hexamethylpropylene-amine oxime labelled leucocyte with ^{111}-Indium tropolonate labelled granulocyte scanning and ultrasound in the diagnosis of intra-abdominal abscess. *Gut* 37:557–564, 1995.)

great potential for imaging of inflammatory conditions, such as inflammatory bowel disease. Ultrasound and ^{99m}Tc-HMPAO scanning were compared using ^{111}In tropolonate.

Methods.—Ultrasound, ^{111}In tropolonate, and ^{99m}Tc-HMPAO were performed on 50 patients with suspected intra-abdominal abscess. Inflammatory bowel disease was found in 25 patients, 21 of whom had Crohn's disease, and 4 of whom had ulcerative colitis. When focal activity on serial ^{111}In tropolonate and ^{99m}Tc-HMPAO images at 1, 3, and 24 hours resulted in activity at least equal to liver activity at 24 hours, an abscess was diagnosed. Because of the continued recruitment of labeled white blood cells into the abscess site, focal, fixed uptake is intense on later images than on early images after reinjection (Fig 2).

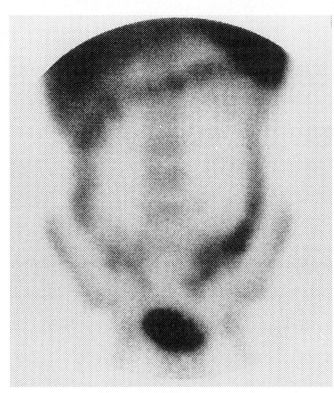

FIGURE 1.—Initial technetium-99m–hexamethylpropyleneamine oxime scan showing total Crohn's colitis and terminal ileitis at 1 hour. Prominent bladder activity is shown. (Courtesy of Weldon MJ, Joseph AEA, French A, et al: Comparison of [99m]Technetium hexamethylpropylene-amine oxime labelled leucocyte with [111]-indium tropolonate labelled granulocyte scanning and ultrasound in the diagnosis of intra-abdominal abscess. *Gut* 37:557–564, 1995.)

Results.—Using each type of white blood cell scanning, 13 abscesses were diagnosed. There was a 100% sensitivity for ^{99m}Tc-HMPAO compared with ^{111}In tropolonate. A total of 17 abscesses were found. Twelve abscesses were detected by ultrasound, including 4 liver abscesses that had not been detected by white blood cell scanning. Using all confirmed abscesses as the reference standard, ultrasound had a specificity of 87% and a sensitivity of 71%. For white blood cell scanning, there was a specificity of 100% and a sensitivity of 76%.

Conclusion.—[111]In tropolonate and ^{99m}Tc-HMPAO were comparably accurate; however, ^{99m}Tc-HMPAO has the advantages of being simpler, more available, superior in image quality, and requiring less radiation. However, its disadvantages include renal excretion resulting in a bladder image and nonspecific intestinal activity (Fig 1). For intra-abdominal abscess detection, both white blood cell scanning methods are more sensitive and specific than ultrasound; however, if neutrophil infiltrate is not suspected, ultrasound is recommended. ^{99m}Tc-HMPAO should be the second-line investigation of choice.

▶ Please notice that the sensitivity in this paper has dropped into the 70-percent range. Actually, these folks did very well looking at the gut, but they had trouble with liver abscesses. I think it is quite understandable that white blood cells have a problem in the liver because the liver is normally so hot. I suspect they could improve their results by doing a technetium colloid template study. Lesions that are "cold " with colloid that became isointense with white blood cells in the rest of the liver represent a positive result, and that would probably improve the statistics.

A. Gottschalk, M.D.

Investigating Inflammatory Bowel Disease—White Cell Scanning, Radiology, and Colonoscopy
Jobling JC, Lindley KJ, Yousef Y, et al (Great Ormond Street Hosp for Children NHS Trust, London; Inst of Child Health, London)
Arch Dis Child 74:22–26, 1996   7–3

Introduction.—Recently, white blood cell scanning has been recommended for demonstrating areas of inflamed bowel. This may be useful in determining inflammatory bowel disease in children, as this diagnosis is difficult to ascertain in this cohort. Thirty-nine children were prospectively evaluated for possible inflammatory bowel disease using the technetium-99m–hexamethylpropyleneamine oxime white cell scan (Tc-WCS), and findings were compared with those of barium follow-through examination (Ba-FT) and colonoscopy plus biopsy.

Methods.—The mean patient age of 20 males and 19 females was 12.1 years. All children underwent Tc-WCS, colonoscopy with endoscopic biopsy, Ba-FT, and erythrocyte sedimentation rate.

Results.—Inflammatory bowel disease was confirmed by biopsy in 31 of 39 children. Imaging modalities indicated positive findings of inflammatory bowel disease in 16 patients (41%) and negative findings in 5 patients (13%). In the remaining 18 patients (46%), there was at least 1 disagreement between histologic findings and imaging modalities. The Tc-WCSs were positive in 28 of 31 children with histologically proven inflammatory bowel disease and negative in 6 of 8 histologically negative biopsies. The sensitivity of Tc-WCS, Ba-FT, and colonoscopy in the detection of inflammatory bowel disease was 90%, 42%, and 87%, respectively. The specificity of Tc-WCS, Ba-FT, and colonoscopy was 100%, 71%, and 88%, respectively.

Conclusion.—The Tc-WCS is a sensitive, specific, and noninvasive technique with a low radiation burden. The role of Ba-FT, with its high radiation burden and low sensitivity, should be reevaluated. Colonoscopy with biopsy remains the method of choice in diagnosing inflammatory bowel disease in children.

▶ These authors took on a somewhat different task, in that they only tried to find abnormality in the entire colon rather than in a specific colonic region.

Clearly, Tc-WCS did very well. These authors emphasize that the study must be done with Tc-WCS because the radiation dose from indium-111 white blood cells is higher and thus not recommended for screening.

I suspect that most places will interact colonoscopy, barium enema, and Tc-WCS based largely on what is available and who is doing it. However, if all are available and done well, these authors make a good argument that there is a solid place for Tc-WCS to screen the child in whom inflammatory bowel disease is suspected, and further, that the Tc-WCS is preferable to the barium enema study.

A. Gottschalk, M.D.

Computed Tomography and Granulocyte Scintigraphy in Active Inflammatory Bowel Disease: Comparison With Endoscopy and Operative Findings
Kolkman JJ, Falke THM, Roos JC; et al (Free Univ, Amsterdam)
Dig Dis Sci 41:641–650, 1996   7–4

Purpose.—Various minimally invasive imaging techniques have been proposed for use in the evaluation of patients with acute exacerbations of or severe inflammatory bowel disease (IBD). Both CT and granulocyte scintigraphy (GS) have been suggested for this purpose, but neither imaging study has been prospectively compared with the gold standard techniques of surgery or endoscopy. Computed tomography and [technetium-99m]hexamethylpropyleneamine oxime (HMPAO) GS were studied for their accuracy in patients with acute IBD.

Methods.—Thirty-two patients with an exacerbation of previous IBD, a severe first attack of IBD, or IBD with suspected abdominal complications were studied. There were 17 patients with Crohn's disease (CD) and 15 with ulcerative colitis (UC). Each patient underwent both CT and [99mTc]HMPAO GS. The results of both studies were scored in blinded fashion in each bowel segment. With operation or endoscopy as the gold standard, the 2 techniques were compared for their ability to detect bowel localization, inflammatory activity, and complications.

Results.—In the patients with CD, GS was 79% sensitive and 98% specific in the detection of inflammatory activity, although it was not effective in the detection of complications. Computed tomography was better able to localize active and fibrostenotic bowel disease, as well as to detect abscesses and fistulas. In the patients with UC, GS was better than CT in the prediction of proximal extension of bowel involvement.

Conclusions.—This prospective study suggests that, in patients with CD, CT is better than GS in the detection of bowel wall pathology. It is even possible to assess local inflammatory activity in the bowel wall through the use of CT. In patients with UC, GS is more accurate than CT in demonstrating the proximal extent of disease. The combination of GS and distal sigmoidoscopy may be a useful alternative to total colonoscopy in patients with UC.

▶ You win some, you lose some.

A. Gottschalk, M.D.

Case Report: Chronic Mesenteric Ischaemia as a Cause of Abnormal Bowel Uptake of Labelled Leucocytes
Ingram G, Reeder A, Tait NP, et al (North Tees Gen Hosp, Stockton on Tees, Cleveland, England)
Br J Radiol 68:1126–1127, 1995   7–5

Background.—The diagnosis of chronic mesenteric ischemia may require a high level of clinical suspicion, coupled with invasive diagnostic procedures. A case of chronic bowel ischemia that mimicked inflammatory bowel disease on labeled leukocyte imaging was reported.

> *Case Report.*—Woman, 69, was hospitalized with constant upper abdominal pain, a history of diminishing appetite and a 20-kg weight loss over 1 year. Laboratory studies were normal except for an elevated white blood cell count. Dilated loops of small bowel and gaseous distention of the large bowel were present on an abdominal radiograph, which suggested ileus, obstruction, or pseudo-obstruction. Abdominal scanning with technetium-99m–hexamethylpropyleneamine oxime (HMPAO)–labeled leukocytes showed distinctly increased small bowel uptake, and the patient was started on high-dose oral corticosteroids while further investigations were performed. None of the results were consistent with Crohn's disease or lymphoma. However, the patient seemed to improve with oral corticosteroids and was discharged. Three days later, she returned with an "acute abdomen" and radiographic findings consistent with obstruction or ileus. Sepsis developed and the patient died. Nearly complete necrosis of the small intestine was seen at autopsy, along with thrombotic occlusion of the origin of the superior mesenteric artery. Recent hepatic infarction and necrotizing pancreatitis were apparent as well.

Discussion.—Chronic bowel ischemia can cause a positive result on labeled leukocyte scanning in patients who are suspected to have more common inflammatory bowel disease or infection. The possibility of ischemic bowel disease should be considered in patients with positive results on labeled leukocyte imaging studies and a consistent history.

▶ If you do inflammatory bowel scintigraphy, or if the other articles on this subject we have cited in this volume make you want to start, you should know about this pitfall.

A. Gottschalk, M.D.

Hemobilia Presenting as Intermittent Gastrointestinal Hemorrhage With Sincalide Confirmation: A Case Report

Spieth ME, Hou CC, Ewing PD, et al (King/Drew Med Ctr, Los Angeles; Family Health Plan Hosp, Fountain Valley, Calif; Pacific Union College, Angwin, Calif; et al)
Clin Nucl Med 20:391–394, 1995   7–6

Introduction.—Nuclear medicine is helpful in localizing the cause of gastrointestinal bleeding. The use of technetium-99m sulfur colloid has given way to ^{99m}Tc-labeled red blood cell (RBC) imaging. The former has only a 2- to 3-minute blood pool window to localize the site of bleeding, and the latter allows imaging for almost 24 hours after a single injection. The patient presented had hemobilia, a finding physicians rarely observe.

Case Report.—Man, 82, was admitted with his third episode of melanotic stools. Two previous workups failed to reveal the source of bleeding. A ^{99m}Tc-labeled RBC scan was ordered after upper and lower endoscopies were negative. The patient denied abdominal discomfort after being injected with 2 mg of stannous pyrophosphate, then 20 mCi of ^{99m}Tc pertechnetate 20 minutes later. The dose was repeated 10 minutes later. Images were taken 5 minutes after each injection and after 4½ hours in the anterior and right lateral views. Five minutes after injection, the physiologic blood pool activity was detected in the liver and major vessels. New activity was seen at 10 minutes at the inferior border of the liver in the region of the gallbladder fossa. Throughout the course of imaging, the gallbladder shape became apparent and the activity continued to increase without excretion to the bowel. The gallbladder activity decreased and there was still no obvious bowel activity after the second injection of sincalide. Bowel activity and continued gallbladder activity were finally observed on delayed images. A laparoscopic cholecystotomy revealed no abnormalities, and the patient was discharged.

He was readmitted 5 days later for rectal bleeding. A second ^{99m}Tc-labeled scan was positive for a bleed, but the source was not identified. Again, upper and lower endoscopies and small bowel study gave no conclusive evidence of the bleeding site. Two months later, he experienced gastrointestinal bleeding and underwent a third ^{99m}Tc-labeled RBC scan with negative results. There was no evidence of thrombosis on color Doppler examination. A fourth ^{99m}Tc-labeled RBC scan, a colloid liver and gastrointestinal bleeding scan, and fluoroscopy to detect gastric varices were negative. He had a severe bleed 5 days later. During surgery, a giant bleeding diverticulum of the jejunum was found and resected. Hepatic metastases were seen. The metastases were poorly differentiated adenocarcinoma from an unknown primary tumor site.

Discussion.—After a labeled RBC study, the differential diagnosis for gallbladder activity includes: (1) if hemobilia is active at the time of injection, it should be visible before RBC breakdown or plasma protein may occur; (2) in the absence of anemia, renal disease, or free pertechnetate, early gallbladder visualization occurs before IV contrast; and (3) delayed gallbladder visualization at 4–24 hours.

Conclusion.—It is possible that the hepatic activity in this patient was inhomogeneous with at least 2 cold defects that could have represented hepatic metastases. This is the first known report of the use of sincalide in helping localize an unusual gastrointestinal bleeding site in a patient with hemobilia.

▶ This is a succinct review of hemobilia and the use of the RBC study. It also points out the need to look carefully at all the organs that show up on any examination. In this case, to my eye, the mass in the liver looks pretty large. Sometimes it may be somewhat difficult to decide whether the liver is truly intact on an RBC study. Be bold, slip the patient some colloid, and figure out what's going on.

A. Gottschalk, M.D.

Positive Technetium-99m-Red Blood Cell Gastrointestinal Bleeding Scan After Barium Small-bowel Study

Rehm PK, Atkins FB, Ziessman HA (Georgetown Univ, Washington, DC)
J Nucl Med 37:643–645, 1996   7–7

Background.—Gastrointestinal bleeding can be reliably identified and localized with technetium-99m–red blood cell (RBC) scintigraphy. Barium in the small bowel is usually considered a contraindication to doing this diagnostic procedure. However, a scintigraphic examination done 2 hours after a barium small-bowel examination demonstrated bleeding sites.

    Case Report.—Man, 53, was assessed for weakness. He had a history of ethanol-associated cirrhosis and portal hypertension. He had a low hematocrit and guaiac-positive stools. During hospitalization, his gastrointestinal bleeding required the transfusion of 7 units of RBCs and 2 units of plasma during 2 days. There were negative findings on upper and lower endoscopy and on a small bowel follow-through radiographic examination with barium sulfate. However, immediately after the small bowel examination, the patient passed a bloody stool. Within 2 hours, ^{99m}Tc was infused to label his blood, and scintigraphic images were obtained at 5-minute intervals for 90 minutes. Intestinal bleeding was identified and localized in the mid to distal small bowel (Fig 1). Scintigraphy also revealed decreased peripheral activity and increased central abdominal activity, consistent with ascites. The patient continued passing blood-mixed stools and was given 4 units of packed red blood cells during the next 2 days. Angiography of the superior

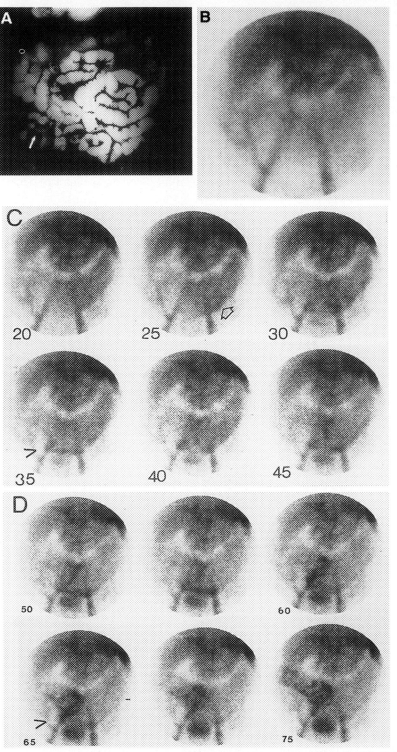

(*Continued*)

mesenteric, inferior mesenteric, and gastroduodenal arteries, done 3 days after the barium examination, revealed portal hypertension related to cirrhosis but no active bleeding or pathology that could explain the bleeding episodes.

Conclusions.—A ^{99m}Tc-RBC scan may identify gastrointestinal bleeding even in the presence of large amounts of intestinal barium. Further study is needed to investigate the influence of barium on scintigraphic accuracy in the detection and localization of bleeding sites.

▶ If you think about it, this should be almost an ideal setup for the detection of small-bowel bleeding. Most of the colon comprises the large photopenic area seen easily on some of the earliest films. In contrast, the small bowel shows up as a hot spot from the tagged red blood cell extravasation. The combination should work well, and these authors have shown that it did. It remains to be seen whether the technique will work as well for large-bowel bleeding in the presence of barium, but I envision a situation where the extravasated blood could pool between areas of residual barium and make it even easier to see. In short, should the occasion arise, give it a shot.

A. Gottschalk, M.D.

Scintigraphic Localization of Recurrent Anastomotic Site Bleeding in the Gastrointestinal Tract

Bagga S, Gupta SM, Johns W (Danbury Hosp, Conn; Univ of Connecticut, Farmington)
Clin Nucl Med 21:296–298, 1996   7–8

Introduction.—Scintigraphy can help to detect and localize gastrointestinal (GI) bleeding before surgery. There are several possible causes of persistent bleeding after colon surgery, which include bleeding from the anastomotic site. The successful use of radionuclide blood pool scintigraphy to localize bleeding from the anastomotic site after colon surgery was reported.

Case Report.—Woman, 67, was admitted with recurrent GI bleeding of unknown cause. Bleeding persisted despite heat coagu-

---

FIGURE 1 (cont.)

   FIGURE 1.—**A,** late image in the small bowel study demonstrates barium in multiple small bowel loops, including the terminal ileum (*arrow*). **B,** immediate image of technetium-99–red blood cell scan shows tubular photopenia caused by barium in the hepatic flexure, transverse colon and distal ileum and a subtle pattern of lower activity peripherally and increased activity centrally, representing ascites. Serial delayed images at (**C**) 20–45 minutes and (**D**) 50–75 minutes show evidence of active gastrointestinal bleeding. Photopenia becomes more obvious in (**C**) and (**D**) (*open arrowheads*), probably resulting from increased contrast caused by intraluminal labeled red blood cells and possibly barium transit during scintigraphy. (Reprinted by permission of the Society of Nuclear Medicine, from Rehm PK, Atkins FB, Ziessman HA: Positive technetium-99m-red blood cell gastrointestinal bleeding scan after barium small-bowel study. *J Nucl Med* 37:643–645, 1996.)

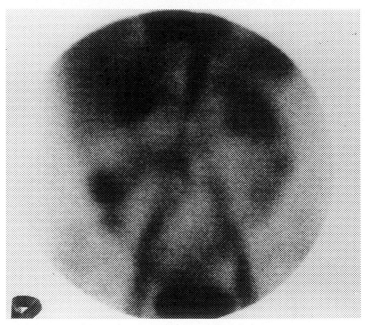

FIGURE 1.—Anterior abdominal image at 5 hours shows intense focal collection of activity in the right midflank (anastomotic site bleeding) with passage of activity through the transverse and descending colon. (Courtesy of Bagga S, Gupta SM, Johns W: Scintigraphic localization of recurrent anastomotic site bleeding in the gastrointestinal tract. *Clin Nucl Med* 21:296–298, 1996.)

lation of 2 small gastric telangiectasias. A technetium-99m–labeled red blood cell scan revealed low-grade GI bleeding from the area of the distal descending colon, but bleeding continued despite heat coagulation of a large vascular angiodysplasia of the cecum. Segmental resection of the ascending colon was performed, and histologic evaluation showed cecal changes consistent with arteriovenous malformation.

Five days after surgery, bleeding began again and the bleeding scan was repeated. Serial images obtained 5.0 to 5.5 hours after injection showed mild activity throughout the colon. Focally intense activity was noted in the right midflank, which suggested that the source of the bleeding was the anastomotic site (Fig 1). Colonoscopy confirmed that this was the bleeding site. Anastomotic revision was required to control the bleeding.

Discussion.—Radionuclide blood pool scintigraphy can help in the diagnosis and management of persistent bleeding after colon surgery. Correct scan interpretation requires knowledge of the precise extent of resection and the site of anastomosis. In the authors' experience, the finding of grade III activity on delayed views—i.e., activity greater than the hepatic blood pool—is more often associated with correct localization than are lesser grades of activity.

▶ We have stressed and cited articles in the past to point out that, once the camera leaves the abdomen on a red blood cell bleeding study after tracer injection, subsequent precise localization of the bleeding site is fortuitous because it is difficult to know how the blood got to where you currently see it. In short, the later-stage red blood cell study becomes a very expensive "stool guaiac."

These authors contradict this through the presentation of a case in which they localize the bleeding site at 5 hours (see Fig 1). As they say, it is always better to be lucky.

A. Gottschalk, M.D.

Scintigraphy of Incidentally Discovered Bilateral Adrenal Masses
Gross MD, Shapiro B, Francis IR, et al (Univ of Michigan, Ann Arbor; Catherine McAuley Health Ctr, Ann Arbor, Mich)
Eur J Nucl Med 22:315–321, 1995   7–9

Introduction.—In this era of sophisticated high-resolution imaging, it is not uncommon to detect a unilateral adrenal mass on a CT scan ordered for reasons other than adrenal dysfunction. Most of these lesions are benign. Bilateral adrenal masses are much less common and have only been reported anecdotally. The use of iodine-131 6β-iodomethylnorcholesterol (NP-59) was analyzed in 29 patients with incidentally discovered, bilateral adrenal masses.

Methods.—A 16-year retrospective review indicated that 29 of 258 patients with adrenal masses detected incidentally during CT scans of the abdomen or chest had bilateral involvement. Patients underwent NP-59 scintigraphy and various combinations of blood and urine laboratory analysis to exclude the presence of adrenal cortical or medullary dysfunction. A qualitative assessment of the relationship of relative NP-59 uptake between the adrenals was determined. Bilaterally symmetric NP-59 uptake was considered a normal finding.

Results.—The indication for all 29 patients with bilateral adrenal masses on CT was: 17 metastases, 9 abdominal pain, and 1 each ascites, renal failure, and pneumonia. The mean lesion diameter was 3.3 cm and

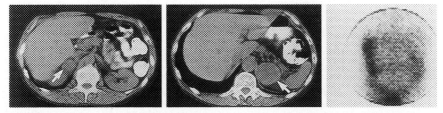

FIGURE 1.—CT scans (**left and center panels**) depict bilateral adrenal metastases (*arrows*) from lung carcinoma. Posterior iodine-131 6β-iodomethylnorcholesterol scan (**right panel**) shows bilateral nonvisualization of the adrenals. (Courtesy of Gross MD, Shapiro B, Francis IR, et al: Scintigraphy of incidentally discovered bilateral adrenal masses. *Eur J Nucl Med* 22:315–321, 1995. Copyright Springer-Verlag.)

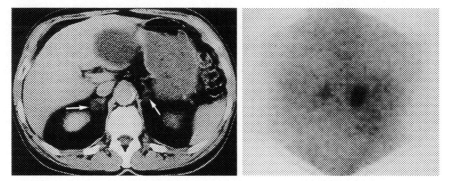

FIGURE 2.—CT scan (**left panel**) depicts bilateral adrenal masses (*arrows*) in a patient with metastatic adrenocarcinoma of the colon. Posterior iodine-131 6β-iodomethylnorcholesterol scan of the abdomen (**right panel**) demonstrates asymmetric tracer (right→left) uptake. The CT-guided adrenal biopsy of the right adrenal was benign, whereas that of the left adrenal disclosed adenocarcinoma. (Courtesy of Gross MD, Shapiro B, Francis IR, et al: Scintigraphy of incidentally discovered bilateral adrenal masses. *Eur J Nucl Med* 22:315–321, 1995. Copyright Springer-Verlag.)

3.4 cm, respectively, on the right and left. Nineteen of 29 patients underwent CT-guided adrenal biopsies. In 13 patients, metastases were found—5 were lung carcinoma, 3 were lymphoma, 3 were adenocarcinoma of the colon, 1 was laryngeal carcinoma, and 1 was anaplastic carcinoma of unknown origin. The NP-59 uptake showed variable patterns in the 29 patients with bilateral adrenal masses. In 8 patients in whom CT-guided adrenal biopsy confirmed metastatic involvement in 1 or both glands, bilateral nonvisualization was observed (Fig 1). Five of 8 patients with asymmetric NP-59 uptake had benign cytology compatible with adenoma determined by CT-guided adrenal biopsy. During a 6-month follow-up, the remaining 3 patients showed no change in adrenal contour. Two patients, respectively, with markedly asymmetric NP-59 uptake had an adenoma in 1 adrenal that coexisted with a contralateral metastatic lung or colon deposit (Fig 2). At 6-month follow-up, 7 of 8 remaining patients had no change in adrenal contour. The remaining patient had bilateral 2-cm-diameter adrenal masses with CT-guided biopsy evidence of adenoma.

Conclusion.—The algorithm used in scintigraphic evaluation of unilateral discovered adrenal masses is more problematic with bilateral lesions. Findings lead to the following conclusions: (1) bilateral masses in patients with malignancies are somewhat more likely to be adenomas than metastases; (2) size is a poor discriminator of malignancy in patients with bilateral lesions in the range of 2–5 cm; (3) it is possible for an adrenal adenoma and contralateral adrenal malignancy to coexist; and (4) NP-59 does have a use in functionally characterizing both unilateral and bilateral lesions and in selecting masses for further diagnostic evaluation.

▶ In these times of managed health care, I suspect these data will be commonly bypassed in favor of direct adrenal biopsy. However, it is good that you know about them, because somewhere down the line a patient will show up in whom a biopsy becomes a last rather than an intermediate step.

Or, you may find someone in whom biopsy may be somewhat hazardous and it may be very important to know which side to biopsy. These data then become invaluable.

A. Gottschalk, M.D.

Hepatocellular Adenoma: Case Report With Tc-99m SC Uptake and Radiologic Correlation

Davis DC, Wulfeck D, Donovan MS (Naval Hosp Jacksonville, Fla)
Clin Nucl Med 21:8–10, 1996   7–10

Background.—The common use of oral contraceptives has increased the prevalence of hepatocellular adenoma. The diagnosis of hepatocellular adenoma can be inferred from technetium-99m sulfur colloid (SC) scintigraphy, ultrasound, and CT. Classically, hepatocellular adenomas had no uptake on ^{99m}Tc SC scintigraphy, but radionuclide uptake may occur with as many as 20% of these tumors. The radiologic findings in a patient with hepatocellular adenoma were described.

> *Case Report.*—Woman, 30, was referred for infertility. She had a palpable abdominal mass, extending from the right upper quadrant toward the lower pelvis, which had been present for 2 years but had caused no symptoms. She had a history of long-term oral contraceptive use. An isodense, homogeneous mass extending along the inferior aspect of the liver to the superior aspect of the urinary bladder was seen on CT, which showed no other liver abnormalities. Ultrasound revealed a slightly hypoechoic pedunculated mass, with large vessels revealed on color Doppler examination. The mass demonstrated radionuclide uptake, which was decreased from normal liver uptake, on ^{99m}Tc SC scintigraphy. The hepatocellular adenoma was removed surgically without complications and measured 13 cm × 11 cm × 7 cm.

Discussion.—Radiographic evidence of a single liver mass in a young woman with a history of long-term oral contraceptive use suggests a diagnosis of either a hepatocellular adenoma or focal nodular hyperplasia. Radionuclide uptake is typically absent in hepatocellular adenomas, but may occur in 20%, whereas uptake is increased in 10% of the cases of focal nodular hyperplasia, normal in 50%, and decreased or absent in 40%. Hepatocellular adenomas can be differentiated from focal nodular hyperplasia by their greater tendency to be detected during physical examination or to cause symptoms and by their substantially greater likelihood of histologic evidence of hemorrhage.

▶ This case reminds us that the differential diagnosis between hepatocellular adenoma and focal nodular hyperplasia is imperfect using conventional imaging criteria.

A. Gottschalk, M.D.

2-(Fluorine-18)-Fluoro-2-Deoxy-D-Glucose PET in Detection of Pancreatic Cancer: Value of Quantitative Image Interpretation
Stollfuss JC, Glatting G, Friess H, et al (Univ of Ulm, Germany; Univ of Berne, Switzerland)
Radiology 195:339–344, 1995   7–11

Introduction.—One of the greatest challenges of pancreatic carcinoma is the lack of an early and accurate method of diagnosing the disease. Recent PET investigations with small populations have found high FDG accumulation in pancreatic carcinoma. Images obtained with FDG PET were compared with CT scans to evaluate the value of quantitative and visual interpretation of images of each in differentiating between chronic pancreatitis and pancreatic adenocarcinoma.

Methods.—Seventy-three patients with suspected pancreatic carcinoma or chronic pancreatitis underwent surgery at a mean of 8 days after FDG PET and contrast-enhanced CT evaluations. Histologic examination revealed that 30 patients had chronic pancreatitis and 43 had pancreatic carcinoma. Six patients with bronchial carcinoma and 4 with stage I or II malignant lymphoma acted as controls. Three observers were blinded to PET and CT findings.

Results.—There was FDG uptake in the liver and kidney parenchyma but no substantive uptake in pancreatic tissue in controls. In 27 of 30 patients (90%) with chronic pancreatitis, images were similar to those of controls and there was no or slight uptake in the pancreatic bed. Forty-one of 43 patients (95%) with pancreatic cancer showed focally increased FDG uptake in the pancreatic bed. The sensitivity of visual interpretation of PET by the 3 observers for detecting pancreatic cancer was 95%. Using standardized uptake values with a cutoff value of 1.53, the sensitivity and specificity of FDG PET for detecting malignant disease were both 93%. There were significant differences in standardized uptake values between patients with chronic pancreatitis and pancreatic carcinoma. The sensitivity and specificity of CT in diagnosing malignancy in 33 of 41 patients were 80% and 74%, respectively.

Conclusion.—Visual interpretation and quantitative analysis of FDG PET indicated accurate differentiation between pancreatic adenocarcinoma and chronic pancreatitis. This tool may prove helpful when CT or ultrasound findings are negative or nondiagnostic.

▶ I have never been convinced that you do a patient any favors by diagnosing pancreatic cancer before it becomes obvious to one and all. However, in this series from Germany, the visual (not quantitative) detection rate was very good, and as high-energy collimators become available for standard SPECT units, it seems these results could be translated into routine SPECT studies using FDG without the need for acquisition of a positron camera.

Ahlström and associates looked at neuroendocrine tumors with PET, using levodopa and hydroxytryptophan tracers labeled with carbon-11.[1] They did all right unless the tumor was nonfunctional. Furthermore, false positives are possible. For example, FDG in infections such as enterocolitis could be a problem.[2] In short, although there is promise for tumor imaging here, the waters may be somewhat muddier than they seem at first glance.

A. Gottschalk, M.D.

References

1. Alhström H, Eriksson B, Bergström M, et al: Pancreatic neuroendocrine tumors: Diagnosis with PET. *Radiology* 195:333–337, 1995.
2. Meyer MA: Diffusely increased colonic F-18 FDG uptake in acute enterocolitis. *Clin Nucl Med* 20:434–435, 1995.

Prominent Uptake of Tl-201 by Duodenal Leiomyosarcoma After Exercise Myocardial Perfusion Study
Shuke N, Tonami N, Takahashi I, et al (Kanazawa Univ, Japan; Komatsu Municipal Hosp, Japan)
Clin Nucl Med 20:299–301, 1995   7–12

Introduction.—The tracer of choice in the evaluation of myocardial perfusion is thallium-201. Extra cardiac uptake of ^{201}Tl recently has been reported to be useful in the evaluation of tumor blood flow or viability. An experience with a man in whom a duodenal leiomyosarcoma was discovered after an exercise myocardial perfusion study using ^{201}Tl SPECT was described.

> *Case Report.*—Man, 72, underwent abdominal ultrasonography for gross hematuria. Bilateral renal stones were seen. An abnormal 3-mm mass near the head of the pancreas was also detected. A CT scan confirmed the mass near the pancreatic head. A gallium-67 scan showed no abnormal uptake. A hypervascular tumor supplied from the arcade of both the posterior and anterior pancreaticoduodenal arteries was seen on celiac angiography. The differential diagnoses included pancreatic acinar cell tumor, islet cell tumor, and duodenal leiomyosarcoma. A preoperative ECG detected positive ST segment depressions in the II, III, and a Vf lead. This finding prompted an exercise ^{201}Tl SPECT study to screen for myocardial ischemia. An abnormal uptake of ^{201}Tl was discovered in the upper abdomen while the projection images were being processed. Reconstruction was performed at the level of the upper abdomen, and abnormal, intense ^{201}Tl uptake was seen clearly in the location corresponding to the tumor observed on CT scan. The delayed SPECT, done 3 hours after injection, clearly showed ^{201}Tl uptake by the tumor. At this time, intestinal activity was more prominent. The patient underwent a pancreatoduodenectomy. Pathologic examination showed large and irregular smooth muscle cells with hyperchromatic nuclei growing into adjacent tissue. The diagnosis was

low-grade leiomyosarcoma originating from the muscular layer of the second portion of the duodenum.

Conclusion.—Abdominal tumor uptake is difficult to differentiate from normal intestinal uptake, even if a tumor accumulates ^{201}Tl well. Fasting for several hours and exercising—the routine protocol for exercise myocardial perfusion—minimizes normal intestinal uptake. It is likely that fasting and exercise are practical ways to accomplish an ideal condition for ^{201}Tl abdominal tumor imaging.

▶ A few more cases like this and we'll have the cardiovascular nucs actually studying the infradiaphragmatic area.

A. Gottschalk, M.D.

Primary Hypothyroidism as a Consequence of 131-I-Metaiodobenzylguanidine Treatment for Children With Neuroblastoma
Picco P, Garaventa A, Claudiani F, et al (G Gaslini Inst for Children, Genoa, Italy; Galliera Hosp, Genoa, Italy)
Cancer 76:1662–1664, 1995   7–13

Introduction.—Cure rates are high in infants and children with localized operable neuroblastoma who are treated with surgery, often without adjuvant therapy. However, patients with disseminated neuroblastoma have a poor prognosis. Preliminary studies have shown promising results of treatment with iodine-131–metaiodobenzylguanidine (MIBG) in patients with disseminated neuroblastoma. However, there is little information about the effects of this treatment on the thyroid gland. Therefore, thyroid function was studied prospectively in children with disseminated neuroblastoma treatment with ^{131}I-MIBG.

Methods.—During a 7-year period, 58 children with unresectable or disseminated neuroblastoma that either did not respond to chemotherapy or had relapsed were treated with ^{131}I-MIBG in doses ranging from 2.5 to 5.5 gigabecquerels (GBq). Patients were also given oral iodide for 7 days before and 7 days after ^{131}I-MIBG administration to inhibit thyroid uptake of radioiodine. The patients were followed every 3–6 months, with assessments of height, weight, and pubertal stage. Before and 6, 12, and 24 months after treatment, serum concentrations of thyroid hormones and thyroid-stimulating hormone were measured.

Results.—The 2-year follow-ups in 14 survivors showed decreased thyroid function in 12 patients. Thyroid dysfunction developed within 6 months in 5 patients, with 2 of these patients having overt hypothyroidism. Eight of the 14 patients demonstrated overt primary hypothyroidism at 2 years. These patients were treated with L-thyroxine, which resolved the hypothyroidism-related symptoms and signs. The cumulative dose of ^{131}I-MIBG ranged from 0.25 to 1.2 GBq/kg in patients with overt hypothyroidism and from 0.15 to 0.87 GBq/kg in patients with compensated hypothyroidism.

Conclusions.—Infants and children treated with ^{131}I-MIBG for neuro-blastoma must be closely monitored for thyroid function. To more effectively inhibit thyroid uptake of radioiodine, it may be necessary to increase the oral iodide doses, prolong administration of iodide doses, and/or investigate alternative methods.

▶ For fun, I did a quick calculation. I assumed (1) that the Lugol's suppressed thyroid uptake could be as high as 4%, (2) that the maximum dose given was about 150 mCi; (3) an effective half-life of 5 days; (4) a child's thyroid weight of about 10 g; and (5) (most important) that all the ^{131}I ultimately comes off all of the ^{131}I-MIBG. With these assumptions, I get a thyroid dose of about 45,000 rads. That is not enough to ablate an adult thyroid remnant (usually about 80,000 rads). If—as I suggest above—the dose is not enough to really wipe out the thyroid, we have to assume that either previous chemotherapy, the juvenile state, or some type of toxic medication reaction occurred. Because we do not know the answer, we should all be forewarned that kids receiving any type of ^{131}I may be at risk for significant thyroid dysfunction in the future, and it is probably worth following them very carefully until this is all clarified.

In the meantime, one would think these authors would easily help solve this problem by doing something mundane like radioactive thyroid uptakes after therapy to further determine what is really going on here.

A. Gottschalk, M.D.

Superselective Intra-arterial Radiometabolic Therapy With I-131 Lipiodol in Hepatocellular Carcinoma
Maini CL, Scelsa MG, Fiumara C, et al ("Regina Elena" Natl Cancer Inst, Rome)
Clin Nucl Med 21:221–226, 1996   7–14

Background.—Various unsealed sources have been used in systemic and intra-arterial radiometabolic therapy for primary and metastatic liver cancer, but the radiation burden has been unacceptably high. The hepatic artery has been used for transarterial tumor embolization with iodine-131–labeled lipiodol in patients with unresectable hepatocellular carcinoma (HCC), with encouraging results. However, portal hypertension continues to be a problem, and there is substantial liver irradiation. If lipiodol could be administered directly into the artery feeding the tumor in superselective fashion, it could improve the tumor-to-background radioactivity ratio while avoiding adverse effects on portal hemodynamics. The clinical results of superselective transcatheter arterial radioembolization with ^{131}I lipiodol in patients with HCC were reported.

Methods.—Eleven patients with unresectable nodular HCC and associated cirrhosis were studied. The HCCs were hypervascular, permitting a superselective arterial approach. Thirteen nodules were treated with ^{131}I,

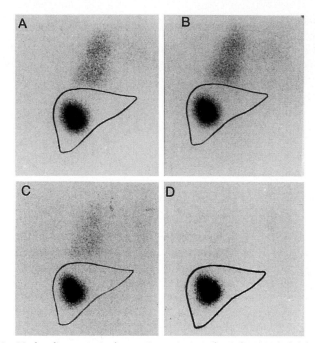

FIGURE 1.—Nuclear liver scans in the anterior projection after iodine-131 lipiodol radiometabolic therapy at **(A)** 1 hour, **(B)** 1 day, **(C)** 7 days, and **(D)** 21 days. The high radiotracer uptake and delayed washout from tumor, with faint visualization of normal liver, are evident. (Courtesy of Maini CL, Scelsa MG, Fiumara C, et al: Superselective intra-arterial radiometabolic therapy with I-131 lipiodol in hepatocellular carcinoma. *Clin Nucl Med* 21:221–226, 1996.)

TABLE 1.—Findings in Patients With Hepatocellular Carcinoma

Patient No.	Nodule	Diameter (cm)	I-131 LDP (MBq)	Dose to Tumor (cGy)	Tumor Size Decrease	Cirrhosis Evolution From/To	Outcome
1†	1	5.0	1480	22,800	no	A/B	living
	2	2.5	259	30,400	no		
2	3	4.0	1110	32,500	no	B	died#
3	4	6.5	1665	10,500	no	A	died##
4	5	7.5	2220	9,200	yes	A/A	living
5	6	4.5	1480	27,200	yes	B/B	living
6	7	4.5	1480	29,000	yes	A/A	living
7	8	5.0	2035	28,600	no	B	died###
8‡	9	3.5	740	30,200	yes	B/B	living
	10	3.0	444	31,500	no		
9	11	4.0	1110	32,800	yes	A/A	living
10	12	7.0	2035	10,200	no	B/C	living
11	13	3.5	740		*	A	*

*Patient excluded from the study.
†2 sessions 6 months apart.
‡In the same session.
Abbreviations: LDP, lipiodol; #, at 3 months; ##, at 20 months; ###, at 2 months.
(Courtesy of Maini CL, Scelsa MG, Fiumara C, et al: Superselective intra-arterial radiometabolic therapy with I-131 lipiodol in hepatocellular carcinoma. *Clin Nucl Med* 21:221–226, 1996.)

259–2,220 MBq, followed by gelatin sponge. All patients were reevaluated at least 2 years after ^{131}I lipiodol therapy.

Results.—Twelve lesions in 10 patients demonstrated intense uptake of lipiodol, with a mean 52% fraction of injected radioactive dose (Fig 1). The mean effective half-life was approximately 5 days. Mean nontumor liver uptake was 30%, compared with 15% in the lung. Radiotolerance was well tolerated clinically and biologically—cirrhosis remained stable in 5 patients and progressed in 2. Five of the 12 lesions decreased in size, and the other 7 did not increase. Two-year survival was 70%; 3 patients died of hepatic failure at 2–20 months after treatment (Table 1).

Conclusions.—In patients with unresectable HCC, superselective arterial radioembolization with ^{131}I lipiodol is an effective palliative approach. It offers long-term local control without progressive cirrhosis. Using the superselective technique described, it is possible to deliver the maximal radiation dose to the tumor without exceeding acceptable systemic radiation levels.

▶ This technique comes up from time to time, and these folks have done it quite well. The data tend to support my personal bias that it takes about 18,000 beta rads (a.k.a. cGy) to kill a cancer. But, as you can see, there were exceptions.

A. Gottschalk, M.D.

Scintigraphic Diagnosis of Protein Losing Enteropathy Using Tc-99m Dextran
Bhatnagar A, Lahoti D, Singh AK, et al (Inst of Nuclear Medicine and Allied Sciences, Delhi, India; RML Hosp, New Delhi, India; MCD Hosp, New Delhi, India)
Clin Nucl Med 20:1070–1073, 1995   7–15

Introduction.—The currently accepted radiolabeled macromolecule for imaging studies of patients with protein-losing enteropathy (PLE) is technetium-99m human serum albumin (HSA). Technetium-99m dextran—a nonprotein macromolecule, molecular weight 60,000 to 90,000, with a long stay in the intravascular compartment—may offer some advantages over ^{99m}Tc HSA. The use of ^{99m}Tc dextran in the imaging of PLE was reported.

Case Report.—Woman, 37, was referred for scintigraphic evaluation of suspected protein loss. Abdominal scintigraphy was performed with ^{99m}Tc dextran through the use of previously reported kit method. The patient was given 555 MBq of ^{99m}Tc dextran intravenously, after which anterior abdominal scintigraphy was performed every 15–30 minutes. Within 15 minutes, abnormal radiotracer concentration was noted in the left lumbar area. Luminal transit in the small intestinal loops was eventually confirmed;

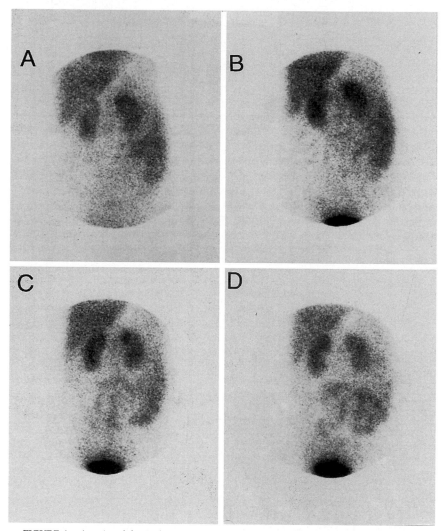

FIGURE 1.—Anterior abdominal images at **(A)** 15 minutes, **(B)** 30 minutes, **(C)** 1 hour, and **(D)** 2 hours after injection of technetium-99m dextran. Intestinal leakage and luminal transit of the radiotracer is seen. Duodenal biopsy showed intestinal lymphangiectasis. (Courtesy of Bhatnagar A, Lahoti D, Singh AK, et al: Scintigraphic diagnosis of protein losing enteropathy using Tc-99m dextran. *Clin Nucl Med* 20:1070–1073, 1995.)

the imaging findings suggested that tracer leakage had occurred in a group of bowel loops in the subsplenic area (Fig 1). Visualization of the large intestine occurred after 4 hours, and the study was ended. Other imaging studies were performed to exclude local causes of lymphedema and intestinal protein loss. Intestinal lymphangiectasia was confirmed by duodenal endoscopic biopsy.

Discussion.—Technetium-99m dextran appears to be a useful alternative to conventional ^{99m}Tc HSA for the diagnosis of PLE. This nonprotein macromolecule is water soluble, does not bind to plasma proteins, and is noncolloidal, which makes it nearly perfect as a plasma pool agent. The ^{99m}Tc dextran kit is easy and inexpensive, with labeling efficiency of greater than 95% and good in vitro and in vivo stability.

▶ Nice case—this suggests that any sizable radiolabeled macromolecule should work.

A. Gottschalk, M.D.

Hepatic Hydrothorax: Diagnosis and Management
Giacobbe A, Facciorusso D, Barbano F, et al (Casa Sollievo della Sofferenza Hosp IRCCS, San Giovanni Rotondo (Foggia), Italy)
Clin Nucl Med 21:56–60, 1996   7–16

Objective.—Pleural effusions can complicate cirrhosis even in patients without ascites. This condition, known as hepatic hydrothorax, results from the passage of ascitic fluid into the pleural cavity through microscopic defects in the diaphragm. The finding of radioactivity in the thorax on radionuclide imaging studies is specific for hepatic hydrothorax because radioactivity in the pleural cavity does not occur with other forms of pleural effusion. The diagnosis and management of 12 patients with hepatic hydrothorax were reported and the role of radionuclide studies was examined.

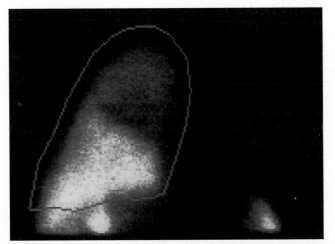

FIGURE 1.—Static scan of the thorax acquired 30 minutes after intraperitoneal injection of 111 MBq of technetium-99m sulfur colloid. The radioactivity flows through the diaphragm and is mainly evident in the lower half of the right pleural cavity. (Courtesy of Giacobbe A, Facciorusso D, Barbano F, et al: Hepatic hydrothorax: Diagnosis and management. *Clin Nucl Med* 21:56–60, 1996).

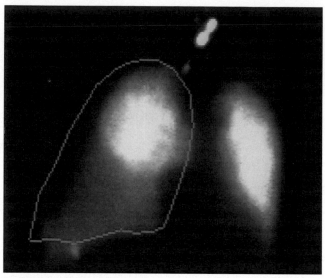

FIGURE 2.—Static scan of the thorax of the patient in Fig 1 acquired 3 minutes after intravenous administration of 74 MBq of technetium-99m macroaggregated albumin. The investigation is performed just after the Fig l scan with the patient remaining in the same position. Technetium-99m macroaggregated albumin is evident only in the upper moiety of the right lung because of atelectasis of the lower right lung. The region of interest outlines the whole lung. (Courtesy of Giacobbe A, Facciorusso D, Barbano F, et al: Hepatic hydrothorax: Diagnosis and management. *Clin Nucl Med* 21:56–60, 1996.)

Findings.—In each patient, the pleural fluid had a slightly higher protein concentration than the ascitic fluid. Thoracic and upper abdominal images were obtained, with dynamic studies performed after intraperitoneal injection of 111 MBq of technetium-99m sulfur colloid (SC). Within 10–15 minutes, the tracer was seen to pass into the right pleural cavity (Fig 1). With the patient in the same position, 74 MBq of ^{99m}Tc macroaggregated albumin (MAA) was injected intravenously to confirm the pleural location of the tracer (Fig 2). The imaging findings suggested that the pleural fluid originated in the abdomen and passed through a 1-way communication through the diaphragm from the peritoneal to the pleural cavity. In 8 of the 12 patients, the hydrothorax did not respond to sodium restriction, diuretics, or repeated thoracenteses. These patients required endopleural tetracycline instillation.

Conclusions.—For cirrhotic patients with suspected hepatic hydrothorax, scintigraphy with intraperitoneal injection of ^{99m}Tc SC provides a rapid and specific diagnostic technique. Confirmation can be obtained by scintigraphy with intrapleural introduction of ^{99m}Tc MAA. Tetracycline pleurodesis may be effective in patients with resistant hydrothorax.

▶ We have brought cases of hepatic hydrothorax to your attention in the past, but they have always been associated with marked ascites. The authors of this article point out that this need not be the case and that ascites need not be present. We also like the use of ^{99m}Tc MAA to confirm that the fluid is clearly in the chest. I suggest that it would be even easier to do this with a transmission scan if you have the sheet source available.

A. Gottschalk, M.D.

Detection of Early Asymptomatic Esophageal Dysfunction in Systemic Sclerosis Using a New Scintigraphic Grading Method

Kaye SA, Siraj QH, Agnew J, et al (Queen Mary's Univ, London; Royal Free Hosp, London)
J Rheumatol 23:297–301, 1996   7–17

Background.—Esophageal involvement is common in patients with systemic sclerosis (SSc); however, as many as 40% of patients with abnormal motility studies will be asymptomatic. Manometry is sensitive in the detection of esophageal hypomotility, but it is not widely available. Radionuclide scintigraphy can detect esophageal dysmotility and acid reflux as well as provide information on morphology. The use of radionuclide scintigraphy to screen patients with SSc for esophageal involvement and the development of a new grading system were reported.

Methods.—Esophageal scintigraphy was performed to detect esophageal dysfunction and gastroesophageal reflux in 301 patients with SSc. The motility results were scored as follows: grade 0, normal erect and supine scans; grade 1, normal erect scan and mildly abnormal supine scan; grade 2, mildly abnormal erect scan and moderately abnormal supine scan; grade 3, moderately abnormal erect scan and severely abnormal supine scan; or grade 4, severely abnormal supine and erect scans. The degree of hypomotility was correlated with the symptom of dysphagia in a retrospective study of 50 patients.

Technique.—The radionuclide studies are performed through the use of a semisolid radioactive meal, activity concentration 1 MBq/mL^{-1}, composed of technetium-99m tin colloid and pineapple puree. With the camera head oriented vertically, the patient sits up with his or her back to the camera in 35-degree left posterior oblique projection. The field of view ranges from the pharynx to the upper stomach, with the positions of the jugular and xiphoid marked with cobalt-57 markers. After a practice run, the patient performs a swallow in the seated position. Another swallow is then performed as the patient lies supine on the imaging table with the camera underneath. With regions of interest outlined for the mouth, stomach, and esophagus, a temporal display of spatial distribution activity in the esophagus is created.

Results.—Esophageal hypomotility was apparent in 82% of patients and gastroesophageal reflux in 28%. The motility abnormality was grade 2 in 33% of patients, grade 3 in 25%, and grade 4 in 8%. Reflux was present in 35% of patients with grade 2 motility, compared with 13% of those with grade 4 motility. In the symptom study, the severity of grade increased along with increasing mean duration of SSc. Disease subset was not significantly related to the presence or severity of esophageal hypomotility. Dysphagia was not a problem for 60% of patients with grade 1 or 2 motility but was more common for patients in grades 3 and 4.

Conclusions.—Esophageal scintigraphy is a useful technique to screen asymptomatic patients with SSc for esophageal involvement. The procedure is well-tolerated and easily performed on an outpatient basis. The frequency of asymptomatic dysmotility, coupled with the growing evidence for an early neuropathic phase of SSc, suggests that interventional studies of promotility agents are warranted.

▶ I am sold. Who can argue with this dynamite series of 301 patients with systemic sclerosis (a.k.a., scleroderma)? I am ready to bring it into my place and use their grading system. Let me see—I need to know what mildly abnormal supine esophageal dysmotility looks like—I'll go to this article and find a picture that tells me. Whoops, there is no picture. That dynamite explosion just turned into a loud burp.

A. Gottschalk, M.D.

8 Vascular

Introduction

My comments last year were devoted to the lack of articles in vascular imaging and the potential for exploration of this field. Although this continues to be an underutilized area, there is some evidence of increasing work during the past year. It is encouraging to see that there are several reports, some using recombinant techniques, that deal with imaging of venous thrombosis. The interpretation of the lung scan has always been an extremely difficult area. This is largely caused by the great gap in the consumer's understanding when it comes to the reporting of indeterminate or intermediate results. Physicians turn to diagnostic tests to resolve dilemmas. When a diagnostic test simply confounds that dilemma, it can be of little help. This has led many physicians to believe that although a negative lung scan is of great value in ruling out pulmonary embolism, any other lung scan is of dubious use. Hopefully, with the development of positive thrombus imaging agents we will be able not only to diagnose pulmonary emboli by direct hot spot imaging and avoid the complicated diagnostic procedures now used, but we will also be able to detect associated peripheral thromboses and the origin of this problem.

The other area of vascular application of radionuclides relates to mainly peripheral vascular disease. Although there are continuing innovations, the practical application of nuclear medicine techniques has not come close to fulfilling its potential. Hopefully, the increase in the number of reports dealing with vascular disease this year will represent the beginning of an upward trend and increased applications and use of nuclear medicine methodology in this very important area, which is very common in older and elderly patients and can lead to significant morbidity and mortality without proper detection and therapy.

M. Donald Blaufox, M.D., Ph.D.

A New Thrombus Imaging Agent: Human Recombinant Fibrin Binding Domain Labeled With In-111

Rosenthall L, Leclerc J (McGill Univ, Montreal)
Clin Nucl Med 20:398–402, 1995
8–1

Background.—Animal studies of human fibronectin labeled with iodine-131 have suggested that this may be useful in imaging atherosclerotic

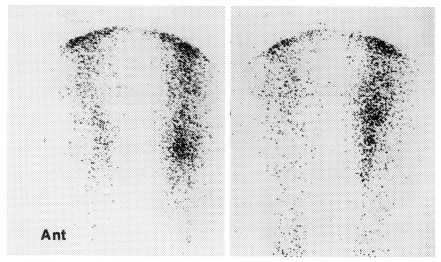

Ant

FIGURE 1.—Positive indium-111 fibrin binding domain scan showing increased uptake in the left thigh and calf and a normal right lower extremity. Impedance plethysmography and duplex ultrasound results were also abnormal for the region. (Courtesy of Rosenthall L, Leclerc J: A new thrombus imaging agent: Human recombinant fibrin binding domain labeled with In-111. *Clin Nucl Med* 20:398–402, 1995.)

plaques and thrombi. A human recombinant fibrin binding domain (FBD) with a 31-kd molecular weight was produced, labeled with indium-111, and investigated in a pilot study.

Methods.—Sixty-two patients were studied. Thirty were patients believed to have deep vein thrombosis, and 32 were control subjects. The patients underwent impedance plethysmography, duplex ultrasonography, contrast venography, or various combinations of these modalities.

Findings.—The results of the FBD imaging and the other modalities were discordant in 8 patients. Three patients with negative scan results had clots that were 1 week old or older. In another 3 patients with negative scan results but positive alternative studies, a history of previous episodes of deep vein thrombosis could have caused the false negative findings. There was 1 documented false negative scan in a new clot. The scans of lower extremities in the control group produced normal results for all but 2 subjects, whose scans showed uptake at the sites of insulin injections (Fig 1).

Conclusion.—Although the results of this study are not definitive, ^{111}In FBD appears to be a promising new imaging agent for patients with thrombi. Further investigations are warranted.

▶ Positive imaging of blood clots is a technique that has been sought for several decades in nuclear medicine, but it has consistently eluded us. Although, as the authors themselves point out, the use of human recombinant FBD labeled with ^{111}In is not definitively shown to be of value in this study, the results are suggestive and encouraging. Hopefully, further use of this technique will define its place in nuclear medicine diagnosis. Not only would it be helpful to have a peripheral vascular thrombosis imaging agent, but I am sure most of us would be very grateful if such a technique could be extended to the diagnosis of pulmonary embolism and begin to help us emerge from the quagmire of indeterminate and intermediate probability studies.

M.D. Blaufox, M.D., Ph.D.

Technetium-99m-modified Recombinant Tissue Plasminogen Activator to Detect Deep Venous Thrombosis
Butler SP, Boyd SJ, Parkes SL, et al (St George Hosp, Sydney, Australia)
J Nucl Med 37:744–748, 1996   8–2

Introduction.—Several radionuclide techniques have been proposed as possible alternatives to venography for the detection of deep venous thrombosis (DVT). The clot-localizing properties of radiolabeled recombinant tissue plasminogen activator (rt-PA) scintigraphy were investigated in 79 patients with suspected DVT.

Methods.—Patients underwent contrast venography and scintigraphy with technetium-99m–rt-PA. The mean time between the 2 tests was 20 hours. The plasminogen binding site of rt-PA was permanently inhibited without inactivating the fibrin and radiolabeled with ^{99m}Tc. Scintigraphy was performed using a gamma camera interfaced to a computer. Results were compared with those of contrast venography.

Results.—Results of venography could not be used in 13 patients. Contrast venography indicated that of 67 proximal vein segments of diagnostic quality, 14 were thrombosed; and 36 of 66 evaluable calf vein segments were thrombosed. Scintigraphy showed that 13 of the 14 thrombosed proximal vein segments had positive scans and that 49 of the 53 nonthrombosed proximal segments had negative scans. For proximal vein thrombosis, the sensitivity was 93% and the specificity was 92%. Scintigraphy indicated that 31 of the 36 thrombosed calf veins had positive scans and 28 of the 30 nonthrombosed calf veins had negative scans. For calf vein thrombosis, the sensitivity was 86% and specificity was 93%.

Conclusion.—Scintigraphy using ^{99m}Tc–rt-PA has promise as a reliable technique for detecting proximal and calf vein thrombosis. It is simple to perform, is not operator dependent, is sensitive to fresh and aged thrombi, and is unaffected by heparin administration.

▶ Modified rt-PA labeled with ^{99m}Tc has proceeded to the point of clinical trial. This reasonably sized study of 79 patients has provided extremely promising results. The authors suggest that ^{99m}Tc-labeled modified rt-PA can be used to detect thrombus in both proximal and calf veins in patients. Although it is the rule in medicine that early promising reports soon become tempered by reality, these excellent results certainly warrant further evaluation of this technique, which has the potential to be extremely valuable.

M.D. Blaufox, M.D., Ph.D.

Difference Analysis of Antifibrin Images in the Detection of Deep Venous Thrombosis

Line BR, Neumann PH (Albany Med Ctr, NY)
J Nucl Med 36:2326–2332, 1995   8–3

Background.—The T2G1s Fab' antifibrin antibody attaches to an epitope on fibrin in acute, newly formed venous thrombi. Technetium-99m T2G1s Fab' scintigraphy is useful for localization of acute thrombi in the

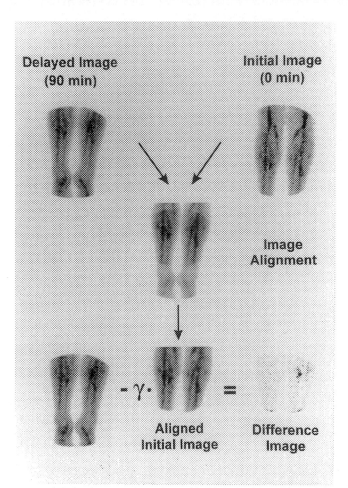

FIGURE 2.—Image manipulations that produce the difference image. The initial and delayed images must be superimposed anatomically point for point for quantitative comparisons. Each limb in the initial image is shifted and rotated until it is anatomically congruent with the limb location in the delayed image. The aligned image is checked by rapidly alternating its display with the 90-minute image (*center*). Once properly aligned, initial blood-pool distribution is multiplied by its fractional change factor (γ) and subtracted from the 90-minute delay image to produce the difference image. The hot spot remaining in the difference image represents a venogram positive thrombus in the right posterior tibial vein. (Reprinted by permission of the Society of Nuclear Medicine, from Line BR, Neumann PH: Difference analysis of antifibrin images in the detection of deep venous thrombosis. *J Nucl Med* 36:2326–2332, 1995.)

lower extremities. However, visual clot detection involves comparisons and decisions about differential uptake and clearance in vascular regions. The hypothesis that computer-assisted differential uptake analysis should increase both the speed and accuracy of interpretations by novices was investigated.

Methods.—Twenty-five patient studies that included immediate blood-pool and 90-minute delayed images were paired into 125 image sets (5 per patient). After aligning the image pairs spatially, a "clot only" image was produced by removing the blood-pool activity in the immediate image from the delayed image. (Fig 2). As part of a receiver operator characteristic (ROC) comparison study, 7 novice readers were presented with both unprocessed data and computer-processed images. Using both sets of data, the novice readers were asked to make independent diagnostic assessments at 250 limb sites. Although image intensity and color scale mappings were freely adjustable, 3 readers were presented with images adjusted with optimal image contrast.

Results.—The area under the ROC curve (Az) for these novice readers was similar for unprocessed data (88.5%) and for computer-processed images (88.8%). However, the 4 readers whose images were not optimized showed a significant difference in the Az between unprocessed data (79.1%) and computer-processed images (90.7%). For all 7 readers, the average diagnostic decision time per limb site was 18 seconds for unprocessed data and 7 seconds for computer-processed images.

Conclusions.—Computer processing of lower-extremity ^{99m}Tc T2G1s Fab' scintigraphy images provides "clot" images that minimize nonspecific blood background activity. At least with novice readers, this allows greater interpreter decision speed and confidence. When image intensity and contrast factors are important, the accuracy of novice readers is improved by using computer-processed images.

▶ In general, the use of computer enhancement procedures has been relatively disappointing in that it has not resulted in very great improvement in diagnostic accuracy. In this study of the imaging of deep venous thrombosis, the investigators have shown that difference analysis can indeed help improve the diagnostic accuracy of novice readers. As with most nuclear medicine techniques, it seems likely that with increasing experience, the observer probably is able to subconsciously carry out the processing that the computer is doing for the novice. It is an amazing fact that in spite of the enormous progress that has been made in computing, the human brain still is able to compete effectively. The major asset of the computer, in general, appears to be a tremendous increase in speed, which is confirmed in this study, in which computer processing more than halved the time required to make a diagnostic decision.

M.D. Blaufox, M.D., Ph.D.

Thrombus Imaging With a Technetium-99m-labeled, Activated Platelet Receptor-binding Peptide

Lister-James J, Knight LC, Maurer AH, et al (Temple Univ, Philadelphia)
J Nucl Med 37:775–781, 1996   8–4

Introduction.—Pulmonary embolism (PE) and deep vein thrombosis (DVT) are both associated with serious morbidity and mortality. An estimated 70% of all pulmonary emboli are the result of lower-extremity DVTs, necessitating the need for both an accurate and timely diagnosis of this clinical condition. Current methods either lack accuracy (duplex ultrasonography) or cause complications (venography). Recently, radiolabeled platelets and antibodies have been investigated as thrombosis-imaging agents, but they fail to provide information in a timely manner and have a potential for inducing an immune response. A preclinical evaluation was conducted to determine whether technetium-99m–P280, a ^{99m}Tc-labeled peptide with high infinity and specificity for the GPIIb/IIIa receptor, is able to detect thromboembolism.

Methods.—Technetium-99m–glucoheptonate was used as a ligand exchange reagent to label P280 peptide with ^{99m}Tc. The inhibition of ADP-stimulated human platelet aggregation, the inhibition of the binding of fibrinogen to the GPIIb/IIIa receptor, and the inhibition of the binding of vitronectin to the vitronectin receptor were used to assess the affinity and specificity of P280 peptide for the GPIIb/IIIa receptor. A canine venous thrombosis model was used for in vivo assessment of the ability of ^{99m}Tc-P280 to detect thrombi. Rats and rabbits were used to test the biodistribution of ^{99m}Tc-P280.

Results.—The P280 peptide was readily labeled by ligand exchange when using ^{99m}Tc-glucoheptonate. It inhibited the aggregation of human platelets in platelet-rich plasma with a concentration that inhibits 50% (IC_{50}) of 79 nM, the fibrinogen binding to the GPIIb/IIIa receptor with an IC_{50} of 6.8 nM, and the vitronectin binding to the vitronectin receptor at an IC_{50} of 13 µM, indicating a high in vitro receptor-binding affinity and specificity of the peptide. Images of the femoral vein thrombi in the canine model showed thrombi and thrombus-to-blood ratio of 4.4 at 1 hour and thrombus-to-muscle ratio of 11 at 4 hours (Table 1). The radiotracer was rapidly cleared from the blood and urine in the dog, rat, and rabbit investigations.

Conclusion.—The high in vitro receptor-binding affinity and specificity, the in vivo thrombus imaging, and fast clearance indicate that ^{99m}Tc-P280 may be a useful thrombus imaging agent. These findings warrant an evaluation of ^{99m}Tc-P280 as a clinical imaging agent.

▶ This article reports a study in animals using peptide P280 labeled with ^{99m}Tc. The authors report in vivo visualization of thrombi with high thrombus-to-blood and thrombus-to-muscle ratios of activity. They suggest that the results that would be obtained in human beings would be even better than those obtained in the dog model because the characteristics of the agent in humans are more suitable to this study. We await clinical application of this

TABLE 1.—Percent Injected Dose per Gram in Selected Tissue and Regions-of-Interest Data at 4 Hours in the Canine Venous Thrombosis Model

Compound	% ID/g Thrombus	% ID/g Blood	Thrombus-to-Blood	Thrombus-to-Muscle	Thrombus/ Vessel (ROI)	Thrombus/ Muscle (ROI)
^{99m}Tc-P280	0.0059 ± 0.0025	0.0012 ± 0.0003	4.4 ± 0.74	11.0 ± 7.0	2.0 ± 0.1	1.9 ± 0.1
^{99m}Tc-glucoheptonate	0.0026 ± 0.0002	0.0015 ± 0.0007	2.2 ± 0.8	4.3 ± 2.4	1.5 ± 0.0	1.6 ± 0.1
^{99m}Tc-platelets	0.18 ± 0.08	0.037 ± 0.006	5.4 ± 3.2	230.0 ± 100.0	1.8 ± 0.6	5.0 ± 2.2

Note: Values are means ± SE.
Abbreviation: ROI, region of interest.
(Reprinted by permission of the Society of Nuclear Medicine, from Lister-James J, Knight LC, Maurer AH, et al: Thrombus imaging with a technetium-99m-labeled, activated platelet receptor-binding peptide. *J Nucl Med* 37:775–781, 1996.)

agent to see whether it lives up to this early potential. It appears that a positive thrombus imaging agent in nuclear medicine is very close to reality.

M.D. Blaufox, M.D., Ph.D.

Detecting Deep Venous Thrombosis With Technetium-99m-labeled Synthetic Peptide P280

Muto P, Lastoria S, Varrella P, et al (Natl Cancer Inst, Naples, Italy; Univ "Federico II" Naples, Italy; Diatech Inc, Londonderry, NH; et al)

J Nucl Med 36:1384–1391, 1995   8–5

Objectives.—An attempt was made to evaluate the imaging of deep venous thrombosis with technetium-99m–P280 and to analyze the relationship between thrombus age and its influence on identifying deep venous thrombosis.

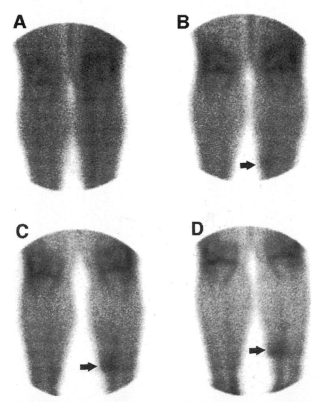

FIGURE 7.—Serial images of the calves acquired 30 (A), 60 (B), 120 (C), and 240 (D) minutes after technetium-99m–P280 administration. The thrombus, located in the left calf, is visualized by 1 hour but is better defined in the later scans when the background activity has cleared. (Reprinted by permission of the Society of Nuclear Medicine, from Muto P, Lastoria S, Varrella P, et al: Detecting deep venous thrombosis with technetium-99m-labeled synthetic peptide P280. *J Nucl Med* 36:1384–1391, 1995.)

Background.—Deep venous thrombosis is difficult to diagnose because more than 50% of patients can be asymptomatic and only 30% of symptomatic patients have objective evidence of the disease. None of the current detection methods is ideally accurate, and none can differentiate acute or active thrombosis from the residual from prior episodes of the disease. Radiolabeled monoclonal antibodies recently have been used to identify acute thrombi. Preliminary studies have shown that ^{99m}Tc-P280 selectively accumulates in fresh thrombi.

Methods.—In 9 patients with evidence of deep venous thrombosis, scintigraphy with ^{99m}Tc-P280 was performed. Images of the head, chest, abdomen/pelvis, and lower extremities were obtained immediately after and 1, 2–4, and 24 hours after injection.

Results.—In 8 of 9 patients with confirmed deep venous thrombosis, there was positive visualization of thrombi within 1 hour of injection. Most patients had recent onset of symptoms. Technetium-99m–P280 did not localize in the femoral thrombus of 1 patient who had had deep venous thrombosis diagnosed by ultrasound 42 days earlier; the patient's history suggested that deep venous thrombosis had developed 7 months previously. Thrombi-to-background ratios were constant throughout the study. Accumulation of ^{99m}Tc-P280 was also noted in 2 patients with pulmonary embolism and in 1 patient with a cerebellar hemangioblastoma. The optimum time for imaging was between 1 and 3 hours after injection (Fig 7). There were no adverse effects.

Conclusion.—Technetium-99m–P280 may be safe and effective for deep venous thrombosis and pulmonary embolism and for monitoring active venous thrombosis. It may be superior to other imaging modalities because of its binding affinity and molecular size, which promotes rapid blood clearance. Further research is needed to evaluate its accuracy in a variety of patients and thrombus ages, sizes, and locations.

▶ Having despaired last year because of the lack of investigations of the vascular system using nuclear medicine, I am delighted by the number of developments in this area this year. It appears that we are moving toward the introduction of a practical imaging technique for venous thrombosis and, hopefully at some point, for pulmonary emboli. The invention and perfection of such a technique will be an extremely valuable addition to routine clinical nuclear medicine. This is especially true because this is an extremely important and life-threatening disease for which simple diagnostic techniques are lacking.

M.D. Blaufox, M.D., Ph.D.

Scintigraphic Recording of Blood Volume Shifts

Baccelli G, Pacenti P, Terrani S, et al (Univ of Milan, Italy; Nuclear Polytechnic, Milano, Italy; Fatebenefratelli Hosp, Milano, Italy)
J Nucl Med 36:2022–2031, 1995
8–6

Background.—A scintigraphic device that permits intravascular blood volume shifts to be continuously and simultaneously measured at several sites has been developed. The reliability of this device was evaluated. Blood shifts caused by common daily activities were also assessed, as were the mechanisms responsible for hemodynamic changes.

Participants and Methods.—The scintigraphic device consists of small scintillation probes that are tightly fixed to the skin (Fig 1). The device was used on 16 healthy men (mean age, 46 years), and measurements were made in 3 fields of the right lung, the liver, and thighs and calves during the Valsalva maneuver, hyperventilation, various posture changes, and treadmill walking.

Results.—Blood volume shifts were always in the expected direction and were consistent with previously published reports. Lung blood volume was increased by leg elevation, compression of the thighs while standing, lying down after sitting and standing, and changing posture from standing to sitting and walking. Conversely, lung blood volume was decreased by the Valsalva maneuver, hyperventilation, sitting or standing from reclining positions, and by standing from sitting.

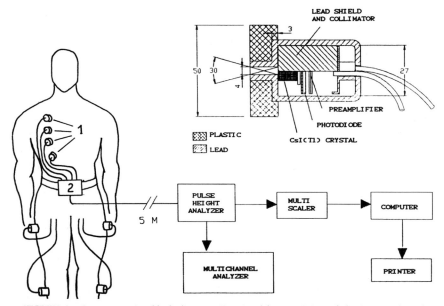

FIGURE 1.—Instrumentation block diagram. (Reprinted by permission of the Society of Nuclear Medicine, from Baccelli G, Pacenti P, Terrani S, et al: Scintigraphic recording of blood volume shifts. *J Nucl Med* 36:2022–2031, 1995.)

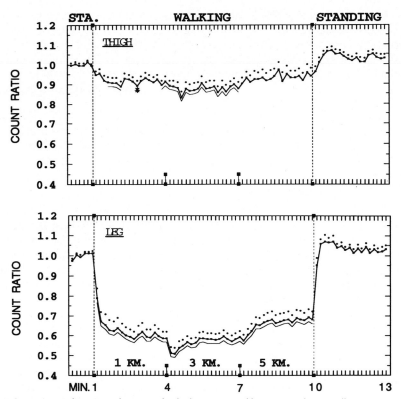

FIGURE 8.—Radioactivity changes in the thigh (*n* = 22) and leg (*n* = 22) during walking at increasing speeds. (Reprinted by permission of the Society of Nuclear Medicine, from Baccelli G, Pacenti P, Terrani S, et al: Scintigraphic recording of blood volume shifts. *J Nucl Med* 36:2022–2031, 1995.)

Blood volume changes recorded in the thigh and calf during posture changes and walking were consistent with previously reported values (Fig 8) and were in the opposite direction of blood shifts in the lung.

Hepatic blood volume was typically unaffected by posture changes. During walking, hepatic blood volume tended to increase slightly with increased speed but decreased progressively thereafter to baseline once speeds of 6 km per hour were reached.

Conclusion.—This noninvasive device is able to reliably and continuously measure blood volume changes at various sites in freely moving individuals. All repeated experimental conditions led to blood volume shifts that were similar in direction, scope, and time course in each of the several fields where radioactivity was measured, indicating that these measurements were reproducible.

▶ I have commented frequently on the lack of attention to the potential role of nuclear medicine in vascular disease. This paper introduces an interesting device that may have a particular role in patients with peripheral vascular disease in whom there is a significant need for a simple, objective measurement of changes induced by various interventions. The technique may also have some potential for use in the evaluation of the severity of disease, especially with various types of interventions. The authors point out other potential uses, including studies of arterial hypotension, but the use in peripheral vascular disease appears to have the greatest potential.

M.D. Blaufox, M.D., Ph.D.

Evaluation of Tissue Perfusion by the Xe-133 Washout Method in Lower Limbs of Patients With Noninsulin-dependent Diabetes Mellitus

Lin W-Y, Kao C-H, Hsu C-Y, et al (Taichung Veterans Gen Hosp, Taiwan, Republic of China)
Clin Nucl Med 20:449–452, 1995   8–7

Background.—Foot problems are the leading cause of hospital admission among patients with diabetes and often result in limb amputation. Because ischemia may play a role in the pathogenesis of diabetes-related foot problems, the xenon-133 washout method was used to assess changes of tissue perfusion in the lower limbs of patients with non–insulin-dependent diabetes mellitus (NIDDM).

Patients and Methods.—Eighty-five patients with NIDDM (mean age, 66 years) and 47 age-matched nondiabetic controls were enrolled in the study. There were no history or findings of peripheral vascular disease in the lower limbs of the patients with diabetes. Patients were grouped according to disease duration and condition of blood sugar control. The ^{133}Xe washout method was performed in the anterior tibial muscle of all study participants.

Results.—In the control group, the mean blood perfusion of muscle tissue (Q value) was 2.85 mL/100 mg per minute vs. 1.98 mL/100 g per minute among the NIDDM patients. This difference was significant (Table 1). Forty-seven of the patients with NIDDM had regular and good control of blood sugar, and 38 had poor control. Significant Q-value differences were noted between groups. In patients with good blood sugar control, the mean Q value was 2.36 mL/100 g per minute, compared with 1.51 mL/100 g per minute among those in the poor-control group. Significant Q-value differences were also observed among the NIDDM patients according to

---

TABLE 1.—Blood Perfusion of Muscle Tissue in Patients With Non–insulin-dependent Diabetes Mellitus

	Number of Patients	Age (Mean ± SD) (yrs)	Q Value (Mean ± SD) (ml/100 g/minutes)
Diabetics	85	66.5 ± 4.8	1.98 ± 1.39
Controls	47	64.5 ± 6.2	2.85 ± 1.35

Note: The difference is significant by unpaired Student's *t*-test ($P < 0.05$)
(Courtesy of Lin W-Y, Kao C-H, Hsu C-Y, et al: Evaluation of tissue perfusion by the Xe-133 washout method in lower limbs of patients with noninsulin-dependent diabetes mellitus. *Clin Nucl Med* 20:449–452, 1995.)

disease duration. Among the 48 patients with a disease duration of less than 10 years, the mean Q value was 2.35 mL/100 g per minute vs. 1.50 mL/100 g per minute among the 37 patients with disease duration of 10 or more years.

Conclusion.—Among patients with NIDDM, tissue perfusion in the lower legs may be significantly decreased and is associated with disease duration and state of blood sugar control. Use of the ^{133}Xe washout method may assist with early identification of diabetic microangiopathy.

▶ This article is gratifying in two respects. First, it is another encouraging effort to extend nuclear medicine studies back into the area of vascular disease. Second, it shows a very significant potential value for the technique in a very prevalent disease condition. Unfortunately, the authors chose to use blood sugar levels as a measure of control of diabetes. This observation would have been more powerful, and probably more reliable, had hemoglobin A_{1C} levels been used instead. Further extension and refinement of these studies should prove to be a valuable aid in the management of patients with NIDDM.

M.D. Blaufox, M.D., Ph.D.

Management of Systemic Vasculitis: Contribution of Scintigraphic Imaging to Evaluation of Disease Activity and Classification
Reuter H, Wraight EP, Qasim FJ, et al (Univ of Cambridge, England)
Q J Med 88:509–516, 1995   8–8

Objective.—In a retrospective study of 50 patients with systemic vasculitis, the sensitivity and specificity of radioisotope-labeled leukocyte scans in the detection of active vasculitis were evaluated. Early determination of the nature and extent of the vasculitis process would allow prompt, appropriate intervention.

Patients and Methods.—The 50 consecutive patients received their diagnosis on the basis of clinical, serologic and histologic features. Thirty-two had Wegener's granulomatosis (WG), 12 had microscopic polyangiitis (MPA), 4 had Churg-Strauss syndrome (CSS), and 2 had temporal arteritis (TA). Leukocyte scans were usually performed within 2 or 3 days of referral to the vasculitis clinic. Sera were assayed for antineutrophil cytoplasmic autoantibodies activity by solid-phase enzyme-linked immunosorbent assay and tested for autoantibody reactivity to a panel of antineutrophil cytoplasmic antigens. Whole-body scans were performed at 3 hours and repeated at 20–24 hours after IV injection of the isotope-labeled leukocytes. Two nuclear medicine physicians performed a blinded review of all 127 leukocyte scans.

Results.—Increased diffuse uptake in the lungs was present in 46 patients on the early scan but had disappeared in 26 of these patients by the time of the later scan. The remaining 20 patients (17 WG, 2 MPA, 1 CSS) had increased uptake of labeled leukocytes on the delayed scan. This uptake was localized in 12 cases and generalized and diffuse in 8. Nasal or paranasal uptake was present in 32 patients on the late scan. Other areas of leukocyte uptake included the bowel, kidneys, meninges, ureter, and vagina. In addition to detecting unsuspected sites of disease, leukocyte imaging was useful for monitoring disease activity and results of treatment (Fig 2). Increased nasal activity was found on the late scans of 12 of 14 anti–proteinase 3–positive, 3 of 5 antimyeloperoxidase-positive, and 1 of 2 anti–human leukocyte elastase–positive patients. Leukocyte scans

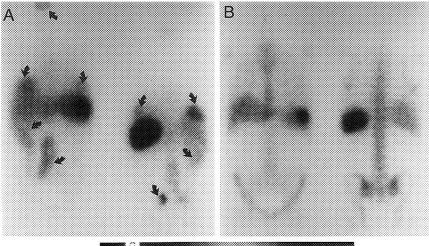

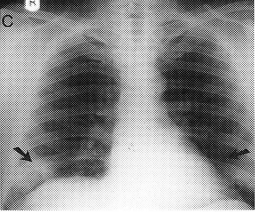

FIGURE 2.—Sequential scintiscans 3 months apart in patient with Wegener's granulomatosis. *Arrows* show abnormal distribution before treatment: anterior view (left side of **upper left panel**) in paranasal areas, lungs (bilateral basal), right kidney/ureter (positive biopsy of ureter) and ascending colon; the posterior view (right side of **upper left panel**) shows additional abnormal uptake in left sacroiliac joint. Chest radiograph (**bottom**), also pretreatment, shows opacities at the lung bases that match the scintiscan abnormalities. Three months after treatment (cyclophosphamide and steroids), both scan (**upper right panel**) and chest radiographs were normal. (Courtesy of Reuter H, Wraight EP, Qasim FJ, et al: Management of systemic vasculitis: Contribution of scintigraphic imaging to evaluation of disease activity and classification. *Q J Med* 88:509–516, 1995 by permission of Oxford University Press.)

yielded more information than CT or conventional radiography and were useful for differentiating between WG and MPA.

Conclusion.—The most consistent scintigraphic feature in these patients with systemic vasculitis was diffuse lung activity. The presence of nasal uptake strongly suggests WG but may occur as well in other vasculitides. There was a significant correlation between anti–proteinase 3 autoantibody specificity and nasal uptake of labeled leukocytes.

▶ This study introduces another innovative and interesting approach to vascular disease. In this situation, the investigators have shown that leukocyte imaging can be of value in patients with systemic vasculitis. They suggest that it may be useful in differentiating microscopic polyangiitis from Wegener's granulomatosis. The signs and symptoms of vasculitis under some conditions can be difficult to classify and as the investigators point out, the extent of deep tissue involvement or progression of disease may be particularly difficult to assess.

A note of caution is warranted, however, as the most useful scintigraphic finding was increased activity in the nasal and paranasal region. The authors do not present specific data on the frequency with which this uptake may occur in patients with clinical or subclinical sinusitis. It is possible that in a larger series of patients, the finding may become less clear. However, this remains an interesting and new application of leukocyte scanning.

M.D. Blaufox, M.D., Ph.D.

Assessment of Peripheral Vascular Effects of Antimigraine Drugs in Humans
van Es NM, Bruning TA, Camps J, et al (Univ Hosp Leiden, The Netherlands; Erasmus Univ, Rotterdam, The Netherlands)
Cephalalgia 15:288–291, 1995   8–9

Background.—Sumatriptan, a selective agonist for $5HT_1$ receptors, has antimigraine effects that may partially result from constriction of cranial arteriovenous anastomoses (AVAs). The vascular beds of the forearm and finger can be used to assess the peripheral effects of antimigraine drugs under normal and pathologic conditions; thus, a forearm and finger blood flow model was used to evaluate the peripheral vascular effects of this novel antimigraine drug.

Participants and Methods.—Twelve healthy male volunteers participated in the study. Among these, 6 men (mean age, 24 years) received sumatriptan, given in cumulative-dose infusions of 10, 100, and 1,000 ng/kg per minute, and 6 (mean age, 23 years) received saline infusions. Experimental and control agents were infused into the brachial artery. All infusions were given during a continuous-infusion of sodium nitroprusside, 5 ng/kg per minute, to ensure adequate baseline blood flow values. The peripheral vascular effects of sumatriptan were assessed by measuring forearm blood flow (FBF) and finger blood flow (FiBF) using venous occlu-

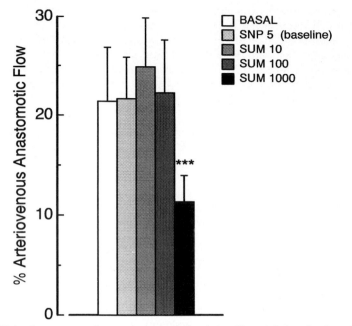

FIGURE 4.—Percentage arteriovenous anastomotic flow induced by an infusion of sodium nitroprus-side (*SNP*) and an infusion of sumatriptan (*SUM*) in cumulative doses of 10, 100, and 1,000 ng/kg per minute. The radioactivity counted over the lungs after an IV bolus injection with microspheres is considered as 100% arteriovenous anastomosis flow. ***$P < 0.001$. (Courtesy of van Es NM, Bruning TA, Camps J, et al: Assessment of peripheral vascular effects of antimigraine drugs in humans. *Cephalalgia* 15:288–291, 1995. By permission of Scandinavian University Press.)

sion plethysmography. The effects of sumatriptan on the patency of finger AVAs were also determined using radiolabeled human albumin aggregates. Experiments were initiated at least 45 minutes after brachial artery can-nulation, and the various infusions were separated by a period of 40–60 minutes to permit FBF and FiBF to return to baseline levels.

Results.—Sodium nitroprusside increased FBF but did not alter FiBF. Dose-dependent reductions in both FBF and FiBF were noted with subse-quent infusion of sumatriptan. Reductions in AVA flow were observed only with the administration of sumatriptan, 1,000 ng/kg per minute. The mean reduction of the shunted fraction of radiolabeled microspheres was 57% (Fig 4). Repeated sumatriptan infusion resulted in a less pronounced response in FBF and FiBF, which was considered indicative of tachyphy-laxis.

Conclusion.—In previous investigations, resting values of FiBF were found to be elevated during migraine attacks compared with values noted between attacks. Subcutaneous administration of therapeutic sumatriptan doses resulted in significant reductions (approximately 35%) in FiBF both during and between migraine attacks. Because FiBF is primarily deter-mined by AVAs, human peripheral AVAs exhibit a similar response to sumatriptan, as noted in animal and in vitro studies. This finding supports the theory that AVAs may play a role in the pathophysiology of migraine.

▶ This interesting report takes advantage of the fact that technetium-labeled spherical human albumin aggregates will be trapped in capillaries, but in the presence of arterial venous anastomosis, which is present in skin vessels, they will pass through and ultimately be trapped in the lung, creating a model for the determination of similar pathways in the brain that are related to migraine disease. Of particular interest is the use of this methodology to evaluate drug effects and potential optimization of drug therapy. Although the authors address themselves solely to pharmacologic evaluation of antimigraine drugs, there are undoubtedly other drugs with vascular activity for which this method may have potential value.

M.D. Blaufox, M.D., Ph.D.

9 Central Nervous System

Introduction

In the 1996 YEAR BOOK OF NUCLEAR MEDICINE, I indicated in the introduction to this chapter that I hoped I could present clinical articles relating to iodine-123–labeled β-CIT for you. The first 3 articles in this year's section do just that. We continue with papers on Parkinson's disease, segue to Parkinson's with Alzheimer's, and then on to papers concerning Alzheimer's disease. Evaluation of the seizure patient remains popular, and this year's selection deals with the ictal vs. interictal approach to seizure diagnosis. You should know that at this time, my own bias is in the ictal camp, which you should take into account when reading my editorial comments. The section concludes with a potpourri of articles involving such diverse topics as schizophrenia, stroke, and the appearance of the SPECT scan in pugilists. It ends with what may become a very important evaluation of brain SPECT utilization by the American Academy of Neurology. You should find this useful in any of the managed care wars you have to fight.

Alexander Gottschalk, M.D.

Reproducibility of Iodine-123-β-CIT SPECT Brain Measurement of Dopamine Transporters

Seibyl JP, Laruelle M, van Dyck CH, et al (Yale Univ, New Haven, Conn; Dept of Veterans Affairs Med Ctr, West Haven, Conn; Research Biochemicals Internatl, Natick, Mass)
J Nucl Med 37:222–228, 1996
9–1

Background.—Iodine-123–labeled β-CIT binds to dopamine and serotonin transporters with high affinity. It has been used as a SPECT probe in humans and other primates. The value of this tracer in measuring striatal dopamine transporters in human disease was investigated.

Methods.—Seven healthy subjects, aged 19–74 years participated in 2 studies of [^{123}I]β-CIT SPECT. The test/retest variability and reliability of SPECT measures obtained after bolus injection of [^{123}I]β-CIT 0–7 hours (day 1) and 18–24 hours (day 2) after administration were documented. The 2 outcome measures were the ratio of specific striatal to nondisplaceable uptake (V"$_3$) and the total specific striatal uptake expressed as a percentage of injected radiotracer dose.

Findings.—The test/retest reproducibility of both outcome measures was excellent in the day 2 study. The variability of V"$_3$ was 6.8%, and that of percent striatal uptake, was 6.6%. The test/retest variability for the day 1 kinetic modeling data differed substantially, depending on the fitting strategy and assumptions about the reversibility of [^{123}I]β-CIT in striatum. A model that assumed a low, fixed value for reversible striatal binding demonstrated low variability.

Conclusion.—Single-photon emission CT imaging done at 0–7 or 18–24 hours after [^{123}I]β-CIT injection enables reliable, reproducible measures of dopamine transporters to be calculated. The use of [^{123}I]β-CIT in the serial assessment of human neuropsychiatric disease is feasible.

▶ As the readers of this YEAR BOOK know, I think this tracer is a real winner. These data do absolutely nothing to change my mind.

A. Gottschalk, M.D.

[^{123}I]β-CIT/SPECT Imaging Demonstrates Bilateral Loss of Dopamine Transporters in Hemi-Parkinson's Disease
Marek KL, Seibyl JP, Zoghbi SS, et al (Yale Univ, New Haven, Conn)
Neurology 46:231–237, 1996   9–2

Background.—Parkinson's disease (PD) usually begins with unilateral symptoms that gradually involve both sides. Identifying patients very early in the course of PD, with only hemiparkinsonism, helps establish the threshold of early clinical detection. Contrasting the symptomatic with presymptomatic sides provides a model in which to assess methods for detecting presymptomatic PD. In vivo SPECT and PET imaging of the dopamine transporter can be used to assess mesencephalic dopamine neuronal projections in early PD. This study determined the extent of transporter loss in patients with minimal symptoms and the efficacy of SPECT imaging with iodine-123–labeled β-CIT in identifying striatal dopamine transporter loss in hemiparkinsonism in the striatum contralateral to and ipsilateral to symptoms.

Methods and Findings.—Eight patients with hemiparkinsonism and 8 age- and sex-matched healthy subjects were studied. Compared with mean [^{123}I]β-CIT striatal uptake in the control group, striatal uptake in the patients was decreased by about 53% contralateral to and 38% ipsilateral to the clinically symptomatic side. The patients' relative decrease in uptake was greater in the putamen than in the caudate (Figs 2 and 3).

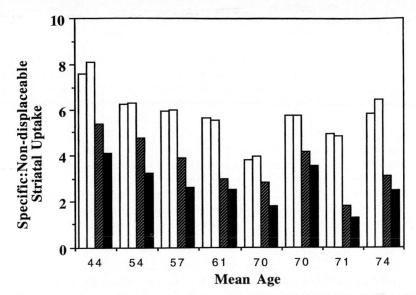

FIGURE 2.—Iodine-123–labeled β-CIT striatal uptake in 8 hemi-Parkinson's disease/healthy subject pairs (mean age of pair indicated). For each pair, the ratio of the specific to nondisplaceable striatal uptake is compared in right and left striatum in the healthy subjects with striatum ipsilateral to symptoms and contralateral to symptoms in the hemi-Parkinson's disease patients. *Open squares* indicate right and left; *cross-hatched squares*, ipsilateral; and *solid squares*, contralateral. (Courtesy of Marek KL, Seibyl JP, Zoghbi SS, et al: [^{123}I]β-CIT/SPECT imaging demonstrates bilateral loss of dopamine transporters in hemi-Parkinson's disease. *Neurology* 46:231–237, 1996. By permission of Little, Brown and Co.)

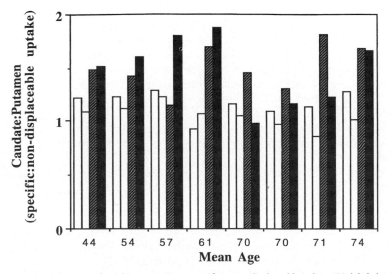

FIGURE 3.—The ratio of caudate to putamen specific to nondisplaceable iodine-123–labeled β-CIT uptake is compared in right and left striatum of healthy subjects with striatum ipsilateral to symptoms and contralateral to symptoms in the hemi-Parkinson's disease patients. *Open squares* indicate right and left; *cross-hatched squares*, ipsilateral; and *solid squares*, contralateral. (Courtesy of Marek KL, Seibyl JP, Zoghbi SS, et al: [^{123}I]β-CIT/SPECT imaging demonstrates bilateral loss of dopamine transporters in hemi-Parkinson's disease. *Neurology* 46:231–237, 1996. By permission of Little, Brown and Co.)

Conclusion.—Single-photon emission CT imaging of the dopamine transporter with [^{123}I]β-CIT seems able to identify patients with PD at the onset of motor symptoms. This modality may also be valuable in identifying individuals with developing dopaminergic abnormalities before the onset of motor symptoms.

▶ I have argued in this YEAR BOOK for years that it should ultimately be possible—using tracer imaging techniques and analysis—to figure out not only which patients have early PD, but those who are at risk to get it. These data suggest that [^{123}I]β-CIT may be the tracer that will do both. If we develop good therapy to keep the disease from progressing, you may find long lines of middle-aged patients lined up outside your office waiting for this test.

A. Gottschalk, M.D.

Striatal Opioid Receptor Binding in Parkinson's Disease, Striatonigral Degeneration and Steele-Richardson-Olszewski Syndrome A [^{11}C]Diprenorphine PET Study
Burn DJ, Rinne JO, Quinn NP, et al (Hammersmith Hosp, London; Natl Hosps for Neurology and Neurosurgery, London; Univ of Turku, Finland)
Brain 118:951–958, 1995   9–3

Introduction.—It is difficult to make a clinical differentiation between Parkinson's disease, striatonigral degeneration (SND), multiple system atrophy (MSA), and Steele-Richardson-Olszewski syndrome (SRO), as evidenced by a nearly 25% misdiagnosis rate. The caudate and putamen contain a dense population of opioidergic neurons and receptors with a close anatomical and physiologic relationship with the dopaminergic system. Striatal opioid receptor binding in groups of patients with clinically defined Parkinson's disease, SND and SRO, was evaluated using PET with [carbon-11]diprenorphine. This ligand was chosen to reflect overall striatal opioid receptor binding changes in these 3 groups of akinetic-rigid patient groups.

Methods.—There were 8, 7, and 6 patients, respectively, with clinically probable Parkinson's disease, SND type MSA, and SRO. The [^{11}C]diprenorphine uptake data for these patients were compared with those of 8 healthy controls with no evidence of neurologic disease.

Results.—The mean patient ages in all groups were comparable. The mean disease duration for patients with Parkinson's disease was significantly shorter (2.6 years) than those of patients with SND (4.9 years) and SRO (3.5 years). Compared with controls, there was no significant difference in the Parkinson's group between mean ligand binding in the putamen and caudate. The mean putamen:occipital cortex ratios for the SND and SRO groups were significantly reduced compared with those seen in the control and Parkinson's groups. When compared with the control and Parkinson's groups, patients in the SRO group had a mean caudate:occipital cortex activity that was significantly reduced. No patients in the

Parkinson's group or the SND group, but 4 of 6 patients in the SRO group, had caudate opioid receptor binding that was well below the normal range. For putamen opioid receptor binding, no patients in the Parkinson's group, 3 patients in the SND group, and all patients in the SRO group were well below the normal range.

Conclusion.—Findings indicate that there are differences in the pattern of opioid receptor binding in the 3 patient populations investigated. The patient probably has Parkinson's disease if there is no significant difference from normal in caudate and putamen ^{11}C activities. The most likely diagnosis is SND if the opioid receptor binding is diminished in the putamen but not the caudate. A patient is likely to have SRO if there is significantly reduced opioid receptor binding in both caudate and putamen.

▶ These authors point out that the diagnosis of Parkinson's disease may be incorrectly made in some 25% of cases that should be properly spread between SND, MSA, and SRO. We are entering an era in which receptor imaging either by PET or by SPECT (using [iodine-123]β-CIT) makes it possible to make the distinction. The authors also note that some of these characteristic receptor binding changes are temporally related to the course of the patient's disease, because any study really represents a disease "snapshot" at the instant the study was made. Nevertheless, as we begin to read more and more about therapeutic approaches to Parkinson's disease, these distinctions of Parkinson-like entities become very important. In this instance, it is interesting that the opioid receptor binding used here for SRO had marked decreased affinity for the caudate compared with normals, SND, and Parkinson's disease.

Laihinen and colleagues found that [^{11}C] β-CIT accumulated significantly less in the putamen in patients with Parkinson's disease, whereas there was no difference between the caudate uptake in patients with Parkinson's disease and that in normal subjects.[1] Another Finnish group tried using these cocaine analogues and iodinated analogues of β-CIT with somewhat disappointing results compared with those of the iodinate β-CIT itself.[2]

A. Gottschalk, M.D.

References

1. Laihinen AO, Rinne JO, Någren KÅ, et al: PET studies on brain monoamine transporters with carbon-11-β-CIT in Parkinson's disease. *J Nucl Med* 36:1263–1267, 1995.
2. Kuikka JT, Åkerman K, Bergström KA, et al: Iodine-123 labelled N-(2-fluoroethyl) I 2β-carbomethoxy-3β-(4-iodophenyl) nortropane for dopamine transporter imaging in the living human brain. *Eur J Nucl Med* 22:682–686, 1995.

Clinical Correlates of [¹⁸F]Fluorodopa Uptake in Five Grafted Parkinsonian Patients

Remy P, Samson Y, Hantraye P, et al (Service Hospitalier Frédéric Joliot, Orsay, France; INSERM Unité 421, Créteil, France; CHU Tenon, Paris; et al)
Ann Neurol 38:580–588, 1995   9–4

Introduction.—To confirm the benefits of fetal mesencephalic grafts in Parkinson's disease (PD), the survival and development of grafted cells must be monitored in large groups of patients in controlled studies. The role of PET using [fluorine-18]fluorodopa ([¹⁸F]dopa) in monitoring graft survival and function and in correlating changes in grafted striatum with motor function was evaluated.

Methods.—Study subjects were 5 patients with severe PD and a mean age of 56 years at the time of the graft. All were grafted unilaterally in the most affected striatum and given immunosuppressive therapy. Patients were examined using PET before the graft and at 3, 6, and 12 months after grafting, and by MRI on the same day as the pregraft PET study and before one of the postgraft examinations. Positron emission tomographic regions of interests were determined using a newly developed method based on the anatomical images acquired by MRI.

Results.—The patients exhibited a progressive and significant increase of [¹⁸F]dopa uptake in the grafted putamen. This increase reached a mean of 63% 12 months after the graft and was maintained at 18 and 24 months in 2 patients with longer follow-up. No significant changes were observed in the caudate when grafted. For the patient group as a whole, correlations were demonstrated between clinical status and uptake in the putamen. Motor improvement was based on 2 different tests: a global scale that is the percentage of daily time spent "on" as rated subjectively by the patient and lateralized time tests that are quantitative and allow a distinction between grafted and nongrafted sides. Values of [¹⁸F]dopa uptake were correlated with the contralateral finger dexterity to the same extent in both grafted and nongrafted putamen, indicating that uptake reflects the motor function of the opposite side of the body.

Conclusion.—Findings in this small group of patients offer insights on potential relationships between [¹⁸F]dopa uptake in the grafted putamen and motor status. Clinical optimal results of fetal mesencephalic grafts might be achieved if the graft brings uptake values in the putamen to about 2 standard deviations of mean control values.

▶ As noted in past issues of the YEAR BOOK OF NUCLEAR MEDICINE, the problem faced with this type of therapy is determining whether any success has been achieved in the face of a progressive, relentless downhill disease. In short, how do you tell whether a patient who is getting worse after a graft is progressing downhill slowly because the graft failed or is in fact better and would have fallen off the edge of a cliff without the therapy. These authors provide data that may help answer this troubling question both subjectively and objectively. We hope this type of study continues in the future.

A. Gottschalk, M.D.

A SPECT Study of Parkinsonism in Alzheimer's Disease

Starkstein SE, Vazquez S, Merello M, et al (Raúl Carrea Inst of Neurological Research, Buenos Aires, Argentina)
J Neuropsychiatry Clin Neurosci 7:308–313, 1995   9–5

Background.—A substantial subgroup of patients with Alzheimer's disease (AD) exhibit extrapyramidal signs (EPS), such as hypokinesia, rigidity, and tremor. Previous studies using SPECT have shown that specific regional cerebral blood flow (rCBF) deficits are associated with specific clinical signs, including predominant language-related cognitive deficits, predominant visuospatial deficits, disinhibition syndrome, and anosognosia. Two groups of patients with AD, with and without EPS, were studied with SPECT to examine differences in rCBF abnormalities.

Methods.—Thirty-five consecutive patients with probable AD were examined with the Unified Parkinson's Disease Rating Scale. Nine patients with EPS and 9 patients with no EPS were identified. These patients underwent a SPECT examination with technetium-99m–hexamethylpropyleneamine oxime. Anterior, medial, and posterior measurements of rCBF were determined in each of the following cortical areas: frontal inferior, frontal superior, temporal inferior, temporal superior, and parietal.

Results.—There were no significant differences in age, sex, education, duration of illness, severity of cognitive deficits, or daily living functional impairments between the 2 groups. All of the patients with EPS had bilateral signs, with no significant side-to-side differences except in 1 patient. Compared with the patients without EPS, those with EPS demonstrated significantly less rCBF in the frontal superior, temporal superior, and parietal regions of the left hemisphere.

Conclusions.—Extrapyramidal signs were associated with CBF deficits lateralized to the left hemisphere in the frontal superior, temporal superior, and parietal regions. These lateralized deficits were, however, associated with bilateral clinical signs, which differentiates AD EPS from unilateral Parkinson's disease, characterized by CBF changes contralateral to the clinical manifestations. Therefore, the mechanism governing EPS in patients with AD is different from that governing Parkinson's disease.

▶ This study is concerned with a difficult problem to solve, and I am not sure the authors have solved it. Selecting only 18 of the 35 patients recruited because they represent polar ends of the spectrum makes me nervous that those patients in between won't fit in either group. Furthermore, the SPECT camera used had a resolution of 34 mm. Subtle (or even not so subtle) changes are not likely to show up on that system. In short, I find the data interesting but far from definitive.

A. Gottschalk, M.D.

High-resolution SPECT to Assess Hippocampal Perfusion in Neuropsychiatric Diseases

Ohnishi T, Hoshi H, Nagamachi S, et al (Miyazaki Med College, Japan)

J Nucl Med 36:1163–1169, 1995   9–6

Introduction.—Because the hippocampus is so highly associated with memory disturbance, this region may be the earliest and most sensitive to be assessed by regional cerebral blood flow (rCBF) SPECT in demented patients. A study of patients with a variety of neuropsychiatric diagnoses used high-resolution SPECT to clarify changes in hippocampal perfusion and the correlation between hippocampal perfusion and memory deficits.

Methods.—Forty-five patients and controls, all right-handed, were investigated. Diagnoses in the patient group included dementia (13 with dementia of the Alzheimer type) in 23, transient global amnesia in 3, and Parkinson's disease in 2. Fourteen controls were also studied. All demented patients and those with Parkinson's disease underwent neuropsychological testing. In all subjects, rCBF in the parietal cortex and hippocampus was evaluated using high-resolution SPECT with HMPAO.

Results.—Compared with controls, patients with dementia of the Alzheimer type and those with multi-infarct dementia had lower rCBF measurements in the parietal cortices and hippocampus bilaterally. Hippocampal hypoperfusion was observed in undemented patients with memory disturbance as well as in those with dementia of any cause, but it was not present in controls. Hypoperfusion in the hippocampus was a more sensitive marker for dementia of the Alzheimer type than was hypoperfusion in the parietal cortex. The severity of dementia and memory disturbance was reflected in degree of hippocampal hypoperfusion, whatever the cause of the patient's dementia.

Conclusion.—Hippocampal perfusion can be evaluated by hexamethylpropyleneamine oxime rCBF high-resolution SPECT. Aging itself had no effect on hippocampal perfusion in normal controls, but patients with memory disturbance had hypoperfusion that correlated with the severity of dementia and deficits in memory. Hippocampal hypoperfusion in patients with dementia of the Alzheimer type was significantly lower than that of nondemented neuropsychiatric patients.

▶ For years, I have occasionally heard neurologists say that the hippocampus is the site where the earliest Alzheimer's changes take place. These authors present data to indicate that we may not have paid enough attention to this region of the brain in the past.

A. Gottschalk, M.D.

Preserved Pontine Glucose Metabolism in Alzheimer Disease: A Reference Region for Functional Brain Image (PET) Analysis
Minoshima S, Frey KA, Foster NL, et al (Univ of Michigan, Ann Arbor)
J Comput Assist Tomogr 19:541–547, 1995   9–7

Background.—When analyzing nonquantitative SPECT or PET data from patients with Alzheimer's disease (AD), examiners often normalize regional metabolic or blood flow values to a reference area that is least affected by or independent of the disease processes. Selecting a reference region, however, may be problematic, as patients with AD have global reductions in cerebral metabolism and blood flow. The regional preservation of energy metabolism in AD and the effects of PET data normalization to reference regions were assessed.

Methods.—Thirty-seven patients with probable AD and 22 healthy individuals were investigated. Regional metabolic rates in the pons, thalamus, putamen, sensorimotor cortex, visual cortex, and cerebellum were determined stereotaxically based on quantitative FDG-PET measures. The metabolic rates of the parietotemporal association cortex and whole brain were normalized to each reference region.

Findings.—The best preservation of glucose metabolism was found in the pons. Metabolism in the other reference regions was relatively preserved compared with the parietotemporal association cortex and whole brain, but metabolism was significantly reduced. Data normalization to the pons increased the significance of metabolic reduction in the parietotemporal association cortex and preserved the presence of global cerebral metabolic decreases indicated in the analysis of the quantitative data.

Conclusion.—In patients with probable AD, energy metabolism is well preserved. The use of the pons as a reference for data normalization will improve diagnostic accuracy and the efficiency of quantitative and nonquantitative functional brain imaging.

▶ Life in the Alzheimer's business used to be relatively easy. Using your old SPECT or PET camera and examining patients with AD (usually highly selected), all you had to find was a hole in the parietotemporal region that you could drive a train through and the diagnosis was secure. Then life got more complicated. Imaging devices got better, the patient selection got more sophisticated, and other diseases that suggested AD but were not began to creep into the patient group.

These authors may have made a key contribution to sorting everything out by providing what seems to be a reasonably constant reference standard (the pons) in brains that are otherwise deteriorating in all directions. They point out that their work, although designed for PET analysis, may apply equally to SPECT.

The same group has developed a 3-dimensional stereotaxic surface system for AD diagnosis,[1] whereas Dr. Page and colleagues from King's Hospital in London use a neural network and brain SPECT to diagnose AD.[2] A group from Perugia in Italy used MR spectroscopy, MRI-based hippocampal volume assessment, and hexamethylpropyleneamine oxime–SPECT for diagnosis.[3] A group from Germany compared PET and SPECT in AD and vascular dementia,[4] and the effect of the region-of-interest selection was studied by a group from Holland.[5]

A. Gottschalk, M.D.

References

1. Minoshima S, Frey KA, Koeppe RA, et al: A diagnostic approach in Alzheimer's disease using three dimensional sterotactic surface projections of fluorine-18-FDG PET. *J Nucl Med* 36:1238–1248, 1995.
2. Page MPA, Howard RJ, O'Brien JT, et al: Use of neural networks in brain SPECT to diagnose Alzheimer's disease. *J Nucl Med* 37:195–200, 1996.
3. Parnetti L, Lowenthal DT, Presciutti O, et al: ¹H-MRS, MRI-based hippocampal volumetry, and ^{99m}Tc-HMPAO-SPECT in normal aging, age-associated memory impairment, and probable Alzheimer's disease. *J Am Geriatr Soc* 44:133–138, 1996.
4. Mielke R, Pietrzyk U, Jacobs A, et al: HMPAO SPECT and FDG PET in Alzheimer's disease and vascular dementia: Comparison of perfusion and metabolic pattern. *Eur J Nucl Med* 21:1052–1060, 1994.
5. Claus JJ, vanHarskamp F, Breteler MMB, et al: Assessment of cerebral perfusion with single-photon emission tomography in normal subjects and in patients with Alzheimer's disease: Effects of region of interest selection. *Eur J Nucl Med* 21:1044–1051, 1994.

Functional MR in the Evaluation of Dementia: Correlation of Abnormal Dynamic Cerebral Blood Volume Measurements With Changes in Cerebral Metabolism on Positron Emission Tomography With Fludeoxyglucose F 18

González RG, Fischman AJ, Guimaraes AR, et al (Massachusetts Gen Hosp, Boston; Harvard Med School, Charleston, Mass; Massachusetts Alzheimer's Disease Research Ctr, Boston)
AJNR 16:1763–1770, 1995

9–8

Introduction.—In differentiating Alzheimer's disease (AD) from other causes of dementia, PET and SPECT are superior to routine anatomical CT and MR. The newly emerged functional MR may provide information similar to that of PET and SPECT. Ten patients with clinical evidence of dementia underwent both PET and functional MR evaluation.

Methods.—The mean patient age was 70.3 years. Patients were injected with between 200 and 300 MBq of FDG during PET scans. Patients undergoing functional MR were injected with 0.2 mmol of gadopentetate dimeglumine per kg. The PET and functional MR studies were quantitatively and qualitatively evaluated.

Results.—After co-registration of the images for each patient, quantitative comparisons were made between the PET and functional MR scans. There were significant correlations in 72 of 74 brain sections. For qualitative analysis, brain images from each patient were categorized into 8 regions. Each region was visibly inspected to determine normal and abnormal PET and functional MR images. Of 80 brain regions, 16 were determined to be abnormal on both PET and functional MR, 46 were normal on both examinations, 10 were judged to be abnormal on PET alone, and 8 were considered abnormal with functional MR alone. The overall agreement between PET and functional MR was highly significant (78%).

Conclusion.—The dynamic cerebral blood volume images obtained from functional MR gave information similar to that of FDG PET images in patients with evidence of dementia. If additional research proves that functional MR is helpful in differentiating between AD and other forms of dementia, this examination could easily be included in standard brain MR evaluation.

▶ For the past few years, functional MR studies that show data similar to those found with FDG have appeared. Note that these authors believe that by correlating MRI with FDG they are demonstrating cerebral metabolism. I suspect this is a major oversimplification. I worry that FDG uptake is primarily related to brain blood flow. If this is true, it is not a very specific indicator of anything, but it may be a common indicator of many types of abnormality. For instance, a South American group found a high frequency of lesions involving the frontal lobe in trauma patients. They discuss this frontal lobe dementia for those of you who are interested.[1] A group from Japan provides data to let you calibrate a standard brain input function using venous blood sampling.[2]

A. Gottschalk, M.D.

References

1. Starkstein SE, Migliorelli R, Teson A, et al: Specificity of changes in cerebral blood flow in patients with frontal lobe dementia. *J Neurol Neurosurg Psychiatry* 57:790–796, 1994.
2. Ito H, Koyama M, Goto R, et al: Cerebral blood flow measurement with iodine-123-IMP SPECT, calibrated standard input function and venous blood sampling. *J Nucl Med* 36:2339–2342, 1995.

SPECT in the Localisation of Extratemporal and Temporal Seizure Foci
Newton MR, Berkovic SF, Austin MC, et al (Univ of Melbourne, Australia)
J Neurol Neurosurg Psychiatry 59:26–30, 1995   9–9

Background.—The surgical treatment of epilepsy is most effective in patients with unilateral temporal lobe epilepsy. In almost all such patients, localizing the focus preoperatively can be done noninvasively. Such localization is difficult in patients with extratemporal and temporal lobe epilepsies with unusual seizure patterns, who must undergo intracranial electroencephalography recordings. The value of SPECT in one series of patients with refractory partial seizures examined by ictal, interictal, or postictal SPECT was explored.

Methods and Findings.—One hundred seventy-seven patients were included. In 119 patients with known unilateral temporal lobe epilepsy, ictal SPECT localization was correct in 97%, compared with 71% with postictal SPECT, and 48% with interictal SPECT. Among patients with known or suspected extratemporal epilepsy, the yield of ictal SPECT was 92%, compared with 46% with postictal studies. Usually, only very early postictal examinations were diagnostic. Interictal SPECT was of little use in this patient group.

Conclusion.—In addition to its value in localizing temporal lobe seizures, ictal SPECT has a high diagnostic yield in a wide range of extratemporal epilepsies. Although true ictal SPECT can be difficult to achieve because of the brevity of many extratemporal seizures, the efforts needed to use it in this setting are justified.

▶ In a large series, these authors clearly demonstrate the value of ictal SPECT for identifying both the temporal and extratemporal seizure foci. They also show that interictal SPECT has very little value. They make no comment about the equipment they use, although the only image they show looks quite crude to me by today's standards using high-resolution multidetector SPECT scanning systems. As a result, we might hope that these excellent results could be improved still further. The interested reader may wish to review an article on the surgery for epilepsy.[1]

A. Gottschalk, M.D.

Reference

1. Engel J: Surgery for seizures. *N Engl J Med* 334:647–652, 1996.

Increased Interictal Cerebral Glucose Metabolism in a Cortical-Subcortical Network in Drug Naive Patients With Cryptogenic Temporal Lobe Epilepsy
Franceschi M, Lucignani G, Del Sole A, et al (Inst H San Raffaele, Milan, Italy; Univ of Milan, Italy; Epilepsy Centre HS Paolo, Milan, Italy)
J Neurol Neurosurg Psychiatry 59:427–431, 1995   9–10

Background.—Although PET with FDG has been used to study cerebral metabolism patterns in different types of epilepsies, its use has not been reported in drug-naive patients with cryptogenic temporal lobe epilepsy. The mechanism of origin and diffusion of the epileptic discharge may differ in these patients from those in patients with other epilepsies.

Methods and Findings.—Thirteen patients aged 17–53 years with cryptogenic temporal lobe epilepsy never treated with antiepileptic agents and 13 age-matched healthy volunteers were assessed. The patients had significant interictal glucose hypermetabolism in a bilateral neural network, including the temporal lobes, thalami, basal ganglia, and cingular cortices. Metabolism in these regions and in the frontal lateral cortex could be used in a discriminant function analysis to correctly classify patients and controls. Bilateral increases in glucose metabolism, ranging from 10% to 15% that of controls (although nonsignificant), occurred in the frontal basal and lateral, temporal mesial, and cerebellar cortices.

Conclusion.—These patients differed from those in previous studies in that the former group had cryptogenic rather than symptomatic temporal lobe epilepsy, had mild illness, and were not taking medication. These differences may explain discrepancies between the current findings and previous ones. The finding of a bilateral hypermetabolic network is not consistent with the notion of well-localized epileptogenic zones in the pathophysiology of cryptogenic temporal lobe epilepsy.

▶ These authors show us that patient selection may have a major impact on the PET (or SPECT) findings in epilepsy.

A. Gottschalk, M.D.

Interictal Metabolism and Blood Flow Are Uncoupled in Temporal Lobe Cortex of Patients With Complex Partial Epilepsy
Gaillard WD, Fazilat S, White S, et al (NIH, Bethesda, Md)
Neurology 45:1841–1847, 1995   9–11

Background.—The relationship of regional cerebral blood flow (rCBF), cerebral glucose metabolic rate (CMRGlc), and oxygen utilization in brain tissues, which are usually tightly coupled, may be altered in some pathologic conditions. It was hypothesized that perfusion and metabolism are uncoupled in interictal epileptogenic temporal cortex.

Methods.—Twenty patients with complex partial seizures underwent PET with FDG and ^{15}O water. Glucose metabolism and blood flow in temporal lobe epileptic foci were identified by ictal scalp-sphenoidal video-electroencephalograph (EEG) telemetry. Twenty minutes after blood flow, glucose metabolism was measured without moving the patient from the scanner. Eleven patients also underwent technetium-99m–hexamethylpropyleneamine oxime (HMPAO) SPECT.

Findings.—The local cerebral metabolic rates of glucose and rCBF were reduced significantly in temporal cortex ipsilateral to the EEG focus. In the inferior lateral and inferior mesial temporal cortex, the local CMGClc was reduced by 11.2% and 11.1%, respectively, whereas rCBF was decreased by only 3.2% and 6.1%, respectively. The ratio of local CMRGlc to rCBF in inferior mesial temporal cortex ipsilateral to the ictal focus was decreased significantly. Blinded raters using standardized criteria found focal FDG-PET hypometabolism in 16 patients, all in the epileptogenic area. Ten patients had focal ^{15}O water PET hypoperfusion, although in 2 patients it was falsely lateralized. Five of 11 patients had focal ^{99m}Tc-HMPAO SPECT hypoperfusion, also falsely lateralized in 2.

Conclusion.—Interictal metabolism and blood flow appear to be uncoupled in epileptic temporal regions. The degree of local CMRGlc reduction and of rCBF in all temporal regions were strongly correlated, but the local CMRGlc-to-rCBF ratio in ipsilateral inferior lateral temporal cortex differed significantly from that in the contralateral region. The difference between mesial and lateral temporal lobe local CMRGlc-to-rCBF may be the result of mesial volume averaging, a greater inclusion of white matter in mesial temporal regions of interest, or the effect of lost projections from sclerotic hippocampus on lateral temporal cortex. Despite reduced metabolism, perfusion is maintained.

▶ More data to further muddy the interictal waters.

A. Gottschalk, M.D.

Role of I-123-Iomazenil SPECT Imaging in Drug Resistant Epilepsy With Complex Partial Seizures

Sjöholm H, Rosén I, Elmqvist D (Univ Hosp, Lund, Sweden)
Acta Neurol Scand 92:41–48, 1995   9–12

Background.—Recent research has shown that benzodiazepine receptors can be imaged with SPECT iodine-123–I-Iomazenil (I-IOM). However, ^{123}I-IOM SPECT does not appear to have any advantages over technetium-99m–hexamethylpropyleneamine oxime (HMPAO) SPECT in patients with focal epilepsy. Sequential ^{123}I-IOM imaging optimized for specific imaging of receptor distribution and maximal contrast between focus and nonfocus locations was described.

Methods.—Fifteen patients with treatment-resistant partial complex seizures and no structural lesions underwent interictal ^{123}I-IOM to assess benzodiazepine receptor distribution and ^{99m}Tc-HMPAO SPECT to assess cerebral blood flow distribution. Scans were obtained immediately, 1 hour and 2 hours after IV injection of ^{123}I-IOM. The relationship between regional abnormalities and seizure onset patterns in electroencephalograms recorded later with implanted subdural strips was determined.

Findings.—Within the first 2 hours after injection, there was a continuous change from an immediate flow-related distribution toward a more specific receptor distribution. Over time, the radioactive decay of ^{123}I in the brain was linear. Elimination was much faster in 2 patients receiving benzodiazepines, who also had no focal abnormalities. Concordant focal benzodiazepine defects were observed in 8 patients with obvious unifocal seizure onset. In these patients, the ^{123}I-IOM scans showed a progressive focus/homotopic nonfocus enhancement over time that was much greater than that on the HMPAO scans. In addition, the estimated focal area of abnormality on the ^{123}I-IOM scans was more restricted than that on the HMPAO scans. Seizure onset patterns were more complex in 5 patients. These patients often had a mismatch between the locations of abnormalities on ^{123}I-IOM and HMPAO scans, but benzodiazepine receptor abnormalities were also more circumscribed.

Conclusion.—Single-photon emission CT with ^{123}I-IOM appears to be more useful than ^{99m}Tc-HMPAO SPECT used interictally in patients with partial complex epilepsy. In addition to showing the hemispheric laterality of the epileptogenic zone, ^{123}I-IOM may demonstrate its anatomical location with greater confidence.

▶ Considering the difficulties encountered in identifying the epileptogenic brain with interictal SPECT using ^{99m}Tc-HMPAO, these authors could be presenting us with a potential tracer improvement. However, with only 15 patients, this should just be considered a good start. I hope these folks will enlarge this series in the future.

A. Gottschalk, M.D.

Single-photon Emission Computed Tomography Using Hexamethylpropyleneamine Oxime in the Prognosis of Acute Cerebral Infarction
Bowler JV, Wade JPH, Jones BE, et al (Charing Cross Hosp, London; Westminster Med School, London)
Stroke 27:82–86, 1996   9–13

Background.—Although SPECT is less useful than CT and MRI in the diagnosis of cerebral infarction, several studies have reported that SPECT provides useful prognostic information. However, the prognostic usefulness of SPECT has not been critically evaluated to determine the uniqueness of this information. Therefore, data from several prognostic tools were collected and analyzed in unselected patients with acute cerebral infarction to determine whether SPECT adds new prognostic information.

Methods.—Fifty consecutive patients with their first cerebral infarction were admitted into the study. Of the 50 patients, 33 completed the study, 10 died during the study, and 7 withdrew. Clinical examinations, using the Canadian Neurological Scale and the Barthel Index (BI), and SPECT were done as soon as possible after admission and repeated at 1 week and 3 months after the onset of the cerebral infaction. Computed tomographic scanning was also done, usually 3–7 days after the infarct. Prediction of the clinical outcome at the third evaluation, as reflected by the Canadian Neurological Scale and BI scores, was analyzed in relation to the Canadian Neurological Scale and BI scores at the first 2 evaluations and CT and SPECT infarct volumes.

Results.—There were significant correlations between clinical outcome and all of the prognostic indicators. However, the correlation coefficients were not high, ranging from 0.57 to 0.74. The Canadian Neurological Scale score at 1 week was the best prognostic indicator and the only significant independent predictor in forward stepwise multiple logistic regression analysis. The SPECT infarct volumes had less predictive power, and CT infarct volumes had the least predictive power.

Conclusions.—Although SPECT findings of infarct volumes did provide prognostic information, it was only slightly more predictive of clinical outcome than CT data and was less accurate than simple clinical assessments. Therefore, SPECT scanning is not recommended in the routine evaluation of patients with cerebral infarction.

▶ This is discouraging news with obvious implications in these times of managed care.

A. Gottschalk, M.D.

Hypofrontality Revisited: A High Resolution Single Photon Emission Computed Tomography Study in Schizophrenia

Ebmeier KP, Lawrie SM, Blackwood DHR, et al (Royal Edinburgh Hosp, Scotland)
J Neurol Neurosurg Psychiatry 58:452–456, 1995   9–14

Background.—Hypofrontality, defined as reduced perfusion or glucose uptake in the prefrontal cortex, has been accepted as a finding diagnostic of schizophrenia. However, this established paradigm has been questioned by some recent evidence. To characterize prefrontal cortical activity in schizophrenia, trace activity in the frontal regions was quantified using SPECT in subgroups of psychotic patients and a control group.

Methods.—Single-photon emission CT was performed with a technetium-99m exametazime tracer in 20 drug-free schizophrenic and schizophreniform patients, 40 neuroleptic-treated patients with schizophrenia or schizophreniform disorder (including 20 with and 20 without a good treatment response), and 20 healthy community volunteers. Uptake count densities were analyzed in several frontal regions in comparison with count densities in the occipital cortex.

Results.—Among the control subjects, there was increased tracer uptake in most of the prefrontal regions, especially on the right side. Among the untreated schizophrenic patients, similar hyperfrontality, particularly on the right side, was found, with reduced uptake in the left inferior cingulate cortex. The treated schizophrenic patients had comparatively nonsignificantly reduced uptake in the frontal areas with significantly reduced uptake only in the mesial frontal regions.

Conclusions.—Global or prefrontal hypofrontality at rest is not a common finding in chronic schizophrenia, regardless of whether it is treated. Localized reduced activity in the mesial frontal and/or anterior cingulate cortex seems a more accurate characteristic of schizophrenia.

▶ Throughout the years that I have reviewed articles for this section of the YEAR BOOK, the relationship between hypofrontality and schizophrenia has been a controversial subject. Consequently, I have always taken definitive arguments on the subject with a grain or two of salt. These folks have a large series going and certainly put a dent in the hypofrontality thesis. However,

I am not convinced that the Strichman scanner used in this study is quite the high-resolution device they think it is. Consequently, I am not putting my salt shaker away just yet.

A. Gottschalk, M.D.

Parieto-occipital Hypoperfusion in Late Whiplash Syndrome: First Quantitative SPET Study Using Technetium-99m Bicisate (ECD)
Otte A, Ettlin T, Fierz L, et al (Univ Hosp Basel, Switzerland; Rehabilitation Clinic, Rheinfelden, Switzerland; Bern, Switzerland)
Eur J Nucl Med 23:72–74, 1996   9–15

Introduction.—Late whiplash syndrome may persist for years after injury. Characteristics of the condition are head and neck pain, visual problems, and cognitive disturbances. A previous report found that most patients with the syndrome exhibit parieto-occipital hypoperfusion. A quantitative study was conducted to compare patients and controls for the presence of parieto-occipital hypoperfusion.

Methods.—Ten patients with whiplash injury resulting from a rear-end car collision had persistent concentration and memory disturbances 1–4 years after the injury. The 11 controls were age-matched normal individuals. Both patients and controls were studied with brain single-photon emission tomography with N,N"-1,2-ethylene-diylbis-L-cysteine diethyl ester dihydrochloride. The patients had normal cranial CT or MRI scans, no clinical evidence of brain injury, no signs of neurovascular or neurodegenerative diseases, and were not receiving vasoactive or neuroactive drugs.

Results.—Imaging results had enabled 2 independent readers unaware of the clinical diagnosis to separate patients from controls on the basis of bilateral parieto-occipital hypoperfusion, observed in all patients. Confirmation was obtained by calculating the perfusion rate of parieto-occipital over global (perfusion index), after drawing elliptical regions of interest in transversal-oblique slices. The difference in perfusion indices between the 2 groups was significant.

Conclusion.—This quantitative study proved that patients with late whiplash syndrome have parietal-occipital hypoperfusion. There was a statistically significant difference between patients and controls in perfusion indices.

▶ Personal injury lawyers might have a love-hate relationship with this type of data. Lawyers whose clients have this problem will love it; those whose do not (possibly with the pecuniary whiplash syndrome) may not be so thrilled.

A. Gottschalk, M.D.

Cerebral Perfusion and Psychometric Testing in Military Amateur Boxers and Controls

Kemp PM, Houston AS, Macleod MA, et al (Royal Naval Hosp, Gosport, Hampshire, England; Inst of Naval Medicine, Alverstoke, Gosport, Hampshire, England)
J Neurol Neurosurg Psychiatry 59:368–374, 1995   9–16

Background.—Dementia pugilistica is characterized by dementia and disordered movement caused by widespread damage throughout the brain. Early subtle damage can be detected with technetium-99m–hexamethyl-propyleneamine oxime (HMPAO) SPECT cerebral perfusion imaging. To assess changes associated with boxing, psychometric testing results and cerebral perfusion were compared in amateur boxers and nonboxing athletes.

Methods.—Thirty-four military amateur boxers and 34 military nonboxing amateur athletes underwent ^{99m}Tc-HMPAO scanning. The images were compared with normal findings derived from images of 50 healthy subjects. In addition, 41 boxers and 27 controls underwent a battery of psychometric tests assessing reaction time, psychomotor learning, reasoning, perception and comparison, short-term memory, and motor function.

Results.—Abnormal perfusion scans were found in 41% of the boxers and 14% of the controls. The abnormalities were typically singular in the control group and multiple in the boxers. The boxers also performed significantly less well on 4 of the 5 psychometric tests, even after adjustment for age and education. Boxers who had fought in more bouts had significantly poorer performance on reaction time and pattern recognition tasks than boxers who had fought in fewer bouts.

Conclusions.—Compared with nonboxers, boxers had significantly greater cerebral perfusion abnormalities and significantly poorer psychometric findings, particularly among those who had fought the most bouts. These findings and those of other studies indicate the risk of neurologic and vascular damage associated with multiple blows to the head (Table 6). Further study is needed to determine the long-term significance of these findings.

▶ If you are like me, you were both impressed by the dignity and saddened by the physical changes Muhammad Ali displayed at the 1996 Summer Olympics. These authors point out that it may be true that more cerebral damage occurs from frequent less damaging blows than from the serious knockout blows to the head that are delivered in boxing. In retrospect, it makes you wonder how good a strategy "rope a dope" really was.

At any rate, it also makes you wonder whether nuclear medicine has a major role to play in monitoring boxers. With the potential of tracers used to look at Parkinson's disease (like iodinated β-CIT described in this volume), or simply cerebral perfusion itself, one could easily argue that neuronuclear medicine should do control studies at the beginning of a career and make a pugilist stop when deterioration is noted. If any of you have a direct channel

TABLE 6.—Major Studies Assessing the Safety of Amateur Boxing

Investigators	Participants	Findings	Comments
Thomassen *et al* DENMARK 1979	53 former boxers 53 footballers	No significant differences on clinical examination, EEG, or psychometric testing.	These findings are confounded by the fact that 88% of the controls and 75% of the boxers sustained head injuries outside the ring.
McLatchie *et al* SCOTLAND 1987	20 active boxers Variable number of controls	Abnormal clinical examination in 35% of boxers, abnormal EEG in 40% of boxers, abnormal psychometric testing in 63% of boxers.	No controls had clinical examination or EEG. University staff used as controls for psychometric testing.
Brooks *et al* SCOTLAND 1987	29 active boxers 19 controls	No significant differences on psychometric testing.	Only 39% of invited boxers participated. Controls matched for age, education, and ethnicity.
Haglund *et al* SWEDEN 1990	50 former boxers 50 athletes	No significant differences on clinical examination, CT, MRI. EEG showed significantly greater abnormalities in boxers.	Although the authors concluded that amateur boxing appeared "safe" the differences on EEG examination remained unexplained.
Butler *et al* ENGLAND 1993	86 active boxers 31 water polo and 47 rugby players	Significant differences between boxers and controls on initial psychometric testing to the detriment of the boxers. Improvement noted on longitudinal assessment. No differences on clinical examination, evoked responses, EEG, CKBB isoenzymes, or ophthalmological assessment.	No allowance for the intellectual differences between the controls (some were university students) and the boxers (many early school leavers). Authors concluded no evidence of damage in boxers.
Stewart *et al* USA 1994	484 amateur boxers	Significant tests of trend between psychometric testing ability and number of bouts. No deterioration on 2 year follow up.	Authors urge caution in the interpretation of the longitudinal findings as a longer latency period may be required before effects are manifest.
Kemp *et al* ENGLAND 1994 (This study)	(i) 34 active boxers 34 controls (ii) 41 active boxers 27 controls	Boxers had significantly more abnormalities on Tc-99m HMPAO cerebral perfusion imaging. Psychometric testing revealed boxers to perform significantly worse than controls and, in addition, those boxers with the greater number of bouts performed significantly worse than those with few bouts.	All invitees participated thus reducing selection bias. Subjects with extraneous head injuries were not included. Controls matched for age and education.

Abbreviations: EEG, electroencephalography; *CKBB*, creatine kinase BB band.
(Courtesy of Kemp PM, Houston AS, Macleod MA, et al: Cerebral perfusion and psychometric testing in military amateur boxers and controls. *J Neurol Neurosurg Psychiatry* 59:368–374, 1995.)

into your local boxing commission, sound them out. You never know—they might buy the idea.

A. Gottschalk, M.D.

Heterogeneous Cerebral Glucose Metabolism in Normal Pressure Hydrocephalus

Tedeschi E, Hasselbalch SG, Waldemar G, et al (Natl Univ Hosp, Copenhagen; Univ of Copenhagen; "Federico II", Naples, Italy)
J Neurol Neurosurg Psychiatry 59:608–615, 1995   9–17

Background.—The normal pressure hydrocephalus (NPH) syndrome is a form of dementia that is potentially treatable with CSF shunt surgery or CSF evacuation by repeated lumbar punctures. However, the treatment response is highly variable. It was hypothesized that patients with NPH would have different patterns of regional cerebral glucose ($rCMR_{glu}$) metabolism, as measured by PET with FDG, which would correspond to the underlying degenerative process. To test this hypothesis, patterns of $rCMR_{glu}$ were investigated with PET-FDG in patients with NPH and were correlated with clinical symptom severity, histologic findings, and response to shunting.

Methods.—Eighteen consecutive patients with idiopathic NPH and 11 neurologically normal volunteers underwent cranial PET-FDG. Regional CMR_{glu} was measured and left-right and anterior-posterior asymmetry ratios were calculated in 3 regions: frontal, temporal, and parietal. The patients also underwent clinical examination and a lumboventricular perfusion test. A small biopsy was obtained from the right superior frontal cortex and the underlying white matter in the patients and was examined histologically and immunohistochemically to determine the prevalent pathology. The clinical status of the patients was determined 9 months after they underwent a shunt operation.

Results.—The shunt operation yielded clinical improvement in 6 patients, no clinical change in 8 patients, and symptom progression in 3 patients. In overall comparisons between the patient and control groups, $rCMR_{glu}$ was significantly reduced in the entire cortex; in the frontal, temporal, parietal, and occipital lobes; and in the central gray and white matter. There were no significant differences between the 2 groups in asymmetry ratios. Although there was $rCMR_{glu}$ reduction in the patient group as a whole, this reduction was extremely inhomogeneous. Among individuals, both focal and diffuse significant reductions were seen and asymmetry ratios were unpredictably distributed throughout the cortex. No characteristic patterns of metabolic abnormalities could be seen in the patient group, whether classified by histologic findings, lumboventricular perfusion findings, or response to the shunt. There were specific correlations between the severity of dementia and $rCMR_{glu}$ reductions in the central gray matter and the frontal cortex.

Conclusions.—Patients with NPH demonstrate heterogeneous patterns of metabolic abnormalities throughout the cortex as well as heterogeneous histopathologic changes, suggesting that NPH is nonspecifically related to many of degenerative disorders.

▶ For years I have argued that the diagnostic yield from the radionuclide cisternogram was somewhere between very limited and useless. These authors now present data to indicate how this can be true. They conclude that NPH is not specifically associated with a single degenerative change, but rather has multiple metabolic and histopathologic underpinnings. It is no wonder we cannot find a consistent diagnostic set of criteria that work regularly.

A. Gottschalk, M.D.

Abnormal Gallium-67 Skull Uptake: A Sign of Peripheral Marrow Activation in HIV-positive Patients With Disseminated Mycobacterioses
del Val Gomez M, Gallardo FG, Cobo J, et al (Inst of Health Carlos III, Madrid)
J Nucl Med 36:2211–2213, 1995   9–18

Background.—The improved life expectancy in patients with HIV infection has brought an increased incidence of mycobacterioses. The diagnosis of mycobacteriosis is often challenging, particularly in patients with disseminated disease, who may have nonspecific clinical symptoms. The

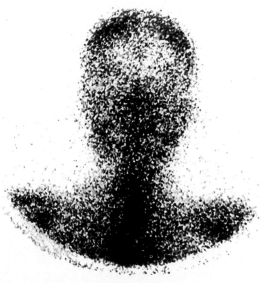

FIGURE 1.—Abnormal gallium-67 skull uptake in an AIDS patient with fever of unknown origin. Bone marrow culture was positive for *Myocobacterium avium*. (Reprinted with permission of the Society of Nuclear Medicine, from del Val Gomez M, Gallardo FG, Cobo J, et al: Abnormal gallium-67 skull uptake: A sign of peripheral marrow activation in HIV-positive patients with disseminated mycobacterioses. *J Nucl Med* 36:2211–2213, 1995.)

diagnostic significance of altered gallium-67 uptake in skull bone marrow was investigated in patients with HIV and disseminated mycobacterial infection.

Methods.—The ^{67}Ga skull scans of 39 HIV-positive patients with mycobacterioses and of 15 HIV-positive patients without mycobacterioses were analyzed. The diagnosis of mycobacteriosis was established by culture, chest roentgenogram, or biopsy. Of the 39 patients with mycobacterioses, disease was disseminated in 29 patients and focal in 10.

Results.—There was skull uptake of ^{67}Ga (Fig 1) in 24 of the 29 patients with disseminated mycobacterioses (82%), 1 of the 10 patients with localized tuberculosis (who was found to have peripheral leukoerythroblastosis), and 1 patient in the control group (who was found to have Burkitt's lymphoma with bone marrow involvement). In the diagnosis of disseminated mycobacterioses in patients with HIV infection, skull uptake of ^{67}Ga had a sensitivity of 82% and specificity of 92%.

Conclusions.—Assessment of bone marrow uptake of ^{67}Ga may have clinical usefulness in the diagnosis of mycobacteriosis, particularly disseminated disease, in patients with AIDS who have a fever of unknown origin. The abnormal skull uptake of ^{67}Ga may indicate peripheral marrow activation and expanded bone marrow, which could also be related to other conditions, including hematologic diseases or leishmaniasis.

▶ The authors present an interesting observation. I suspect the sensitivity and specificity figures given relate to the patient population selected. However, these data would certainly indicate that you should not pass off this finding as a "normal variant." These data certainly indicate that finding the skull uptake has diagnostic utility.

A. Gottschalk, M.D.

Importance of the Lateral View in the Evaluation of Suspected Brain Death
Spieth M, Abella E, Sutter C, et al (Univ of California, Sacramento; King/Drew Med Ctr, Los Angeles)
Clin Nucl Med 20:965–968, 1995   9–19

Background.—The criteria for brain death are met when both cerebral activity and cerebellar activity are absent. Two cases presented here failed to meet criteria for whole brain death when cerebellar activity was demonstrated on lateral images. These cases confirm the importance of technetium-99m–hexamethylpropyleneamine oxime (HMPAO) in evaluating brain death and the need to obtain lateral views before brain death is declared.

Case Report.—Man, 18, was admitted with a self-inflicted gunshot wound to the head. The bullet had lodged in the left parieto-occipital region. After initial improvement, his condition deteriorated 6 days after the injury. The patient met all criteria for clinical brain death the following day and underwent a nuclear medicine cerebral perfusion study using ^{99m}Tc-HMPAO. Flow images indicated no cerebral flow in the anterior and middle cerebral arteries. Although the delayed anterior image revealed no cerebral activity, cerebellar activity was apparent on lateral images. This unusual finding meant that the patient did not meet criteria for whole brain death.

Discussion.—The second patient showed similar cerebellar activity in the lateral images, and there have been other reports of cerebellar activity when cerebral activity was absent. This finding reverses in 24–48 hours, and repeat imaging should confirm brain death. Timing is critical for radionuclide cerebral angiograms, because an image obtained too soon may give a false sense of hope, whereas delay may allow the organs of a potential donor to be damaged. The presence of cerebellar perfusion without cerebral perfusion challenges the current criteria for brain death.

▶ These folks have made a good observation.

A. Gottschalk, M.D.

Assessment of Brain SPECT: Report of the Therapeutics and Technology Assessment Subcommittee of the American Academy of Neurology
Altrocchi PH, Brin M, Ferguson JH, et al (Therapeutics and Technology Subcommittee, American Academy of Neurology, Minneapolis)
Neurology 46:278–285, 1996   9–20

Introduction.—The American Academy of Neurology's Therapeutics and Technology Assessment Subcommittee requested an assessment of the clinical usefulness of brain SPECT. This neuroimaging technique is less expensive, although less accurate, than PET. It measures regional cerebral blood flow, which is typically highly correlated with brain metabolism, providing functional data not assessed by conventional CT or MRI.
Methods.—The current literature on brain SPECT applications in neurologic disorders was reviewed. The comments of 13 reviewers were combined in a preliminary draft, which was modified by a panel of 12 experts and by the opinions of the Academy members.
Findings.—Published studies have reported several established, promising, and investigational uses of SPECT in the evaluation of neurologic disorders (Table). Brain SPECT has good sensitivity and specificity in the localization of ischemic stroke. It shows promise in the classification of stroke subtypes, which has clinical significance, because different subtypes require different management strategies. The detection of vasospasm-related ischemia after subarachnoid hemorrhage is another promising use. Investigational uses of brain SPECT in stroke include prognostic evaluation, therapeutic monitoring, and the diagnosis and prognostic evaluation

TABLE.—Summary of the Effectiveness of SPECT for Brain Applications

Application	Rating	Quality of evidence	Strength of evidence
Stroke			
Detection of acute ischemia	Established	Class II	Type B
Determination of stroke subtypes	Promising	Class II	Type C
Vasospasm following SAH	Promising	Class II	Type B
Prognosis/recovery from stroke	Investigational	Class II	Type C
Monitoring therapies	Investigational	Class III	Type C
Diagnosis of TIA	Investigational	Class III	Type C
Prognosis of TIA	Investigational	Class II	Type C
Neoplasm			
Grading of gliomas	Investigational	Class III	Type C
Differentiating radiation necrosis from tumor recurrence	Investigational	Class II	Type B
HIV encephalopathy	Investigational	Class II	Type B
Head trauma	Investigational	Class II	Type C
Epilepsy			
Presurgical ictal detection of seizure focus	Established	Class II	Type B
Localization of seizure focus	Promising	Class II	Type C
Differential diagnosis of ictus	Investigational	Class III	Type C
Interictal detection of seizure focus	Investigational	Class III	Type C
Determination of seizure subtypes	Investigational	Class III	Type C
Receptor studies	Investigational	Class III	Type C
Monitoring therapy	Doubtful	Class III	Type D
Alzheimer's disease			
To support clinical diagnosis	Established	Class II	Type B
Huntington's chorea	Investigational	Class III	Type C
Persistent vegetative state	Investigational	Class III	Type C
Brain death	Promising	Class III	Type C

Abbreviations: SAH, subarachnoid hemorrhage; *TIA*, transient ischemic attack.
(Reprinted from *Neurology*, Altrocchi PH, Brin M, Ferguson JH, et al: Assessment of brain SPECT: Report of the therapeutics and technology assessment subcommittee of the American Academy of Neurology. *Neurology* 46:278–285, 1996, by permission of Little, Brown and Co.)

of transient ischemic attacks (although this application depends on timely performance). Brain SPECT has been investigated, and should be investigated further, to differentiate between radiation necrosis and tumor recurrence and to determine glioma grading. The early diagnosis of HIV encephalopathy may be possible with SPECT scans. Although further larger studies are needed, SPECT may be useful in the investigation of closed head trauma or postconcussion syndrome. In the evaluation of patients with epilepsy, SPECT has been established in the preoperative detection of a seizure focus and shows promise in localizing the focus. Also being investigated is the use of SPECT in the differential diagnosis in these patients, for the interictal detection of seizure focus, for subtype classification, and for receptor studies, which could improve localization of seizure focus. Use of SPECT has established value in providing supporting evidence of Alzheimer's disease and may differentiate between Alzheimer's disease and the pseudodementia of depression. It is a promising technique in establishing a diagnosis of death on neurologic criteria. Other investigational applications include establishing an early diagnosis of Huntington's chorea and prognostically evaluating patients in a persistent vegetative state.

Conclusions.—Brain SPECT seems to have numerous and evolving clinical applications in the evaluation of neurologic disorders. Its cost-effectiveness should be further studied.

▶ This is not the type of article I usually put in the YEAR BOOK OF NUCLEAR MEDICINE. However, in these days of managed care, this report may be used heavily by health care providers. It could be useful to you because it may provide guidelines for your own institution. On the other hand, if you are now actively involved doing something in the "doubtful" category, you should be prepared to make a good argument explaining why you think this subcommittee was wrong.

A. Gottschalk, M.D.

10 Cardiovascular Nuclear Medicine

Introduction

Nuclear cardiology continues its rapid evolution. Although the dominant procedure is stress perfusion imaging, a topic that occupies most of the abstracts in this chapter, metabolic imaging and evaluation of innervation with metaiodobenzylguanidine are also growing. In this era in which techniques must demonstrate their role in clinical decision making, perfusion imaging is particularly well situated. An article on managed care and the future of nuclear cardiology addresses this issue. Several articles evaluate prognosis and the clinical value of perfusion imaging. Assessment of viability is another area where perfusion imaging excels. Evidence now suggests that radionuclide-determined viability is less specific than echocardiography as a predictor of wall motion improvement after revascularization. However, revascularization of radionuclide viable zones correlates with decreased mortality (confirming once again the importance of ischemia as a prognostic factor in patients with coronary disease).

A thought-provoking article describes a lower contrast between normal and ischemic zones with technetium tetrofosmin. Despite these disturbing findings, many laboratories have switched to this agent. Perhaps this problem can be overcome by increasing the duration of exercise after injection. Enhancements to perfusion imaging, such as attenuation correction, dual tracer imaging, and recording short acquisition gated SPECT studies all attest to the continuing, vigorous health of radionuclide techniques in the evaluation of patients with heart disease.

H. William Strauss, M.D.

Regional Myocardial Blood Flow, Glucose Utilization and Contractile Function Before and After Revascularization and Ultrastructural Findings in Patients With Chronic Coronary Artery Disease

Maes A, Flameng W, Borgers M (KU Leuven, Belgium; Janssen Research Found, Beerse, Belgium; Univ Limburg, The Netherlands)
Eur J Nucl Med 22:1299–1305, 1995   10–1

Background.—Positron emission tomography is a noninvasive tool that can be used in clinical settings to predict improvement in myocardial contractility in poorly contracting myocardial segments. Follow-up measures of myocardial blood flow, metabolism, and function were correlated with histologic findings in patients with chronic coronary artery disease (CAD).

Methods.—Forty-one patients with chronic CAD and a severely stenosed left anterior descending coronary artery underwent PET flow/metabolism study and nuclear angiography just before and 3 months after bypass surgery. At surgery, biopsy specimens were obtained from the left ventricular anterior wall. Control biopsies were obtained from donor hearts used for transplantation and from the hearts of patients with a defect of the atrial septum.

Findings.—The 41 patients were divided into 3 groups: 11 (group A) had apparently normal flow values in the biopsy area; 15 (group B) had a mismatch pattern; and 15 (group C) had a match pattern in the biopsy area. Group B had significantly improved flow and regional contractile function. Compared with preoperative values, glucose utilization was significantly reduced. Groups A and C had no significant changes in flow, metabolism, or function. Control biopsy specimens showed significantly fewer myolytic cells than did specimens obtained from groups B and C. Control specimens also had less fibrosis than those obtained from group C. Linear relationships were documented between flow and both percentage fibrosis and regional anterior ejection fraction after surgery. Significant recovery of flow and function after revascularization, with a disappearance of enhanced glucose uptake, was documented only in mismatch areas.

Conclusions.—After revascularization, mismatched areas showed significant recovery of flow and function and a significant reduction in glucose utilization. In patients with this pattern, flow value improvement resulted in a better linear relationship between flow and percentage fibrosis after surgery. The association of regional ejection fraction and percentage fibrosis after surgery remained low, probably because of delayed functional recovery in viable areas. Before and after surgery, impairment of regional myocardial blood flow, metabolism, and function persisted in match areas.

▶ This article presents more evidence that FDG uptake correlates with tissue that can contract after revascularization. The authors also make the important correlation between flow and percentage fibrosis after surgery. As a result, the percent improvement in function should have a better correlation with the degree of decreased perfusion than with the degree of FDG uptake. However, FDG uptake will be necessary to identify those zones with residual viable myocardium that have severely decreased perfusion.

H.W. Strauss, M.D.

Assessment of Myocardial Perfusion and Viability With Technetium-99m Methoxyisobutylisonitrile and Thallium-201 Rest Redistribution in Chronic Coronary Artery Disease
Rossetti C, Landoni C, Lucignani G, et al (Univ of Milan, Italy; "I Monzino" Found, Milan, Italy)
Eur J Nucl Med 22:1306–1312, 1995   10–2

Background.—Thallium-201, long the tracer used for myocardial perfusion studies in patients with coronary artery disease, is being replaced by other radiotracers such as technetium-99m–labeled methoxyisobutylisonitrile (MIBI). A number of different techniques have been used to identify areas of viable myocardium within perfusion resting defects, with FDG used as the reference method. Thallium-201 rest-redistribution and FDG were compared for their ability to identify areas of viable myocardium within ^{99m}Tc-MIBI perfusion defects.

Methods.—The study included 27 patients with chronic coronary artery disease in stable condition and regional dysfunction of the left ventricular wall. The patients all had more than 50% reduction in the diameter of at least 1 major coronary artery, confirmed Q-wave myocardial infarction more than 4 weeks previously, and moderately depressed left ventricular function. All patients underwent 4 scintigraphic studies: stress and rest ^{99m}Tc-MIBI studies, ^{201}Tl rest-redistribution SPECT, and FDG PET. Matched tomographic images were used to divide the left ventricle into 11 segments, and that showing the greatest activity under stress was used as the reference, i.e., activity = 100%. Any perfusion defects on rest ^{99m}Tc-MIBI scanning were classified as mild, moderate, or severe, i.e., activity = 60% to 85%, 50% to 60%, or less than 50%. If FDG and rest-redistributed ^{201}Tl uptake was greater than 50% of the reference segment, it was defined as significant.

Results.—There were 33 segments with severe ^{99m}Tc-MIBI rest perfusion defects, 37 with moderate defects, and 134 with mild defects. Significant FDG uptake was noted in 64% of severe perfusion defects, 78% of moderate defects, and 96% of mild defects. Significant ^{201}Tl rest-redistributed uptake was observed in 30% of severe defects, 83% of moderate defects, and 98% of severe defects. In the severely impaired segments, ^{201}Tl rest-redistribution was less sensitive but approximately as specific as FDG in detecting viable myocardium.

Conclusions.—In patients with chronic coronary artery disease, the severity of ^{99m}Tc-MIBI perfusion defects is inversely correlated with the uptake of rest-redistributed ^{201}Tl and FDG. In left ventricular segments with mild to moderate perfusion defects, both tracers are adequate markers of myocardial variability. In segments with more severe defects, ^{201}Tl may underestimate viability, compared with FDG.

▶ This paper is important because it evaluates patients with ejection fractions averaging 43%. Previous work has suggested a greater sensitivity of FDG imaging in patients with severely impaired ventricular function compared with studies utilizing Tl redistribution imaging. In this study of patients with moderate impairment of ventricular function, these investigators showed a far lower sensitivity with sestamibi. These data suggest that Tl should be used when an assessment of viability is missing. An alternative may be to administer nitroglycerin before the rest ^{99m}Tc-MIBI scan to enhance the detection of viable tissue.

H.W. Strauss, M.D.

Delineation of Myocardial Stunning and Hibernation by Positron Emission Tomography in Advanced Coronary Artery Disease
Conversano A, Walsh JF, Geltman EM, et al (Edward Mallinckrodt Inst of Radiology, St Louis; Washington Univ, St Louis)
Am Heart J 131:440–450, 1996   10–3

Introduction.—In many patients with chronic coronary artery disease, left ventricular function commonly improves spontaneously or after coro-

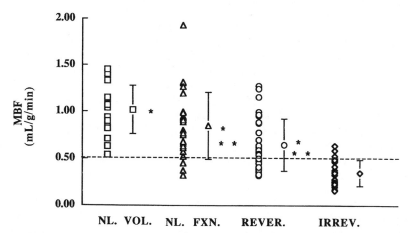

FIGURE 2.—Individual and average values (and 1 standard deviation) for myocardial blood flow (*MBF*) in myocardial segments exhibiting normal function ([*NL FXN*]; *triangle; n* = 25), reversible dysfunction ([*REVER*]; *circle; n* = 32), and irreversible dysfunction ([*IRREV*] *diamond; n* = 23) from assessments of systolic function in response to coronary revascularization. Segmental values for 19 normal volunteers are shown as well (average = 1.02 ± 0.26 mL/mg per minute). *Dotted line* at 0.50 mL/g per minute, 2 SD below mean for controls and was used as a cutoff to define abnormally low values in patients. The range of flow in reversibly dysfunctional segments is wide. Twenty segments exhibited values within the normal range; 12 exhibited flow values > 2 SD below mean for controls. *P < 0.0001 compared with irreversibly dysfunctional segments. **P < 0.0004 compared with normal volunteers. (Courtesy of Conversano A, Walsh JF, Geltman EM, et al: Delineation of myocardial stunning and hibernation by positron emission tomography in advanced coronary artery disease. *Am Heart J* 131:440–450, 1996.)

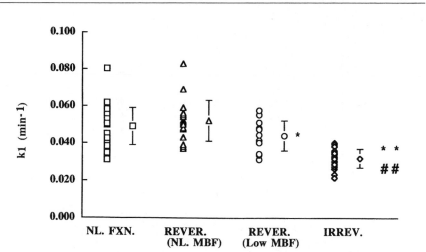

FIGURE 3.—Average values and standard deviations for measurements of myocardial oxygen consumption in reversibly dysfunctional (*REVER*) segments that exhibited normal myocardial blood flow (*NL MBF*) or reduced blood flow (*Low MBF*). Measurements in segments exhibiting normal contractile function (*NL FXN*) or irreversible dysfunction (*IRREV*) are included for comparison. In reversibly dysfunctional segments with preserved perfusion, oxygen consumption was comparable with that measured in segments with normal function. In contrast, in reversibly dysfunctional segments with reduced perfusion (i.e., hibernating), oxygen consumption was reduced compared with that observed in reversibly dysfunctional segments with maintained perfusion. *$P < 0.03$ compared with normal or reversibly dysfunctional segments with normal flow. **$P < 0.0001$ compared with normal segments or reversibly dysfunctional segments with preserved flow. ##$P < 0.001$ compared with reversibly dysfunctional segments with reduced flow. (Courtesy of Conversano A, Walsh JF, Geltman EM, et al: Delineation of myocardial stunning and hibernation by positron emission tomography in advanced coronary artery disease. *Am Heart J* 131:400–450, 1996.)

nary revascularization. However, the precise myocardial perfusion abnormality responsible for this reversible resting systolic dysfunction is unknown. Myocardial hibernation—a proposed adaptive state in which myocardial function is depressed in response to a persistent reduction in myocardial blood flow—has not been definitively demonstrated in humans. Myocardial stunning has been well demonstrated, but its contribution to reversible myocardial dysfunction remains unclear. The flow abnormalities causing reversible left ventricular dysfunction were investigated in PET studies of patients with chronic coronary artery disease.

Methods.—The study included 17 patients with left ventricular wall motion abnormalities resulting from coronary artery disease. All underwent cardiac catheterization and selective coronary angiography, followed by a coronary revascularization procedure. However, before cardiac revascularization, PET was performed to determine regional myocardial perfusion, oxygen consumption, and glucose metabolism at rest. The flow and metabolic characteristics of segments in which mechanical function improved after revascularization were analyzed.

Results.—Of 80 segments available for analysis, 25 were normal, 23 were irreversibly dysfunctional, and 32 were reversibly dysfunctional. The flow rate in the reversibly dysfunctional segments ranged from 0.32 to 1.25 mL/g per minute (Fig 2). Twenty segments showed preservation of

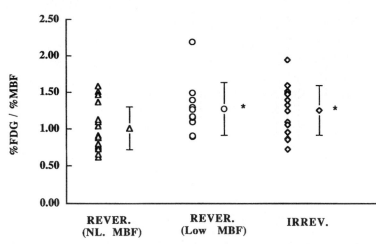

FIGURE 4.—Average values and standard deviations for measurements of myocardial glucose metabolism normalized to flow in reversibly dysfunctional segments (*REVER*) that exhibited normal myocardial blood flow (*NL MBF*) or reduced myocardial blood flow (*Low MBF*). Measurements in segments with irreversible dysfunction (*IRREV*) are included for comparison. By definition, measurements in segments exhibiting normal contractile function exhibited value of 1. In reversibly dysfunctional segments with preserved perfusion, glucose metabolism normalized to flow was comparable with that measured in segments with normal function. In contrast, in reversibly dysfunctional segments with reduced perfusion, glucose metabolism was increased relative to flow compared with that observed in reversibly dysfunctional segments with maintained perfusion. *$P < 0.02$ compared with normal segments or reversibly dysfunctional segments with preserved flow. (Courtesy of Conversano A, Walsh JF, Geltman EM, et al: Delineation of myocardial stunning and hibernation by positron emission tomography in advanced coronary artery disease. *Am Heart J* 131:440–450, 1996.)

flow, which was accompanied by preservation of myocardial oxygen consumption and no changes in myocardial substrate usage. The remaining 12 dysfunctional segments had reduced flow compared with age-matched controls. These segments showed decreased oxygen consumption (Fig 3) and increased myocardial glucose usage (Fig 4).

Conclusion.—In patients with chronic coronary artery disease, reversibly dysfunctional left ventricular segments show a variety of resting flow abnormalities on PET studies. Many of these segments have normal myocardial perfusion at rest, suggesting that the reversibility of their mechanical dysfunction arises not from myocardial hibernation but from intermittent myocardial stunning. Further studies of the flow abnormalities underlying left ventricular mechanical dysfunction will help in the development of new pharmacologic and mechanical treatment approaches.

▶ There are 2 aspects to the Holy Grail of myocardial viability: (1) detection of viable tissue, and (2) prediction of restored function. When perfusion is near normal and myocardium is dysfunctional, revascularization will usually result in improved function. However, when function is impaired, the relationship of FDG uptake to perfusion has been used to identify patients who would benefit from revascularization. This article suggests that oxidated metabolism, derived from carbon-11 acetate measurements, appears to be a better predictor than the relationship of segmental glucose metabolism to myocardial blood flow. As a result, acetate may be the wave of the future.

H.W. Strauss, M.D.

Comparison of Defect Size Between Thallium-201 and Technetium-99m Tetrofosmin Myocardial Single-photon Emission Computed Tomography in Patients With Single-vessel Coronary Artery Disease
Matsunari I, Fujino S, Taki J, et al (Fukui Prefectural Hosp, Japan; Kanazawa Univ, Japan)
Am J Cardiol 77:350–354, 1996   10–4

Background.—Thallium-201 myocardial imaging is an established method for detecting and predicting the prognosis of coronary artery disease. However, its low photon energy and relatively long half-life are disadvantages. Technetium-99m–labeled tetrofosmin has been proposed as an alternative to thallium-201. Whether defect sizes differ between ^{99m}Tc-tetrofosmin and ^{201}Tl myocardial perfusion images in patients with 1-vessel coronary artery disease was investigated.

Methods.—Sixteen men and 4 women aged 46–77 years were included in the study. Exercise-reinjection ^{201}Tl SPECT and exercise-rest ^{99m}Tc-tetrofosmin SPECT imaging were done in each patient. The left ventricular myocardium was divided into 20 segments based on 3 short-axis slices from the apical, middle, and basal ventricular levels for visual analysis. For quantitative analysis, a square region of interest was placed on the center of each segment used in visual analysis. Relative regional activity to the normal reference region was then calculated.

Findings.—Exercise ^{99m}Tc-tetrofosmin imaging depicted a smaller defect size than exercise (6.9 ± 3.9 vs. 8.8 ± 3.0) ^{201}Tl imaging by visual image interpretation. However, the defect size on ^{99m}Tc-tetrofosmin images was similar to that on reinjection ^{201}Tl images. In the quantitative analysis, mean defect sizes during exercise were smaller on ^{99m}Tc-tetrofosmin SPECT than those on ^{201}Tl SPECT at all tested threshold cutoff points, ranging from 50% to 70%. Defect sizes did not differ significantly between rest ^{99m}Tc-tetrofosmin and reinjection ^{201}Tl imaging.

Conclusions.—Exercise ^{99m}Tc-tetrofosmin SPECT defect size in visual or quantitative analyses may be smaller than that on exercise ^{201}Tl SPECT. However, estimated defect sizes between rest ^{99m}Tc-tetrofosmin and reinjection ^{201}Tl imaging are comparable. Thus clinicians must interpret exercise ^{99m}Tc-tetrofosmin images cautiously.

▶ The reason for the smaller lesion size is unclear, but slower blood clearance of tetrofosmin may account for this difference. The lesions might be the same size if exercise were continued for 2 minutes after injection rather than 1 minute. An additional concern with this study is the short duration of exercise. It is likely that the investigators stopped the stress test at the onset of ischemia rather than allowing it to continue. If that is the case, they would have minimized the sensitivity of perfusion imaging.

H.W. Strauss, M.D.

Assessment of Myocardial Area at Risk by Technetium-99m Sestamibi During Coronary Artery Occlusion: Comparison Between Three Tomographic Methods of Quantification

Ceriani L, Verna E, Giovanella L, et al (Ospedale Regionale, Varese, Italy; Univ of Pavia, Italy; Univ of Milan, Italy)
Eur J Nucl Med 23:31–39, 1996   10–5

Background.—Quantifying the degree of myocardium at risk in patients with acute myocardial ischemia is of great value in prognostically stratifying patients with coronary artery disease (CAD). Many quantitative methods for analyzing tomographic images have been described to assess perfusion defect size. The reliability of 3 quantitative methods of technetium-99m–labeled sestamibi image analysis was determined by directly comparing them in patients with selective balloon-induced transmural ischemia.

Methods.—Nineteen patients were included. Single-vessel percutaneous transluminal coronary angioplasty was performed by injecting the ^{99m}Tc-sestamibi at the time of coronary artery occlusion during inflation of the balloon. After imaging, 11 patients were classified as having anteroseptal defects (group 1) and 8 as having posterolateral defects (group 2). The planimetric method based on polar maps proposed by Verani et al. (method A), that described by Tamaki et al. (method B), and that validated by O'Conner et al. (method C) were compared. The limits of the perfusion defect were defined by threshold values of 45%, 50%, and 60% of the maximum left ventricular count.

Findings.—The mean values of the area at risk (AR) determined by the 3 methods using the original cutoff differed significantly. The mean values of the AR estimated by the 3 methods using the same cutoffs did not differ significantly. The best correlation among the techniques resulted from the use of 60% of the maximum left ventricular count. However, a difference of more than 10% between the AR values assessed by the 3 methods was documented in 4 patients. The 3 methods did not differ significantly between groups 1 and 2 in the assessment of AR. All methods had good reproducibility (Fig 5).

Conclusions.—The 3 methods compared in the analysis of the AR by ^{99m}Tc-sestamibi SPECT imaging performed comparably and had good reproducibility when the same cutoff level was used. Defect location did not affect the comparability of the 3 methods. A cutoff level of 60% for all 3 methods was recommended.

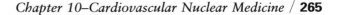

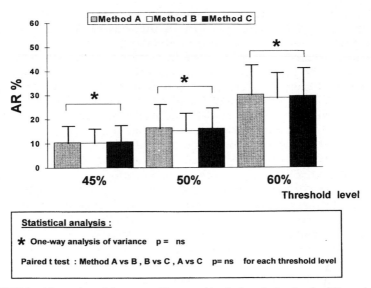

FIGURE 5.—Mean values of the area at risk assessed by the 3 methods using the different threshold levels and results of the statistical analysis. *Abbreviation: AR*, area at risk. (Courtesy of Ceriani L, Verna E, Giovanella L, et al: Assessment of mycocardial area at risk by technetium-99m sestamibi during coronary artery occlusion: Comparison between three tomographic methods of quantification. *Eur J Nucl Med* 23:31–39, 1996. Copyright Springer-Verlag.)

► The authors performed a very interesting study, but they missed a major opportunity to answer a key question about the importance of tracer clearance on lesion size. They could have also correlated the lesion extent with the duration of occlusion and the presence of angiographic collaterals. However, by adjusting the threshold values, lesions can be made to appear of comparable size.

H.W. Strauss, M.D.

Exercise Myocardial Perfusion SPECT in Patients Without Known Coronary Artery Disease: Incremental Prognostic Value and Use in Risk Stratification
Hachamovitch R, Berman DS, Kiat H, et al (Cedars-Sinai Med Ctr, Los Angeles; Univ of California, Los Angeles)
Circulation 93:905–914, 1996   10–6

Background.—Many studies have documented the incremental prognostic value of nuclear testing in patients with coronary artery disease. However, there have been no studies of the incremental prognostic value of myocardial perfusion scintigraphy in a homogeneous population without previously documented coronary artery disease.
Methods.—Two thousand two hundred consecutive patients were studied. None had undergone catheterization, coronary artery bypass surgery,

or percutaneous transluminal coronary angioplasty at the time of dual-isotope SPECT. None had a history of previous myocardial infarction. Patients were followed for a mean of 566 days.

Findings.—Nuclear testing added incremental prognostic value after inclusion of the most predictive clinical exercise variable according to assessment of clinical, exercise, and nuclear models using pre-exercise tolerance testing (ETT), post-ETT, and nuclear information in a stepwise Cox proportional hazards model and receiver-operating characteristic curve analysis. In a multiple logistic regression analysis, scan information contributed 95% of the information on referral to catheterization, with additional data provided by initial symptoms and exercise-induced ischemia. Rates of referral to early catheterization and revascularization paralleled rates of hard event (cardiac death and myocardial infarction) in all scan categories. Referral rates were very low in patients with normal scan results, and the rates of referral as a function of worsening scan results were significantly increased. Even after stratification by clinical and exercise variables, nuclear scan findings further stratified patient subgroups by risk, demonstrating clinical incremental value (Table 9).

Conclusions.—In patients with no evidence of previous coronary artery disease and at low risk overall, myocardial perfusion SPECT provides incremental prognostic information and permits risk stratification, even

TABLE 9.—Hard Event Rates in Patient Subgroups

	Normal	Scan Result Mildly Abnormal	Severely Abnormal
Pre-ETT LK CAD			
Low	0.1% (817)	2.0% (101)	9.2% (65)†
Int	0.1% (724)	6.6% (167)	9.0% (89)†
High	0.0% (79)	3.3% (30)	15% (41)†
Post-ETT LK CAD			
Low	0.1% (892)	2.5% (120)	10.4% (48)†
Int	0.3% (611)	5.2% (134)	7.6% (79)†
High	1.7% (117)	9.1% (44)	13.2% (68)†
Symptoms			
Nonanginal	0.4% (1181)	4.2% (191)	8.0% (113)†
Anginal	0.0% (439)	5.6% (107)	13.4% (82)†
Sex			
Men	0.4% (907)	3.7% (218)	6.3% (207)†
Women	0.3% (710)	7.8% (102)	19.2% (52)*†
Age			
Young	0.0% (378)	4.3% (47)	8.3% (24)†
Middle-aged	0.4% (905)	4.0% (573)	4.6% (131)†
Old	0.6% (341)	7.0% (100)	14.4% (104)†

Note: Values represent hard event rate (N). Young are less than 55 years of age; middle-aged, 55–70 years of age; old, greater than 70 years of age. *Low* <0.15; *Int (intermediate)* 0.15–0.85; and *high*, >0.85.
* Significant difference in hard event rate within group(s) in same scan category (P < 0.05).
† Significant increase in hard event rate as a function of scan result (P < 0.05).
Abbreviations: ETT, exercise tolerance testing; *LK*, likelihood; *CAD*, coronary artery disease.
(Reproduced with permission from Hachamovitch R, Berman DS, Kiat H, et al: Exercise myocardial perfusion SPECT in patients without known coronary artery disease: Incremental prognostic value and use in risk stratification. *Circulation* 93:905–914, Copyright 1996, American Heart Association.)

after clinical and exercise information is available. Referring physicians apparently use this test to select patients to be referred to catheterization or revascularization.

▶ A major point made by this paper is the value of myocardial perfusion data to referring clinicians, when they believe the result. The usefulness of perfusion imaging depends on the quality of the data. Institutions providing consistent high-quality data find that clinicians use the information for key clinical decisions. This is an important paper because of the large number of patients who were included. Although the follow-up time was relatively short (less than 2 years), the data in this population were extremely useful.

H.W. Strauss, M.D.

Impact on Exercise Single-photon Emission Computed Tomographic Thallium Imaging on Patient Management and Outcome

Nallamothu N, Pancholy SB, Lee KR, et al (Presbyterian Med Ctr, Philadelphia, Pa)
J Nucl Cardiol 2:334–338, 1995   10–7

Objective.—Stress perfusion imaging is of prognostic value in patients with known or suspected coronary artery disease—the more severe the abnormality on a stress perfusion scan, the higher the cardiac event rate. In the managed care setting, information on patient outcomes is needed to confirm the value of these tests. The contributions of exercise SPECT thallium-201 scanning to subsequent patient management and outcomes were evaluated.

Methods.—The analysis included 2,700 consecutive patients undergoing exercise ^{201}Tl SPECT imaging for suspected myocardial infarction. There was no history of previous coronary angiography, coronary revascularization, or Q-wave myocardial infarction in any of the patients. The mean follow-up was 37 months. The SPECT scans were classified as normal or abnormal, and their impact on the need for coronary angiography and revascularization and on "hard" cardiac events—cardiac death or nonfatal myocardial infarction—was analyzed.

Results.—The results of ^{201}Tl SPECT scanning were normal in 2,027 patients and abnormal in 673. Coronary angiography was performed within 6 months after the SPECT scan in just 3% of patients with normal scan findings, compared with 36% of those with abnormal scan results. Patients with normal SPECT scan results who underwent coronary angiography had a higher pretest probability of coronary disease than did patients who did not have coronary angiography. Patients with abnormal SPECT scan results who had coronary angiography had more perfusion defects. Only 2% of patients with normal SPECT scan results underwent coronary revascularization within 3 months after coronary angiography, compared with 32% of those with abnormalities on SPECT scans. No "hard" cardiac events occurred in patients whose SPECT scans showed no abnormalities who received medical treatment after coronary angiography, compared with 15 such events in patients with abnormal SPECT scan results.

Conclusions.—In patients with known or suspected coronary artery disease, SPECT thallium scanning plays an important role in terms of patient management and outcome. For a patient whose exercise ^{201}Tl SPECT scan shows no abnormalities, the risk of coronary angiography, coronary revascularization, and "hard" cardiac events is low. The goal should be to optimize the use of imaging modalities to avoid unnecessary coronary angiography and coronary revascularization without increasing risk to the patient.

▶ A normal scan result has excellent prognostic power, because no subjects in this group had hard events. On the other hand, patients with abnormalities on scans have a much higher incidence of hard events, and, as seen in this study, generally have further evaluation in anticipation of revascularization. However, the positive predictive value of an abnormal scan finding is still low.

It is difficult to define the specific role of a process that has become an integral component of patient care. The outcome of an abnormal scan finding is typically a change in therapy. The change in therapy may result in a decrease in events.

H.W. Strauss, M.D.

Management Decisions in Valvular Heart Disease: The Role of Radionuclide-based Assessment of Ventricular Function and Performance
Borer JS, Wencker D, Hochreiter C (Cornell Univ, New York)
J Nucl Cardiol 3:72–81, 1996   10–8

Introduction.—Radionuclide testing is well established in determining the prognosis of patients with regurgitant valvular diseases. Its prognostic value for patients with stenotic lesions is less clear. Radionuclide ventriculography is useful in the evaluation of patients with valvular diseases for several reasons, including its precision, its use for exercise stress testing, and its ability to provide performance information on both ventricles. The current use of radionuclide ventriculography for the evaluation of valvular heart disease was reviewed.

Regurgitant Disease.—Radionuclide cineangiography for left ventricular (LV) performance assessment is of demonstrated prognostic value in patients with aortic valve regurgitation. These studies are commonly used in deciding whether to operate on such patients, although no randomized trials have been or are likely to be performed. Some rest echocardiographic variables and exercise radionuclide cineangiographic descriptors are significant outcome predictors, but their prognostic value compared with other noninvasive variables remains to be determined. One recent study of patients with severe aortic regurgitation found that the change in LV ejection fraction (LVEF) from rest to exercise—normalized for the change in end-systolic LV meridional wall stress—is a very useful prognostic measure. For all outcomes assessed, measures describing radionuclide cineangiographic LV performance provided more efficient prognostic information than resting echocardiographic data.

In patients with mitral regurgitation, which directly affects both the LV and the right ventricle (RV), radionuclide-based determination of RV ejection fraction is of prognostic value. Useful predictive information is also gained from radionuclide studies of LV performance and function. In both types of regurgitant valvular disease, radionuclide studies are useful in assessing the postoperative results and in evaluating the effects of drug therapy.

Valvular Stenoses.—Currently, radionuclide studies have no defined role in management decision making for patients with aortic or mitral stenosis. In aortic stenosis, radionuclide cineangiography has been useful for pathophysiologic studies and in defining the natural history of the LV response to valve replacement. In mitral stenosis, information on right ventricular performance may have prognostic value.

Discussion.—Radionuclide studies have an important role in management decisions in patients with regurgitant valvular diseases and have contributed useful knowledge about valvular stenotic disease. More information is needed to determine the optimal application of radionuclide studies, as well as echocardiography, in valvular diseases. As more information on the cellular and molecular pathophysiology of these diseases becomes available—from radionuclide-based procedures and other sources—new approaches to management decision making will emerge.

▶ This is a well-written, well-referenced review article by a group that has made major contributions to the field of radionuclide angiography.

H.W. Strauss, M.D.

Exercise Thallium-201 Single Photon Emission Computed Tomography for Evaluation of Coronary Artery Bypass Graft Patency
Lakkis NM, Mahmarian JJ, Verani MS (Baylor College of Medicine, Houston)
Am J Cardiol 76:107–111, 1995   10–9

Introduction.—The last 10 years have seen substantial progress in radionuclide assessment of myocardial perfusion and function. In the localization of native coronary stenoses, thallium-201 SPECT is superior to planar imaging. However, there are no data on the use of ^{201}Tl SPECT for assessing graft patency in patients who have undergone coronary artery bypass grafting (CABG). Thallium-201 SPECT was compared with exercise ECG in detecting graft stenoses in the late stages after CABG.

Methods.—The study included 50 patients (mean age, 58 years) who had undergone CABG a mean of 51 months previously. Thirty were being evaluated for angina and 20 for atypical chest pain. Of the patients who

TABLE 2.—Diagnostic Ability of Thallium-201 SPECT to Localize Stenosed Grafts

Graft to:	Stenosed Grafts (No.)	Matching Thallium Defects (No.)	Sensitivity (%)	Specificity (%)	Positive Predictive Value (%)	Negative Predictive Value (%)
Left anterior descending artery	28	23	82	90	85	88
Right coronary artery	12	11	92	91	85	95
Circumflex artery	8	6	75	75	60	86

(Reprinted by permission of the publisher from Lakkis NM, Mahmarian JJ, Verani MS: Exercise thallium-201 single photon emission computed tomography for evaluation of coronary artery bypass graft patency. Am J Cardiol 76:107–111, 1995. Copyright 1995 by Excerpta Medica, Inc.)

had had myocardial infarction, their mean ejection fraction was 58%. All patients underwent symptom-limited exercise ^{201}Tl SPECT within 3 weeks of graft contrast angiography.

Results.—Coronary angiography demonstrated greater than 50% stenosis in 48 of the 119 grafts. Eighty-three percent of the stenotic grafts were detected by ^{201}Tl SPECT. In patients with typical recurrent angina, ^{201}Tl SPECT was 84% sensitive in detecting any graft stenosis, compared with 24% for exercise ECG. The SPECT study was also more sensitive in detecting stenoses in patients with atypical symptoms, 70% vs. 50%. Thallium-201 SPECT was 82% sensitive in localizing graft stenoses in the left anterior descending artery, 92% for those in the right coronary artery, and 75% for those in the circumflex coronary artery (Table 2).

Conclusions.—Late after CABG, bypass graft stenoses can be very effectively detected and localized using exercise ^{201}Tl SPECT. This radionuclide study is significantly more sensitive than symptom assessment or exercise ECG, whether the patients have typical recurrent angina or other symptoms. The effects of ^{201}Tl SPECT scanning on patient management and outcome remain to be determined.

▶ The authors address an important application of perfusion imaging—the follow-up of the revascularized patient. An abnormal scan result can indicate either progression of disease in the native circulation distal to the graft or graft stenoses. In spite of the inability to differentiate these conditions, the scan is useful for separating ischemia as the cause of symptoms from other noncardiac causes. In addition, the scan identifies the territory at risk. Unfortunately, as we become more cost-conscious, the question will be asked about going directly to coronary angiography.

H.W. Strauss, M.D.

Prognostic Value of Iodine-123 Labelled BMIPP Fatty Acid Analogue Imaging in Patients With Myocardial Infarction

Tamaki N, Tadamura E, Kudoh T, et al (Hokkaido Univ, Sapporo, Japan; Kyoto Univ, Japan; Kobe Gen Hosp, Japan)
Eur J Nucl Med 23:272–279, 1996   10–10

Background.—In patients with myocardial infarction, the identification of myocardium that is viable but still at risk is important in determining risk status and appropriate management. Stress thallium-201 imaging tends to underestimate the presence of severe myocardial ischemia. Although PET using FDG is highly predictive, it is not widely available. The authors have studied the use of iodine-123–labeled 15-iodophenyl-3-R,S-methyl pentadecanoic acid (BMIPP), which reflects myocardial usage of fatty acids. They found regions of reduced BMIPP uptake, relative to ^{201}Tl perfusion, at rest in patients with myocardial infarction. The clinical relevance of these discrepancies is unknown. The prognostic value of BMIPP imaging in patients with myocardial infarction was investigated.

Methods.—The study included 50 consecutive patients with chronic myocardial infarction in stable clinical condition. Each patient, having

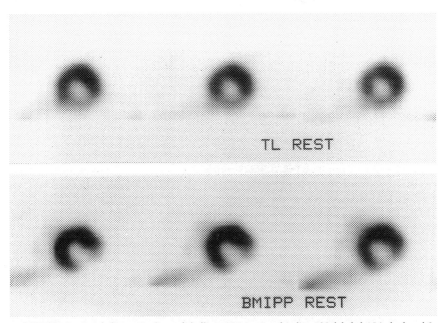

FIGURE 1.—Serial short-axis slices of thallium-201 (**top**) and iodine-123–labeled 15-iodophenyl-3-R,S-methylpentadecanoic acid (*BMIPP*) (**bottom**) images obtained at rest in a patient with inferior wall myocardial infarction, 1 month after onset. Although a similar decrease in both tracers is seen in the inferior region, a definite decrease in BMIPP relative to ^{201}Tl was noted in the lateral region. The patient was in stable condition at the time of the radionuclide study, but reinfarction occurred during the follow-up interval. (Courtesy of Tamaki N, Tadamura E, Kudoh T, et al: Prognostic value of iodine-123 labelled BMIPP fatty acid analogue imaging in patients with myocardial infarction. *Eur J Nucl Med* 23:272–279, 1996. Copyright Springer-Verlag.)

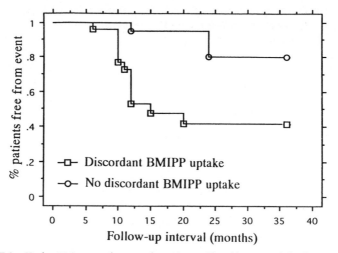

FIGURE 2.—Kaplan-Meier event-free rates for patients with stable myocardial infarction who had a decrease in iodine-123–labeled 15-iodophenyl-3-R,S-methylpentadecanoic acid (*BMIPP*) uptake relative to thallium-201 perfusion (discordant BMIPP uptake) in at least one myocardial segment and for those without such discordant uptake. The event-free rate was significantly lower among patients showing the discordant BMIPP uptake ($P < 0.001$). (Courtesy of Tamaki N, Tadamura E, Kudoh T, et al: Prognostic value of iodine-123 labelled BMIPP fatty acid analogue imaging in patients with myocardial infarction. *Eur J Nucl Med* 23:272–279, 1996. Copyright Springer-Verlag.)

been referred for stress thallium scanning and coronary arteriography, also underwent BMIPP imaging at rest. The patients were followed for a mean of 23 months to assess the ability of the radionuclide studies to predict cardiac events.

Results.—Cardiac events occurred during follow-up in 9 patients. The BMIPP scans provided excellent myocardial images in all cases. Fifty-eight percent of the patients had decreased BMIPP uptake relative to ^{201}Tl perfusion, including 8 of the 9 patients who went on to have cardiac events (Fig 1). The number of segments with such discordances was the best predictor of future cardiac events on univariate analysis, followed by the presence of discordances and the number of ^{201}Tl redistribution segments (Fig 2). The presence of discordant BMIPP uptake was an independent predictor of future cardiac events on Cox regression analysis. It was also the strongest predictor, followed by the number of angiographically demonstrated coronary stenoses.

Conclusions.—In patients with myocardial infarction, discordance between BMIPP uptake and ^{201}Tl perfusion provides a powerful and independent predictor of future cardiac events. The combination of these 2 imaging studies may become a useful part of the prognostic evaluation of patients with myocardial infarction. Discordances in BMIPP uptake may correspond to areas of jeopardized myocardium in which fatty acid usage is severely suppressed relative to myocardial perfusion.

▶ Once again, discordant metabolic and perfusion data identify patients at high risk of events. The etiology of this finding is unclear. Perhaps, once injured, the ability to restore fatty acid metabolism requires greater "healing."

H.W. Strauss, M.D.

Technetium-99m Tetrofosmin Myocardial Perfusion Scan: Comparison of 1-day and 2-day Protocols
Au Yong TK, Chambers J, Maisey MN, et al (Guy's Hosp, London)
Eur J Nucl Med 23:320–325, 1996   10–11

Background.—The myocardial perfusion imaging agent tetrofosmin requires 2 separate injections for stress and rest studies. There are certain presumed advantages to using a rest-stress protocol for tetrofosmin studies, although these have not been proven. A 1-day stress-rest protocol, a 1-day rest-stress protocol, and a 2-day protocol of technetium-99m tetrofosmin single-photon emission tomography were compared.

Methods.—The study included 19 patients with angina, all of whom also underwent coronary angiography, which was used as the gold standard. The 1-day protocols consisted of a stress study followed 4 hours later by a rest study or a rest study followed 4 hours later by a stress study. These studies were performed on 2 consecutive days, with delayed imaging performed before rest injection on the second day; thus, the stress study on the first day and the rest study on the second day made up a 2-day protocol. The 3 protocols were assessed to determine their value in the diagnosis of coronary heart disease and in the detection of myocardial segments with reversible ischemia.

Results.—Sensitivity in diagnosing ischemic heart disease was 100% with the 1-day stress-rest protocol and 94% for the 1-day rest-stress protocol. Accuracy was 100% and 95%. Diagnostic performance was similar for ischemic heart disease overall and in individual coronary artery territories. On analysis of 342 myocardial segments, the 2-day protocol was similar to the stress-rest protocol in overall identification of segments with reversible ischemia and in terms of individual coronary artery territories. The rest-stress protocol and the 2-day protocol were also similar in their ability to identify segments with reversible ischemia. Scan interpretation was affected by abdominal activity in 5 of 36 studies. In 5 patients undergoing 24-hour delayed imaging, 24 segments with washout were identified.

Conclusions.—If ^{99m}Tc single-photon emission tomography for the evaluation of ischemic heart disease can be performed, a 1-day stress-rest protocol and a 1-day rest-stress protocol are just as effective in diagnosing coronary heart disease. Both protocols are similar to a 2-day protocol in identifying myocardial segments with reversible ischemia. The 1-day stress-rest protocol is recommended for routine use because the patient can be discharged if results of the stress study are normal.

▶ The investigators do not comment on the slight increase in bowel activity encountered in some patients imaged immediately after injection. Although this can be annoying, reimaging the patient 30–60 minutes later usually permits the recording of diagnostic quality images.

A major strength of this paper is the striking reproducibility of the exercise result with tetrofosmin. There was no difference between the 1-day and 2-day protocols in sensitivity and accuracy for detecting ischemic heart disease.

H.W. Strauss, M.D.

Impairment of Regional Fatty Acid Uptake in Relation to Wall Motion and Thallium-201 Uptake in Ischaemic But Viable Myocardium: Assessment With Iodine-123-labelled Beta-methyl-branched Fatty Acid
Taki J, Nakajima K, Matsunari I, et al (Kanazawa Univ, Japan)
Eur J Nucl Med 22:1385–1392, 1995   10–12

Background.—Previous studies have noted discrepancies between the uptake of thallium-201 and methyl branched fatty acids at rest in patients with coronary artery disease. Several different fatty acids labeled with iodine-123 have been suggested for clinical use, including 15-(*p*-iodophenyl)-3-*R,S*-methylpentadecanoic acid (BMIPP). Iodine-123–labeled BMIPP was used to study fatty acid myocardial uptake and wall motion in patients with chronic coronary artery disease.

Methods.—Forty-five patients with chronic coronary artery disease, with more than one major coronary artery stenosis of greater than 75%, underwent ^{123}I-BMIPP myocardial tomography at rest. The results were compared with those of exercise-reinjection thallium-201 tomography, with special attention to wall motion at rest in segments with stress-induced ischemia (Fig 2). Thirty-six patients underwent contrast left ventriculography to assess regional wall motion.

Results.—Two hundred thirty-seven segments with reversible ^{201}Tl defects and 90 segments with nonreversible ^{201}Tl defects were identified. Thirty-nine percent of the segments with reversible defects had similarly decreased uptake on the reinjection ^{201}Tl and BMIPP images, 50% had more severe decreases in BMIPP uptake, and 11% had more severe decreases in uptake of reinjection [201]Tl (Table 4). For the nonreversible defects, uptake was equal in 79%, more severely decreased with BMIPP in 7%, and more severely decreased with ^{201}Tl in 14%. Ischemic segments with more severely decreased BMIPP uptake had greater impairment of wall motion than segments with more severely decreased ^{201}Tl uptake (Table 6).

Conclusions.—In patients with coronary artery disease, resting BMIPP and stress-reinjection ^{201}Tl imaging together may help in assessing meta-

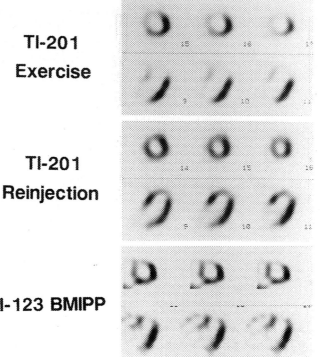

TI-201
Exercise

TI-201
Reinjection

I-123 BMIPP

FIGURE 2.—Stress and reinjection thallium and iodine-123–labeled 15-(*p*-iodophenyl)-3-*R*,*S*-methylpentadecanoic acid (*BMIPP*) tomographic images (short-axis and transverse images) from a 64-year-old male patient with a proximal 99% stenosis of the left anterior descending coronary artery and old anteroseptal myocardial infarction. The thallium study shows severely decreased uptake in the apex to the anteroseptum at stress with fill-in on reinjection images. The BMIPP uptake is more severely decreased than reinjection thallium uptake in these areas, suggesting more impaired fatty acid uptake or metabolic alteration at rest than would be expected from reinjection thallium uptake, which is considered representative of the perfusion at close to the resting condition. (Courtesy of Taki J, Nakajima K, Matsunari I, et al: Impairment of regional fatty acid uptake in relation to wall motion and thallium-201 uptake in ischaemic but viable myocardium: Assessment with iodine-123-labelled beta-methyl-branched fatty acid. *Eur J Nucl Med* 22:1385–1392, 1995. Copyright Springer-Verlag.)

bolic alterations and wall motion abnormalities at rest, regardless of perfusion abnormalities. Segments with stress-induced ischemia are more likely to show greater reductions in resting fatty acid uptake than in reinjection ^{201}Tl uptake. Uptakes of BMIPP and ^{201}Tl decrease similarly in most fixed perfusion defects. Greater wall motion impairments in ischemic myocardium are noted in segments with more severe reductions of BMIPP uptake than of reinjection ^{201}Tl uptake. Uptake of ^{201}Tl is more likely than BMIPP uptake to show metabolic alterations and wall motion abnormalities at rest, independent of perfusion abnormalities.

▶ In 45 patients with ischemic heart disease resulting from one or more coronary stenoses (greater than 75% luminal narrowing), the regional distri-

TABLE 4.—[123]I-BMIPP and Reinjection [201]T1 Findings in Relation to Angiographic and Left Ventriculographic Study in the Segments With Reversible Defects

| | Defect Score | | |
	BMIPP>T1	BMIPP≤T1	Total
Coronary artery stenosis			
<90%	26	27	53
90%–<99%	42	35	77
99%–100%	50	57	107
Total	118	119	237
			(*P*=NS)
Collaterals			
With	26	23	49
Without	105	83	188
Total	131	106	237
			(*P*=NS)
[201]T1 score improvement from stress to reinjection			
1	79	86	165
2	38	33	71
3	1	0	1
Total	118	119	237
			(*P*=NS)

Abbreviation: ^{123}I-BMIPP, iodine-123–labeled 15-(p-idophenyl)-3-R,S-methylpentadecanoic acid.
(Courtesy of Taki J, Nakajima K, Matsunari I, et al: Impairment of regional fatty acid uptake in relation to wall motion and thallium-201 uptake in ischaemic but viable myocardium: Assessment with iodine-123-labelled beta-methyl-branched fatty acid. *Eur J Nucl Med* 22:1385–1392, 1995. Copyright Springer-Verlag.)

TABLE 6.—[123]I-BMIPP and Reinjection Thallium-201 Findings in Relation to Wall Motion in the Segments With Reversible [201]T1 Defects in Patients With and Without Old Myocardial Infarction

| | Defect score | | |
Wall motion	BMIPP>T1	BMIPP≤T1	Total
Patients without old myocardial infarction			
Normal or mild hypokinesis	17	64	81
Severe hypo- or dyskinesis	16	13	29
Total	33	77	110
			(*P*<0.05)
Patients with old myocardial infarction			
Normal or mild hypokinesis	10	22	32
Severe hypo- or dyskinesis	48	11	59
Total	58	33	91
			(*P*<0.005)

Abbreviation: ^{123}I-BMIPP, iodine-123–labeled 15-(p-idophenyl)-3-R,S-methylpentadecanoic acid.
(Courtesy of Taki J, Nakajima K, Matsunari I, et al: Impairment of regional fatty acid uptake in relation to wall motion and thallium-201 uptake in ischaemic but viable myocardium: Assessment with iodine-123-labelled beta-methyl-branched fatty acid. *Eur J Nucl Med* 22:1385–1392, 1995. Copyright Springer-Verlag.)

bution of BMIPP injected at rest was compared with that of ^{201}Tl injected at exercise followed by reinjection at rest and regional wall motion (determined by contrast angiography). Zones of relatively diminished BMIPP compared with rest injected thallium uptake had either normal wall motion or mild hypokinesis, whereas zones of severely depressed wall motion abnormalities were associated with a relative increase of BMIPP. The correlation of altered fatty acid uptake compared with perfusion with the wall motion abnormalities stands in contrast to the lack of correlation with the severity of coronary artery narrowing.

The relationship of BMIPP/perfusion has prognostic significance and, therefore, may have clinical value. On scientific grounds, it is interesting that a metabolic impairment persists at rest in the presence of adequate perfusion.

H.W. Strauss, M.D.

Technetium-99m Tetrofosmin Rest/Stress Myocardial SPET With a Same-day 2-hour Protocol: Comparison With Coronary Angiography: A Spanish-Portuguese Multicentre Clinical Trial
Montz R, Perez-Castejón MJ, Jurado JA, et al (Universidad Complutense, Madrid; Instituto de Cardiología, Madrid; Hosp de Bellvitge, Barcelona, et al)
Eur J Nucl Med 23:639–647, 1996   10–13

Objective.—Technetium-99m–tetrofosmin allows early imaging after injection. Technetium-99m–tetrofosmin myocardial SPECT was compared with coronary angiography in a phase III multicenter clinical trial.

Methods.—Coronary angiography was performed in 144 patients with a history of uncomplicated coronary artery disease (CAD); 78 had no history of myocardial infarction. The ^{99m}Tc-tetrofosmin (300 MBq IV) was administered at rest followed in 5–30 minutes by SPECT, and 1 hour later, ^{99m}Tc-tetrofosmin (900 MBq IV) was administered at peak exercise followed by SPECT. Sixty projections were acquired at 20 or more segments per view.

Results.—Images from 142 patients were suitable for analysis. Rest image and stress image quality was good in 86% and excellent in 95% of patients. Images presented interpretational difficulties in 7% of patients, were poor but evaluable in 5%, and uninterpretable in 2%. Coronary angiography detected stenosis of 75% or more in 109 patients and stenosis of 50% or more in 122 patients. Technetium-99m–tetrofosmin SPECT detected CAD with an overall sensitivity of 93%, a specificity of 38%, and an accuracy of 85%. Sensitivity for detecting single-vessel CAD was 90% and for multivessel disease was 95%. The sensitivity, specificity, and accuracy of CAD detection in the left anterior descending artery were 64%, 84%, and 71%, in the left circumflex artery were 49%, 91%, and 72%; and in the right coronary artery were 86%, 57%, and 73%. The agreement between SPECT and coronary angiography was 62% for single-vessel disease and 68% for multivessel disease.

Conclusion.—Short protocol ^{99m}Tc-tetrofosmin SPECT is a feasible myocardial perfusion imaging technique for evaluating CAD, although the study showed low sensitivity for detection of left anterior descending artery disease and a high number of false positive results for detection of right coronary artery disease.

▶ This article is particularly interesting because of the 14% incidence of low-quality images on the rest injected study. Although the sensitivity for detection of CAD was 93%, the specificity in this trial was exceedingly low (38%). Similarly, the identification of stenosed vessels was only 64% for left anterior descending artery lesions. Unfortunately, the investigators do not comment on the duration of exercise after the injection of tetrofosmin, nor do they have a standardized protocol between institutions for the acquisition of their SPECT images (acquisition times for SPECT range from 13 to 31 minutes). The relatively slower blood clearance of tetrofosmin makes it very important to continue exercise for at least an additional 2 minutes after injection to ensure delivery to tissues before the cessation of the stress test.

H.W. Strauss, M.D.

Adenosine Technetium-99m Sestamibi (SPECT) for the Early Assessment of Jeopardized Myocardium After Acute Myocardial Infarction
Claeys MJ, Vrints CJ, Krug B, et al (Univ of Antwerp, Belgium)
Eur Heart J 16:1186–1194, 1995   10–14

Objective.—Using adenosine rather than dipyridamole for scintigraphic assessment of myocardial perfusion after acute myocardial infarction lessens the risk of prolonged serious side effects. Most studies of adenosine stress scintigraphy have used thallium-201 as a perfusion marker, but technetium-99m–labeled sestamibi may provide better scintigraphic evaluation in this situation. Adenosine ^{99m}Tc-sestamibi SPECT to detect jeopardized myocardium after acute myocardial infarction was studied prospectively.

Methods.—Fifty consecutive patients were studied in the early days after uncomplicated myocardial infarction. Rest ^{99m}Tc-sestamibi SPECT was performed 2–10 days after the infarction, adenosine stress scintigraphy at 4–12 days, and heart catheterization with selective coronary angiography at 4–12 days. If an infarct-related vessel with more than 50% diameter stenosis was found to be supplying an infarct area with residual viable myocardium, that myocardium was considered jeopardized. The safety and diagnostic efficacy of adenosine ^{99m}Tc-sestamibi SPECT were evaluated.

Results.—Half of the patients had reversible perfusion defects in the infarct region, and jeopardized myocardium was almost always present in this situation. When no jeopardized myocardium was present, nonreversible perfusion defects were observed in the infarct region. These patients had either no significant vessel stenosis or no significant residual viable myocardium in the infarct region. Adenosine ^{99m}Tc-sestamibi SPECT correctly identified 88% of patients with jeopardized myocardium. Although 80% of patients had side effects related to adenosine infusion, the side effects caused no major problems.

Conclusions.—In the early stages after acute myocardial infarction, adenosine ^{99m}Tc-sestamibi SPECT is an accurate and relatively safe study to detect jeopardized myocardium. It may provide a useful and noninvasive test to identify patients at high risk of future ischemic events.

▶ The increasing efforts to diminish the cost of care are forcing earlier evaluation of patients with infarction. This study evaluated patients at an average of 3 days after infarction without serious untoward events. A significant fraction of patients had residual ischemia in the infarct zone. Unfortunately, these investigators do not indicate whether therapy for these subjects was altered by this information.

H.W. Strauss, M.D.

Quantitative Exercise Technetium-99m Tetrofosmin Myocardial Tomography for the Identification and Localization of Coronary Artery Disease

Sullo P, Cuocolo A, Nicolai E, et al (Università Federico II, Napoli, Italy)
Eur J Nucl Med 23:648–655, 1996   10–15

Objective.—Although technetium-99m–tetrofosmin distributes proportionately throughout the heart and has high myocardial uptake and retention, its accuracy as a cardiac and myocardial perfusion imaging tracer has not been established. The results of a study evaluating the accuracy of quantitative exercise-rest ^{99m}Tc-tetrofosmin SPECT, performed after a 1-day protocol, in the diagnosis of coronary artery disease and in the detection of individual stenosed coronary vessels, were evaluated.

Methods.—Single-photon emission CT (32 projections at 40 sec/ projection) was performed within 30 minutes after each IV administration of ^{99m}Tc-tetrofosmin, 370 MBq at peak exercise and 1,110 MBq 3 hours

---

TABLE 2.—Sensitivity, Specificity, and Diagnostic Accuracy in the Detection of Stenosed Vessels in Patients With Previous Myocardial Infarction and in Those Without Previous Myocardial Infarction

	Patients with previous myocardial infarction				Patients without previous myocardial infarction			
	LAD	LCX	RCA	All	LAD	LCX	RCA	All
Sensitivity (%)	82	67	71	75	91	86	71	84
Specificity (%)	82	100	83	90	100	93	100	97
Accuracy (%)	82	85	77	81	95	91	91	92

Abbreviations: LAD, left anterior descending artery; *LCX,* left circumflex artery; *RCA,* right coronary artery.
(Courtesy of Sullo P, Cuocolo A, Nicolai E, et al: Quantitative exercise technetium-99m tetrofosmin myocardial tomography for the identification and localization of coronary artery disease. *Eur J Nucl Med* 23:648–655, 1996. Copyright Springer-Verlag.)

TABLE 3.—Sensitivity in the Detection of Stenosed Vessels in Territories Supplied by Arteries With Moderate (50%–75%) and Severe (>75%) Stenosis

	Moderate stenosis (50%–75%)	Severe stenosis (>75%)
LAD	64% (7/11)	93% (27/29)*
LCX	37% (3/8)	88% (15/17)*
RCA	44% (4/9)	84% (16/19)*
All vessels	50% (14/28)	89% (58/65)*

*$P < 0.05$ vs. moderate stenosis.
Abbreviations: LAD, left anterior descending artery; *LCX*, left circumflex artery; *RCA*, right coronary artery.
(Courtesy of Sullo P, Cuocolo A, Nicolai E, et al: Quantitative exercise technetium-99m tetrofosmin myocardial tomography for the identification and localization of coronary artery disease. *Eur J Nucl Med* 23:648–655, 1996. Copyright Springer-Verlag.)

after exercise, to 61 patients (4 women) with suspected coronary artery disease and to 13 healthy volunteers (3 women). All patients and controls also had coronary angiography.

Results.—Results of coronary angiography showed that 50 patients had 50% stenosis or greater, 21 with single-vessel, 15 with 2-vessel, and 14 with 3-vessel disease. Severe stenosis (greater than 75%) was present in at least 1 vessel in 46 patients. All of these patients had abnormal findings on tomograms. Peak exercise was interrupted for 11 patients because of fatigue. Two patients without significant narrowing had abnormal qualitative findings and 1 had abnormal quantitative findings. Sensitivity, specificity, and diagnostic accuracy of individual stenosed vessels were 77%, 93%, and 85%, respectively. Results for patients with and without previous myocardial infarction were analyzed separately (Table 2). The sensitivity of detection of individual stenosed vessels in patients with severe disease was significantly better than in patients with moderate disease (Table 3).

Conclusion.—Quantitative 1-day exercise-rest exercise ^{99m}Tc-tetrofosmin SPECT is a sensitive and specific method for identifying coronary artery disease and is highly accurate in diagnosing individual stenosed vessels.

▶ This investigation, performed at a single institution, found a sensitivity of 77% for the identification of specific stenosed vessels. The investigators observed a significantly reduced sensitivity in territories supplied by vessels with moderate stenosis compared with those supplied by vessels with severe stenosis. These data were encountered despite the fact that patients were exercised for 2 minutes after injection of tetrofosmin before the end of the exercise test. The sensitivity of tetrofosmin overall is somewhat lower than that seen with thallium or sestamibi. The reasons for this lower sensitivity are unclear and may relate to reduced contrasts between lesion and normal myocardium.

H.W. Strauss, M.D.

The Role of Na+/K+ ATPase Activity During Low Flow Ischemia in Preventing Myocardial Injury: A ^{31}P, ^{23}Na and ^{87}Rb NMR Spectroscopic Study

Cross HR, Radda GK, Clarke K (Univ of Oxford, England)
Magn Reson Med 34:673–685, 1995
10–16

Background.—The increase in intracellular Na^+ that occurs during ischemia is believed to result in elevated intracellular Ca^{2+} and myocardial injury. Part of this increase could be related to inhibition of Na^+/K^+ adenosine triphosphatase (ATPase) activity. This hypothesis was studied, along with the ability of glucose to maintain Na^+/K^+ ATPase activity in ischemic perfused rat hearts.

Methods.—Experiments were performed using buffer-perfused rat hearts in which ischemia was produced at a low flow rate of 0.5 mL/min. Alterations in myocardial energetics and intracellular and extracellular volumes were investigated using phosphorus-31 spectroscopy. Changes in intracellular Na^+ were studied by means of sodium-23 NMR spectroscopy, with $DyTTHA^{3-}$ as a shift reagent. The activity of Na^+/K^+ ATPase was estimated by rubidium-87 NMR spectroscopy using Rb^+ influx rates, because Rb^+ is an NMR-sensitive congener of K^+. The effects of glucose infusion, 11 mM, on Na^+/K^+ ATPase activity and related parameters were examined as well.

Results.—Hearts provided with glucose showed continued glycolysis throughout the ischemic period, as well as twice the Na^+/K^+ ATPase activity as in non–glucose-treated hearts. The Rb^+ influx rate was 3 times as high in glucose-treated hearts, and intracellular Na^+ at the end of the ischemic period was 5 times lower. Functional recovery of the myocardium during the reperfusion period was twice as high in the glucose-treated hearts.

Conclusions.—In perfused rat hearts, glucose infusion preserves glycolysis throughout low-flow ischemia. With continued glycolysis, Na^+/K^+ ATPase activity remains sufficient to prevent an increase in intracellular Na^+ and thus to reduce myocardial injury. Inhibition of Na^+/K^+ ATPase activity may also help to prevent ischemic contracture.

▶ This interesting study provides evidence that the old Sodi-Pollaris regimen of infusing potassium and insulin in patients with acute ischemic syndromes may do more than "beautify" the ECG. That old approach to therapy may indeed be placing more glucose into the cell to maintain the sodium potassium ATPase pump and thereby minimize damage to myocardium subjected to ischemia.

H.W. Strauss, M.D.

Tc-99m Sestamibi Myocardial SPECT in Syndrome X

Kao C-H, Wang S-J, Ting C-T, et al (Taichung Veterans Gen Hosp, Taiwan, Republic of China)

Clin Nucl Med 21:280–283, 1996   10–17

Background.—Syndrome X is characterized by chest pain but normal coronary angiographic results. Thallium-201 scintigraphy, used in the assessment of patients with syndrome X, often demonstrates regional defects after stress. However, the lower energy emission of ^{201}Tl as a

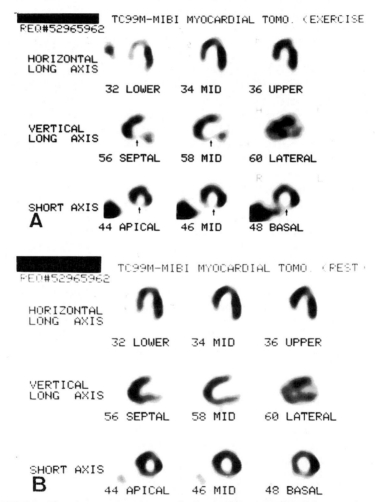

FIGURE 2.—These images represent a case of technetium-99m–MIBI SPECT determined myocardial ischemia: exercise SPECT (**A**) reveals perfusion defects in the inferior wall (*arrows*), and resting SPECT (**B**) is normal. (Courtesy of Kao C-H, Wang S-J, Ting C-T, et al: Tc-99m sestamibi myocardial SPECT in syndrome X. *Clin Nucl Med* 21:280–283, 1996.)

myocardial perfusion agent is a limitation. Higher energy emission technetium-99m–labeled agents, such as ^{99m}Tc-MIBI, significantly improve image quality. Thus, ^{99m}Tc-MIBI SPECT was used to assess myocardial perfusion in patients with syndrome X.

Methods and Findings.—Stress ^{99m}Tc-MIBI SPECT and clinical data on 15 patients with syndrome X were reviewed. Findings on exercise ECG and resting left ventricular ejection fraction (LVEF) were compared with ^{99m}Tc-MIBI SPECT findings. Sixty percent of the patients had normal ^{99m}Tc-MIBI SPECT findings, and 40% had abnormal findings. The results of the exercise ECG were unassociated with perfusion defects on ^{99m}Tc-MIBI SPECT. For patients with abnormal findings on ^{99m}Tc-MIBI SPECT, the incidence of an abnormal resting LVEF and cardiac abnormalities was no higher than in patients with normal findings on ^{99m}Tc-MIBI SPECT (Fig 2).

Conclusions.—These preliminary results suggest that abnormal findings on ^{99m}Tc-MIBI SPECT are common in patients with syndrome X. However, such a result may not be associated with exercise ECG, resting LVEF, or cardiac abnormalities.

▶ Fifteen patients with atypical chest pain, abnormal findings on stress ECG, and no abnormalities on coronary arteriograms (syndrome X) underwent rest and stress sestamibi scans. The investigators found abnormalities on exercise injected scans in 5 subjects. These 5 patients all had involvement of the inferior wall. The lesions extended to the anterior wall in 2 and the septum in 1. Some of the lesions look very striking. Are we looking at abnormal vasoreactivity?

H.W. Strauss, M.D.

Gated Planar Technetium 99m–labeled Sestamibi Myocardial Perfusion Image Inversion for Quantitative Scintigraphic Assessment of Left Ventricular Function
Williams KA, Taillon LA (Univ of Chicago)
J Nucl Cardiol 2:285–295, 1995   10–18

Purpose.—Valuable diagnostic and prognostic information can be obtained by myocardial perfusion scintigraphy and noninvasive studies of left ventricular (LV) function. If perfusion and function could be simultaneously evaluated in a single diagnostic study, it would be very useful for diagnostic evaluation of patients with ischemic heart disease. A new computerized technique for quantitative assessment of LV systolic performance, performed in conjunction with myocardial perfusion scintigraphy, was developed.

Methods.—The study included 264 patients with planar technetium-99m–labeled sestamibi myocardial perfusion images obtained in the best septal left anterior oblique projection. The perfusion images were digitally inverted for semiautomated evaluation of the LV cavity, using edge-detection software developed for use in equilibrium blood pool imaging. The ejection fraction values obtained by this technique were compared with values obtained from other sources: a myocardial perfusion double-chamber phantom, first-pass radionuclide angiography, and contrast ventriculography.

Results.—The new technique was validated in vitro, with linear correlation between the ejection fractions obtained from myocardial perfusion image inversion and the phantom ($r = 0.99$). The in vivo studies demonstrated good linear correlation between the image inversion technique and the first-pass radionuclide angiographic studies ($r = 0.88$). These 2 techniques showed 95% agreement as to whether significant left ventricular systolic dysfunction was present or absent. The values obtained by image inversion and contrast ventriculographic ejection also correlated very well ($r = 0.85$). Intraobserver and interobserver agreement on the image inversion ejection fractions was very good.

Conclusions.—The new image inversion technique, used with gated ^{99m}Tc-labeled sestamibi myocardial perfusion scans, is useful in assessing the dynamics of the LV chamber changes occurring during the cardiac cycle. The new technique can reliably evaluate LV systolic function during myocardial perfusion imaging. The results are highly reproducible and correlate well with the findings of established techniques. The image inversion technique can be used even in the presence of segmental perfusion defects.

▶ The authors have used an interesting approach. Inversion of the gated perfusion images allowed use of existing programs to analyze the data. The correlation between the first-pass ejection fraction and the inverted perfusion imaging injection fraction resulted in an *r* value of 0.77. However, evaluating the scatter shows a mean difference of more than 11%. This could be a substantial drawback to the wide application of this methodology.

H.W. Strauss, M.D.

Simultaneous Transmission/Emission Myocardial Perfusion Tomography: Diagnostic Accuracy of Attenuation-corrected ^{99m}Tc-Sestamibi Single-photon Emission Computed Tomography
Ficaro EP, Fessler JA, Shreve PD, et al (Univ of Michigan, Ann Arbor)
Circulation 93:463–473, 1996   10–19

Background.—Perfusion imaging with SPECT has shown excellent sensitivity but suboptimal specificity in the detection of coronary heart disease (CHD). The specificity may be compromised by the inhomogeneous attenuation of photons in the thorax, which may produce artifactual defects in the images. Therefore, the diagnostic accuracy of a newly developed transmission CT (TCT)/emission CT (ECT) imaging system was evaluated with and without attenuation correction in the detection and localization of CHD.

Methods.—A randomly selected series of 360 patients referred for stress myocardial perfusion imaging underwent both coronary angiography and TCT/ECT imaging. The emission images without attenuation correction (NC) were reconstructed in the conventional fashion. The emission images with attenuation correction (AC) were reconstructed using attenuation maps reconstructed using a penalized, weighted, least-squares algorithm to analyze the truncated transmission data. Both NC and AC images were interpreted for 2 groups of patients: 59 patients with a pretest likelihood for CHD of no more than 5% (group 1) and 60 patients in whom CHD was angiographically verified within 90 days of scintigraphy. The abnormal extent thresholds with each type of image were determined with receiver operating characteristic analysis.

Results.—Compared with the NC images, the AC images yielded significantly better specificity and accuracy for the detection of CHD, the localization of disease overall, and the localization of disease in specific artery territories. There was significant improvement in the detection of CHD with AC images using both the angiographic cutoffs of 50% and 70% stenosis. Maximal diagnostic accuracy for the localization of disease in specific vascular territories occurred as follows: with 12% to 24% stenosis in the left anterior descending coronary artery (LAD), with 12% to 28% stenosis in the left circumflex artery, and with 8% to 12% stenosis in the right coronary artery territories using AC images; and with 12% to 20% stenosis in the LAD, 12% to 28% stenosis in the left circumflex artery, and 0% to 8% stenosis in the right coronary artery with NC images.

Conclusions.—The simultaneous TCT/ECT imaging system, with attenuation correction, improved the diagnostic accuracy of detection and localization of CHD, with the most clinically significant diagnostic improvements occurring in patients with stenoses of intermediate severity. Specificity is substantially improved without diminishing sensitivity with this technique. Further clinical study is warranted.

▶ This excellent article compares attenuation and nonattenuation corrected perfusion images on 60 patients with angiographically documented coronary artery disease to those of 59 patients with less than 5% likelihood of coronary artery disease. Emission and attenuation correction data were acquired simultaneously. Attenuation data were collected using an americium-241 source and fan-beam collimator on one head of a 3-headed camera, while the remaining 2 detectors recorded emission data with high-resolution parallel hole collimators. The striking difference in the appearance of the images after attenuation correction correlates with improved specificity by receiver operating characteristic curve analysis.

H.W. Strauss, M.D.

Attenuation Compensation for Cardiac Single-photon Emission Computed Tomographic Imaging: Part 2. Attenuation Compensation Algorithms

King MA, Tsui BMW, Pan T-S, et al (Univ of Massachusetts, Worcester; Univ of North Carolina, Chapel Hill)
J Nucl Cardiol 3:55–63, 1996   10–20

Background.—Recent years have seen great progress in the ability to estimate attenuation maps in cardiac SPECT. This advance has arisen partly from the increased power of computers in the clinic and partly from improvement in the algorithms used for attenuation correction and in the efficacy of their implementation. Various types of attenuation compensation algorithms were compared, including their implementation, their relative advantages and disadvantages, and their performance.

Attenuation Correction Algorithms.—Three different types of algorithms—intrinsic attenuation-correction methods, iterative filtered backprojection methods, and statistically based reconstruction methods—were compared using a three-dimensional mathematical cardiac torso phantom to create attenuation maps and source descriptions. There is still room for debate regarding which algorithm provides the best attenuation compensation method for cardiac images. Modern intrinsic attenuation correction methods are fast and avoid problems related to the convergence and number of iterations; however, there are potential clinical problems that remain to be identified. Iterative filtered backprojection methods are also fast, but there are problems with mathematical precision and noise characteristics.

In the past, the major factor limiting the use of statistically based reconstruction methods such as the maximum-likelihood expectation-maximization (MLEM) method has been processing time. Now, using a state-of-the-art processing system, the time needed to reconstruct slices with nonuniform attenuation compensation with MLEM is similar to that needed for filtered backprojection reconstructions 10 years ago. This type of reconstruction has several important advantages, especially its good theoretical basis, its convergent method, and its amenability to incorporating the physics of imaging. Further study is needed to determine how best to control noise in MLEM reconstructions and to address the degradations formerly concealed by attenuation. There is also the potential for pitfalls and unexpected complications and artifacts.

Discussion.—Each method of attenuation compensation in cardiac SPECT has its advantages and disadvantages, although increased computing power is eliminating the time problems associated with statistically based reconstruction methods. With further research, nonuniform attenuation correction may one day be a routine part of cardiac perfusion imaging. Still, phantom studies and clinical evaluations should be performed to be sure the system is operating correctly.

▶ This elegant phantom study demonstrates the usefulness of each of these 3 approaches. However, it is clear from clinical data that an important component will also be scatter correction. The very intense activity, typically below the diaphragm, can result in excess attenuation "correction," thereby altering the appearance of the myocardium. As a result, it is not sufficient to just consider the attenuation compensation in isolation; it must also have a component of scatter correction.

H.W. Strauss, M.D.

Improved Left Ventricular Function After Growth Hormone Replacement in Patients With Hypopituitarism: Assessment With Radionuclide Angiography
Cuocolo A, Nicolai E, Colao A, et al (Universitá Federico II, Napoli, Italy)
Eur J Nucl Med 23:390–394, 1996   10–21

Purpose.—Patients with growth hormone deficiency (GHD) commonly have cardiac dysfunction, which has a major negative impact on their prognosis. There is evidence that growth hormone plays an important role in maintaining left ventricular function. It is not known whether growth hormone replacement therapy can reverse the cardiac function abnormalities associated with GHD. This issue was studied using radionuclide angiography.

Methods.—The study included 14 patients with childhood-onset GHD and 12 normal controls. The patients were 9 men and 5 women (mean age, 27 years). The patients and controls were similar in age, sex, and heart rate. Both groups underwent equilibrium radionuclide angiography at rest using technetium-99m–labeled red blood cells. In the patients with GHD, the radionuclide studies were repeated 6 months after treatment with recombinant human growth hormone, 0.05 IU/kg/day.

Results.—Left ventricular ejection fraction was significantly lower in the patients with GHD than in controls, with mean values of 53% vs. 66%. Stroke volume index was 41 vs. 51 mL/m² and cardiac index was 2.8 vs. 3.0 L/min/m². All patients tolerated growth hormone treatment well, and there were no associated changes in heart rate or arterial blood pressure. After growth hormone treatment, mean left ventricular ejection fraction improved from 53% to 59%, stroke volume index from 41 to 47 mL/m², and cardiac index from 2.8 to 3.3 L/min/m².

Conclusions.—Patients with prolonged GHD have impaired ventricular function at rest compared with normal controls. The findings further support the hypothesis that growth hormone plays a physiologic role in maintaining normal left ventricular function and cardiac performance. The cardiac abnormalities associated with GHD are reversed after 6 months of specific hormone replacement therapy.

▶ This paper is important because it identifies the striking enhancement of systolic function in patients who are growth hormone deficient when growth hormone is replaced. Recent studies in patients with cardiomyopathy suggest that growth hormone may have a similar salutary effect.

H.W. Strauss, M.D.

Fast Technetium 99m–labeled Sestamibi Gated Single-photon Emission Computed Tomography for Evaluation of Myocardial Function

Mazzanti M, Germano G, Kiat H, et al (Cedars-Sinai Med Ctr, Los Angeles; Univ of California, Los Angeles)
J Nucl Cardiol 3:143–149, 1996   10–22

Background.—Myocardial function and perfusion can be examined simultaneously with technetium-99m–labeled gated SPECT. The acquisition time of approximately 20 minutes needed with standard gated SPECT protocols can, however, limit the clinical applications. Therefore, the feasibility of the new fast ECG gated sestamibi SPECT protocol was evaluated, and its accuracy was compared with that of the standard protocol in assessing stress myocardial perfusion and function.

Methods.—Fifty consecutive patients referred for myocardial perfusion imaging underwent a 15-minute rest thallium-201 SPECT. The patients then underwent a treadmill stress test and were given an injection of sestamibi at peak exercise. Thirty minutes later, standard gated SPECT was performed, followed immediately by fast gated SPECT. The image sets

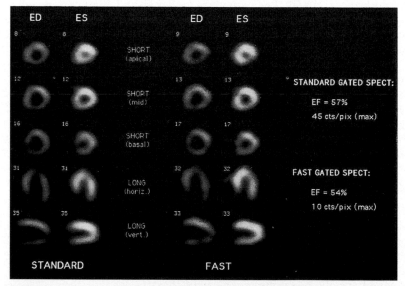

FIGURE 2.—Comparison between standard and fast gated SPECT images at end diastole and end systole in a normal patient. Note essential equivalence of left ventricular ejection fraction values despite a fourfold difference in count statistics. (Courtesy of Mazzanti M, Germano G, Kiat H, et al: Fast technetium 99m–labeled sestamibi gated single-photon emission computed tomography for evaluation of myocardial function. *J Nucl Cardiol* 3:143–149, 1996.)

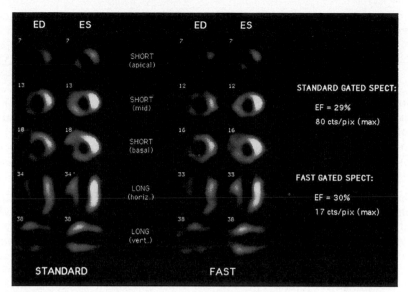

FIGURE 3.—Comparison between standard and fast gated SPECT images at end diastole and end systole in patient with large apical perfusion defect. (Courtesy of Mazzanti M, Germano G, Kiat H, et al: Fast technetium 99m–labeled sestamibi gated single-photon emission computed tomography for evaluation of myocardial function. *J Nucl Cardiol* 3:143–149, 1996.)

were read independently of one another, with scoring of stress perfusion, wall motion, and wall thickening in 20 segments of the left ventricular myocardium.

Results.—Standard gated SPECT images had significantly more myocardial counts per pixel than did the fast gated SPECT images (58 vs. 13). There was no significant difference in heart/lung ratios between the 2 protocols. In comparison of the segmental scores between standard and fast gated SPECT images, there was 92% agreement for myocardial perfusion, 96% agreement for wall motion, and 94% agreement for wall thickening. Agreement on abnormal segments was 95% for perfusions, 92% for wall motion, and 87% for wall thickening. The average left ventricular ejection fractions did not differ significantly (48.1 with standard gated SPECT imaging and 49.3 with fast gated SPECT imaging) (Figs 2 and 3).

Conclusions.—There is good correlation between fast and standard ECG gated acquisition of stress-injected sestamibi in the assessment of stress myocardial perfusion and left ventricular function. The average 6.7-minute acquisition time of fast gated SPECT may expand the clinical applications of this technology.

▶ The investigators observed significant agreement in both the relative distribution of perfusion, segmental wall motion scores, and the calculated ejection fraction of the 2 approaches.

We are now back to exchanging count rate for speed. Although the results look good in this trial, it is unclear whether we are moving forward or backward.

H.W. Strauss, M.D.

Comparison of Single-tracer (Technetium-99m-Sestamibi) and Dual-tracer (Thallium-201 Chloride and Technetium-99m-Sestamibi) Protocols for Identification of Myocardial Ischemia
Loutfi I, Singh A (Univ of Missouri Hosp and Clinics, Columbia)
Invest Radiol 30:367–371, 1995   10–23

Background.—Myocardial perfusion imaging has 2 primary clinical uses: the noninvasive diagnosis of coronary artery disease (CAD) and the differentiation of viable or reversibly ischemic myocardium from nonviable myocardium in patients with diagnosed CAD. It was hypothesized that a dual-tracer technique, using thallium-201 chloride for resting images and ^{201}Tl chloride and technetium-99m–sestamibi (MIBI) for stress images would produce optimal data for the detection of CAD and reversible ischemia. The hypothesis was tested by retrospectively comparing the diagnostic accuracy of this dual-tracer protocol with that of a single-tracer protocol, using only ^{99m}Tc-sestamibi to obtain both rest and stress images.

Methods.—A total of 460 patients with known or suspected CAD underwent myocardial perfusion imaging, including 230 who underwent scintigraphic imaging with the ^{99m}Tc-sestamibi protocol in both the rest and stress conditions (group A) and 230 who underwent imaging with the ^{201}Tl chloride in the rest condition and with ^{99m}Tc-sestamibi in the stress condition (group B). The groups were matched for demographic characteristics and had similar proportions of patients undergoing the treadmill and dipyridamole stress testing. The images were analyzed using a semiquantitative scoring method for determining the presence of reversible ischemia. The ability to detect ischemia was compared in the 2 groups.

Results.—Abnormal myocardial perfusion was diagnosed in 215 patients, including 98 patients (46%) with irreversible defects and 117 (54%) with reversible defects. A significantly greater number of ischemic defects were detected in group B. When the data were analyzed using the ischemia index, the average ischemia index was significantly higher in group B than in group A. There was a highly significant difference between the groups in the detection of more severe ischemia.

Conclusions.—The dual-tracer protocol for myocardial perfusion imaging, using ^{201}Tl chloride at rest and ^{99m}Tc-sestamibi after stress, produces images with significantly greater sensitivity for identifying reversible myocardial ischemia than does the single-tracer protocol, using ^{99m}Tc-sestamibi in both the rest and stress conditions. The dual-tracer imaging protocol appears to produce the optimal imaging data for the evaluation of CAD and myocardial viability.

▶ The investigators studied matched populations with each protocol and found significantly more ischemia in the dual-tracer group. This is another piece of data in favor of the dual-tracer approach.

H.W. Strauss, M.D.

Tc-99m Sestamibi Cardiac SPECT Imaging During Coronary Artery Occlusion in Humans: Comparison With Dipyridamole Stress Studies
Borges-Neto S, Watson JE, Miller MJ (Duke Univ, Durham, NC; VA Med Ctr, Charleston, SC)
Radiology 198:751–754, 1996   10–24

Objective.—Pharmacologic stress testing is a commonly used alternative to exercise stress testing. These tests assume that a deficit of coronary flow is related to the area of myocardium put in jeopardy by coronary occlusion. A previous study of exercise stress testing suggested that stress-induced ischemia does not necessarily reflect the total area of myocardium jeopardized if the coronary artery becomes totally occluded. Changes in regional myocardial perfusion during dipyridamole stress were compared with those occurring during coronary occlusion in humans.

Methods.—The prospective study included 14 men referred for percutaneous transluminal coronary angioplasty, all with greater than 50% stenosis of at least 1 major coronary artery. Twenty-four hours before percutaneous transluminal coronary angioplasty, all patients underwent same-day rest and dipyridamole technetium-99m–labeled sestamibi SPECT. During the procedure, with the vessel occluded by an inflated balloon, 15 mCi of ^{99m}Tc-labeled sestamibi was injected, followed 60 minutes later by SPECT studies. These studies were used to estimate the extent of the perfusion abnormalities.

Results.—The regional perfusion defect was 33% at rest, 53% during dipyridamole infusion, and 47% during occlusion. The estimated SPECT defect during coronary artery occlusion was comparable to that obtained during stress with dipyridamole. The total size of the perfusion defect was significantly larger during dipyridamole infusion than during occlusion, probably because of the effects of multivessel disease.

Conclusions.—The perfusion abnormalities induced by dipyridamole are comparable to those induced by coronary artery occlusion, as defined by ^{99m}Tc-labeled sestamibi SPECT. Thus, dipyridamole stress studies may be useful in estimating the total myocardium in jeopardy from a stenotic lesion. Patients who do not reach an adequate end point on exercise perfusion study may benefit from a repeat perfusion under vasodilator stress.

▶ More evidence that stress perfusion imaging defines the full extent of a perfusion abnormality.

H.W. Strauss, M.D.

Myocardial Viability: Unresolved Issues

Iskandrian AS (Philadelphia Heart Inst)
J Nucl Med 37:794–797, 1996   10–25

Introduction.—Many different techniques have been studied for use in evaluating myocardial viability. Most of these studies have focused on the accuracy of the various techniques, whereas others have assessed the effects on patient outcomes. Some issues related to assessment of myocardial viability are unresolved (Table 1).

Unresolved Issues.—One central issue is the definition of myocardial viability. Whereas normal, hibernating, or stunned myocardium may be viable, nonviable myocardium represents scar tissue. The difference between viability and hibernation is key to understanding the differences between diagnostic methods based on flow, metabolism, or function. Quantitation of the amount of viability is another key issue; any segment can have varying proportions of normal, hibernating, and stunned myocardium. The proportion of hibernating myocardium determines the extent of regional functional recovery after revascularization, and the total extent of hibernation in the left ventricle determines the extent of global functional recovery.

The relationship between regional myocardial perfusion and wall motion is often complex; normal perfusion can be seen in a region with abnormal wall motion for several different reasons. Previous studies have suggested that different techniques may be comparably accurate in predicting functional recovery after revascularization, but this could be because so many studies include only patients with mild to moderate left ventricular dysfunction. Greater differences in accuracy may be seen with worsening left ventricular dysfunction. Although most studies perform follow-up assessments at 8–12 weeks after revascularization, this is not necessarily the optimal time. Recovery may occur later, and it is important to perform serial measurements. Even if an accurate viability assessment is obtained, the degree of left ventricular recovery will depend on the completeness of revascularization, freedom from perioperative myocardial infarction, and continued patency of the grafts or angioplasty. This raises questions about the criteria used to detect postoperative infarction. Finally,

---

TABLE 1.—List of Unresolved Issues in Myocardial Viability

1. Definition of viable myocardium
2. Quantification of viable myocardium
3. Correlation between perfusion and function
4. Patient selection
5. Time of follow-up assessment
6. Completeness of revascularization
7. Perioperative myocardial infarction
8. End points

(Reprinted by permission of the Society of Nuclear Medicine, from Iskandrian AS: Myocardial viability: Unresolved issues. *J Nucl Med* 37:794–797, 1996.)

there are questions about the best end points to use in evaluating the results of coronary revascularization. Improvement in ejection fraction seems to be the best primary end point; however, the secondary end points of survival and reduced symptoms are far more important to the patient.

Discussion.—Many complex issues, independent of the perfusion pattern, will affect the clinical application of myocardial viability assessment, including the various imaging patterns seen. For ethical and other reasons, it will be difficult to test the relatively new concept of reversing left ventricular function to improve survival. Given the high costs of managing patients with congestive heart failure, a large trial in this patient group is needed.

▶ This is an excellent editorial by a knowledgeable clinician-investigator. He highlights the unresolved issues and points out the strengths and weaknesses of each modality. No method is perfect. The clinical issues should define which test is used. It is worth your time to read this one in the original text.

H.W. Strauss, M.D.

The Incidence of Scintigraphically Viable and Nonviable Tissue by Rubidium-82 and Fluorine-18-Fluorodeoxyglucose Positron Emission Tomographic Imaging in Patients With Prior Infarction and Left Ventricular Dysfunction
Go RT, MacIntyre WJ, Cook SA, et al (Cleveland Clinic Found, Ohio)
J Nucl Cardiol 3:96–104, 1996   10–26

Background.—It is necessary to differentiate between viable and nonviable myocardial tissue in patients with previous myocardial infarction being considered for coronary revascularization. Viable tissue can be defined by 2 disease states detected with nuclear imaging techniques: the reversible defect of stress-induced ischemia on the scintigraphic myocardial perfusion scan or the hibernating myocardium, characterized by a perfusion defect at rest with enhanced glucose-load FDG uptake on PET. The incidence of these 2 patterns was determined to assess the clinical need for FDG PET imaging in patients with previous myocardial infarction.

Methods.—A consecutive series of 155 patients with previous myocardial infarction referred for PET imaging before consideration of coronary revascularization were studied. All patients underwent both rest and stress PET perfusion imaging after infusion of rubidium-82, followed by FDG PET imaging after an oral glucose load. The perfusion images were examined first in 24 myocardial regions in the left ventricle to determine whether the perfusion patterns were reversible (ischemic) or irreversible (fixed). Next, the FDG metabolic images were interpreted in conjunction with the perfusion images to facilitate localization of patterns.

Results.—Of the 1,240 segments in the 155 patients, 51% had normal perfusion patterns. Of the segments with abnormal perfusion patterns,

13% were reversible and 87% were irreversible. Of the segments with reversible perfusion defects, 42% demonstrated decreased FDG uptake, 40% demonstrated enhanced uptake, and 18% demonstrated partial uptake. Of the segments with irreversible defects, 18% demonstrated enhanced FDG uptake, 11% demonstrated partial uptake, and 58% demonstrated decreased uptake. Therefore, the following diagnoses were made: stress-induced ischemia with variable FDG uptake in 20%, hibernating myocardium in 29%, and myocardial scar tissue in 51% of the patients.

Conclusions.—Although viable myocardium could be identified in 20% of the patients with perfusion imaging alone, metabolic FDG PET imaging was needed to identify viable myocardium in 29% of the patients who had the perfusion-metabolism mismatch pattern of hibernating myocardium and to confirm the nonviability of myocardium in 51% of the patients who had the perfusion-metabolism match pattern of myocardial scar. Therefore, FDG PET imaging has substantial clinical value in the evaluation of patients with previous myocardial infarction being considered for coronary revascularization.

▶ After infarction, static [82]Rb PET perfusion imaging at rest and stress identified only 20% of the viable segments, whereas metabolic imaging was far more sensitive. It would have been helpful to know whether dynamic rubidium imaging could do as well as FDG imaging.

H.W. Strauss, M.D.

Adenosine Technetium-99m Sestamibi Myocardial Perfusion SPECT in Women: Diagnostic Efficacy in Detection of Coronary Artery Disease
Amanullah AM, Kiat H, Friedman JD, et al (Cedars-Sinai Med Ctr, Los Angeles; Univ of California, Los Angeles)
J Am Coll Cardiol 27:803–809, 1996   10–27

Objective.—Although the incidence of coronary artery disease among women increases dramatically after age 45, and is similar to that for men by age 75, the sensitivity and specificity of myocardial perfusion SPECT has not been studied in women. Technetium-99m, with its lower attenuation by breast tissue, is considered particularly suitable for detection of coronary artery disease in women. The diagnostic efficiency of adenosine ^{99m}Tc sestamibi SPECT was studied in a large number of female patients.

Methods.—Adenosine ^{99m}Tc sestamibi myocardial perfusion SPECT was performed in 71 women with a low risk of coronary artery disease and in 130 catheterized women who also had coronary angiography. In the latter group, 94 had coronary artery narrowing ≥50%, and 83 had narrowing ≥70%; 27 had had a previous myocardial infarction (MI). The catheterized group was further classified as low risk (<25%), intermediate risk (25% to 75%), or high risk (>75%) for coronary artery disease.

Thallium-201 and ^{99m}Tc sestamibi SPECT were performed separately. The 64 SPECT projections were visually interpreted using 20 segments per projection. Uptake was scored on a 0–4 scale in which 0 indicated normal uptake and 4 indicated no uptake.

Results.—In the catheterized group, the overall sensitivity of adenosine ^{99m}Tc sestamibi SPECT for detecting ≥50% stenosis was 93%, the specificity was 78%, and predictive accuracy was 88% and corresponding values for detecting ≥70% stenosis were 95%, 66%, and 85%. The normalcy rate for the low-risk group was 93%. The 103 patients in the catheterized group with no history of MI had respective rates of 91%, 78%, and 86% for ≥50% stenosis and 95%, 67%, and 83% for ≥70% stenosis. The sensitivity (92%) and specificity (83%) for detecting ≥50% stenosis in patients with angina symptoms was similar to the corresponding values, 93% and 69%, for patients without angina symptoms. There were no significant differences in sensitivities and specificities between both subgroups of catheterized patients and the low-risk group. The sensitivity and specificity for the low-risk, medium-risk, and high-risk groups were 82% and 82%, 93% and 73%, and 95% and 100%, respectively. The sensitivities and specificities for detecting ≥50% stenosis were 76% and 81% for the left anterior descending coronary artery, 44% and 99% for the left circumflex coronary artery, and 75% and 77% for the right coronary artery.

Conclusion.—Adenosine ^{99m}Tc sestamibi myocardial perfusion SPECT is a sensitive and specific method for detecting coronary artery disease in both symptomatic and asymptomatic women.

▶ This retrospective analysis of 130 patients who underwent catheterization and 71 patients with a low prescan likelihood of coronary disease adds additional evidence of the usefulness of adenosine imaging with a technetium perfusion agent and subjective interpretation of SPECT perfusion images. This is particularly important because of the potential role of breast attenuation as a cause of false abnormalities. It is particularly interesting that this group, known for their quantitative interpretation, chose subjective interpretation in this group of patients.

H.W. Strauss, M.D.

The Effect of Managed Care on Nuclear Cardiology
Michnich ME, Mills PS, Seidman JJ (American College of Cardiology, Bethesda, Md)
J Nucl Cardiol 3:65–71, 1996   10–28

Objective.—Managed care is becoming the main model of health care delivery in the United States. There are many different forms of managed care, including not only HMOs and preferred provider organizations but also managed fee-for-service and point-of-service plans. Regardless of the type of managed care, it has important implications for the practice of nuclear cardiology. The impact of managed care on nuclear cardiology was reviewed.

Delivery of Nuclear Cardiology.—To remain viable in the managed care environment, nuclear cardiology will have to demonstrate its long-term value in both clinical and economic studies. Some cardiology groups are finding it more effective to send certain patients directly to cardiac catheterization. In addition, some contracting arrangements effectively shut out nuclear cardiologists, such as those in which local radiology networks have contracted to provide nuclear cardiology services as part of the full spectrum of radiology services. As care shifts from inside to outside the hospital, cardiologists perform more and more nuclear cardiology services. The way in which nuclear cardiology procedures and protocols are developed varies considerably between managed care organizations and has a major impact on the practice of nuclear cardiology.

Practice Implications.—The effects of managed care on everyday practice for the nuclear cardiologist will depend on a number of factors, including the practice setting. Large single-specialty group practices can negotiate more and better contracts than smaller practices, although they will still be dependent on the referral patterns of the plan's primary care physicians. Practice location and hospital affiliations will also have an important effect. In deciding which managed care options to pursue, practices must consider a number of factors, such as the impact on referrals, their clinical autonomy, their access to capital, the financial risk involved, and any legal issues.

Discussion.—Managed care is bringing major changes to the practice of nuclear cardiology. Many important issues related to this trend must be considered, including who will deliver nuclear cardiology services, where these services will be made available, and how procedures and protocols will be developed. Efforts are needed on the organizational, local, state, and federal levels to ensure the high quality of cardiovascular care into the next century.

▶ The future of nuclear cardiology will be determined by financial incentives, the structure of referral arrangements, and the effectiveness and cost of the procedures relative to those of other technologies. Capitation of physicians provides incentives to limit referrals for noninvasive procedures, when cardiac catheterization may provide the most cost-effective determination of the need for revascularization. The decision about who will provide the service will be made by the quality of care.

This is an excellent article about a complex topic. The authors present a thoughtful perspective on the delivery of services under various scenarios. This article is well worth reading.

H.W. Strauss, M.D.

Quantitative Myocardial Thallium Single-photon Emission Computed Tomography in Normal Women: Demonstration of Age-related Differences

Cohen M, Touzery C, Cottin Y, et al (Centre-Georges-François-Leclerc, Dijon, France; Universitaire de Dijon, France; Domaine Universitaire du Sart Tilman-B.35, Liege, Belgium)
Eur J Nucl Med 23:25–30, 1996   10–29

Objective.—Because breast tissue can produce more or less attenuation in the activity of thallium-201, myocardial perfusion imaging with ^{201}Tl can lead to false positive or false negative results in women. Although this attenuation is expected to decrease with age, there is no attenuation index available that would increase specificity without sacrificing sensitivity. A database of normal women for quantitative analysis of exercise and reinjection myocardial SPECT was developed.

Methods.—Myocardial stress tests were performed in 40 men and 61 women aged 21–88 years, with no evidence of coronary artery disease, using an ergometric bicycle test ($n = 51$), dipyridamole infusion ($n = 27$), or both ($n = 23$). Thallium-201 was injected at peak exercise and at the end of the stress test, and tomographic imaging was performed. Thallium uptake was quantified and subjected to multivariate analysis of variance.

Results.—Women were significantly older than men, and significantly more women than men had the dipyridamole stress test. Thallium uptake varied widely. The difference in uptake between myocardial regions was significant, although, for both sexes, the region of highest uptake was the lateral wall near the apex and the region of lowest uptake was the basal septum. Stress did not affect uptake. Both at stress and after reinjection, men had less uptake in the 3 areas of the inferior wall, and women had significantly fewer counts in the anteroapical and lateroapical regions. At stress and at reinjection, age was significantly related to uptake in the anteromedian, anterobasal, and anteroapical regions. Anterior wall uptake was significantly reduced by 8% at stress and reinjection for women younger than 55 years. Women older than 55 years had anterior wall uptake similar to that of men.

Conclusion.—Increased breast tissue attenuation of ^{201}Tl uptake in younger women suggests that breast volume, morphologic characteristics, and density account for the decreased uptake. The use of 2 different databases for myocardial SPECT investigation of possible anterior wall ischemia will avoid underestimation of the disease in women older than 55 years.

▶ The investigators present interesting findings, but they missed the most important point. It is not clear whether the differences between zones of uptake are related to sex or attenuation artifacts. No attempt was made to correlate the findings with body build, breast size, or relative fibrous composition of the breast. In addition, the investigators identify a major difference in age between their male and female subjects. As a result, although it is clear that men and women have different normal ranges, it is difficult to know what to make of this report.

H.W. Strauss, M.D.

Thallium-201 Reverse Redistribution at Reinjection Imaging Correlated With Coronary Lesion, Wall Motion Abnormality and Tissue Viability

Marzullo P, Gimelli A, Cuocolo A, et al (CNR Inst of Clinical Physiology, Pisa, Italy; Univ Federico II, Napoli, Italy; Fondazione Clinica del Lavoro IRCCS, Veruno, Italy)
J Nucl Med 37:735–741, 1996   10–30

Objective.—The clinical significance of thallium-201 reverse distribution on stress-redistribution ^{201}Tl scintigraphic studies is uncertain. In most such defects, reinjection is followed by normalization, suggesting that the defects represent viable myocardium. Reverse redistribution at reinjection imaging was studied for its relationship to standard 4-hour redistribution; the presence of coronary lesions, abnormal wall motion, and previous myocardial infarction; and myocardial viability.

Methods.—The analysis included 29 patients, from a series of 270, who had reverse redistribution after reinjection of ^{201}Tl on an exercise study performed because of stable angina. The study definition of reverse redistribution was a region with normal activity in the stress image that showed definitely abnormal ^{201}Tl activity on reinjection, with a greater than 15% decrease in relative tracer uptake. All but 2 of the 29 patients had signs of previous myocardial infarction, all but 1 had coronary lesions, and the average ejection fraction was 0.38.

Results.—Of 377 segments analyzed, 13% showed the pattern of reverse distribution. Seventy-eight percent of the segments with reverse distribution had coronary lesions of 50% or greater. Half of the segments were occluded, with 35% of the occluded vessels showing collateral circulation. Seventy-two percent of the segments were hypokinetic or akinetic. Of these, 44% showed tissue viability, with uptake of greater than 55% of the peak value. Half of the segments with reverse redistribution also showed abnormal uptake at conventional 4-hour redistribution, whereas the other half had reverse distribution at reinjection only. Although the degree of coronary stenosis was greater in the former group, no significant differences were found in rate of coronary occlusion, ventricular dysfunction, or maintained viability.

Conclusions.—In patients with chronic coronary artery disease, the finding of ^{201}Tl reverse redistribution may reflect a significant coronary lesion, dysfunctioning myocardium with a collateral blood supply, and preserved tissue viability. More than 40% of these segments show viable myocardium, with some differences between segments with early vs. late redistribution. Because reverse redistribution can occur after reinjection, viability imaging should be considered for all patients with coronary artery disease and regional wall motion abnormalities who have ^{201}Tl scintigraphy.

▶ The authors provide more data on a controversial topic. Several conclusions can be drawn from this article. Reverse redistribution occurred in about 10% of patients, and those patients who manifest the finding have it in about 13% of segments. The finding often is associated with previous infarction in that territory. The clinical impact of this observation remains murky, however, because reverse redistribution did not signify a higher incidence of viability.

H.W. Strauss, M.D.

Does Positron Emission Tomography Contribute to the Management of Clinical Cardiac Problems?
Camici PG, Rosen SD (Hammersmith Hosp, London)
Eur Heart J 17:174–181, 1996   10–31

Background.—More and more centers are performing PET, which offers improved accuracy in the measurement of regional radioactivity concentrations and permits the use of true biological tracers. Ongoing advances are reducing the cost and increasing the reliability of this technique. There are questions about the "research" and "clinical" uses of PET, although these roles can be regarded as complementary. The current clinical applications of PET in the management of cardiac disease were investigated.

Clinical Applications.—Although PET is capable of identifying viable myocardium that can be revascularized in patients with coronary artery disease and chronic left ventricular dysfunction, the question is whether it offers information superior to that provided by other techniques. Current protocols using FDG can show the presence of metabolically active tissue in the myocardium; however, they cannot determine the amount of viable tissue present within the asynergic region. Measuring FDG uptake during hyperinsulinemic euglycemic clamp can provide high-quality images with uniform tracer uptake and permit the performance of PET studies under standard metabolic conditions. When this technique is used in conjunction with information on myocardial regional wall motion, there is no need for a simultaneous flow tracer.

Many different tracers have been used for measurement of myocardial blood flow with PET. Absolute myocardial blood flow can be measured noninvasively, which is especially useful in assessing the functional significance of coronary stenoses. Positron emission tomography also can evaluate myocardial blood flow in individuals with physiologic vs. pathologic left ventricular hypertrophy. It may be helpful in presymptomatic diagnosis for patients at risk of hypertrophic cardiomyopathy and has recently been used to assess coronary vasodilator reserve in patients with secondary left ventricular hypertrophy.

Discussion.—Achievements to date have made PET the "gold standard" for assessment of myocardial viability in patients with clinical cardiac disease. Ongoing research will refine the techniques used and the clinical application of the data they provide. Positron emission tomography provides a noninvasive technique to obtain absolute measurements of myocardial blood flow, which helps in evaluating the impact of epicardial coronary stenoses on regional microvascular function and in distinguishing benign from pathologic myocardial hypertrophy.

Evaluation of Cardiac Sympathetic Innervation With Iodine-123-Metaiodobenzylguanidine Imaging in Silent Myocardial Ischemia

Matsuo S, Takahashi M, Nakamura Y, et al (Shiga Univ, Japan)
J Nucl Med 37:712–717, 1996   10–32

Objective.—Patients with silent myocardial ischemia (SMI) have no sensation of pain despite having objective evidence of myocardial ischemia. One major cause of SMI is thought to be an autonomic nervous system abnormality caused by diabetic neuropathy. Iodine-123–labeled metaiodobenzylguanidine (MIBG) is useful in assessing the sympathetic innervation of the heart. The presence of SMI was compared with the myocardial [123I]MIBG uptake in patients with diabetes.

Methods.—The study included 14 patients with diabetes and SMI, 14 patients with diabetes and angina pectoris, 8 nondiabetic patients with SMI, and 21 normal controls. Planar and SPECT imaging were done immediately and 3 hours after injection of [123I]MIBG; exercise thallium scintigraphy was performed as well. Uptake of MIBG was expressed as the myocardial-to-mediastinal ratio, the inferior wall to anterior wall count ratio, the relative regional uptake (RRU) washout rate, and the corrected [123I]MIBG defect score.

Results.—The mean myocardial-to-mediastinal ratio was 2.1 in the diabetic SMI group and 2.3 in the nondiabetic SMI group, slightly lower than the 2.6 ratio in the control group. For normal individuals, the lowest RRU value was found in the inferior wall of the left ventricle. The controls had less [123I]MIBG uptake in the interior and apex myocardial segments than in the anterior segments. The RRU in the inferior segment of the distal left ventricle was significantly different between the patients with diabetes who had symptomatic vs. asymptomatic ischemia. Although the patients with diabetes and SMI patients had the smallest inferior wall to anterior wall count ratio, there was no significant difference in the corrected [123I]MIBG score between the 3 patient groups.

Conclusions.—Cardiac sympathetic dysfunction may be signaled by the finding of decreased MIBG uptake in the inferior myocardial wall in patients with diabetes and SMI. Thus, cardiac nervous system abnormalities may play a key role in the development of SMI. The precise diagnostic role of [123I]MIBG remains to be determined. Normal individuals have diverse MIBG uptake values.

▶ Innervation is not the whole story, but it may play a role in the lack of pain often seen in these patients.

H.W. Strauss, M.D.

Dual-tracer Autoradiography With Thallium-201 and Iodine-125-Metaiodobenzylguanidine in Experimental Myocardial Infarction of Rat
Iwasaki T, Suzuki T, Tateno M, et al (Gunma Univ, Japan; Univ of Tokyo)
J Nucl Med 37:680–684, 1996   10–33

Introduction.—In acute myocardial infarction, ischemic damage may have greater effects on cardiac sympathetic nervous system function—as shown by iodine-123 metaiodobenzylguanidine myocardial scintigraphy—than on the myocardium itself—as shown by thallium-201 scintigraphy. Few studies have compared radioiodinated MIBG and ^{201}Tl scintigraphic measurements of infarct size on a histopathologic and biochemical basis. To determine the significance of the discrepancy between [^{125}I]MIBG and ^{201}Tl distribution on dual-tracer autoradiography, a study was done in rats.

Methods.—Experimental myocardial infarction was produced in rats by 30 minutes of left coronary artery ligation followed by reperfusion. Four hours or 2 days after reperfusion, dual-tracer autoradiography of infarcted heart sections was done using [^{125}I]MIBG and ^{201}Tl. The infarcted area was then defined by immunohistochemical staining with myoglobin monoclonal antibody. The infarct region defined by dual-tracer autoradiography and myoglobin immunostaining was investigated for ultrastructural changes and norepinephrine content.

Results.—The region around the experimental infarct was discrepant on dual-tracer autoradiography, with decreased [^{125}I]MIBG uptake but normal ^{201}Tl distribution. The discrepant region resolved after 2 days (Fig 2). Nerve terminals in this region showed loss of granular cores, although normal structures were found between normal myocytes. The mean myocardial norepinephrine level was 255 ng/mg in the discrepant region vs. 550 ng/mg in the nonischemic region.

Conclusions.—In experimental myocardial infarction, the discrepancy in uptake between ^{201}Tl and [^{125}I]MIBG reflects a functional denervation of the regional cardiac sympathetic nerve terminals in the noninfarcted myocardium. This denervation is transient, resolving within 2 days in the rat model used in this study. The autoradiographic and morphologic evidence of functional denervation is supported by the finding of decreased myocardial norepinephrine content in the discrepant region.

▶ Everything in life is transient. Eventually, innervation and perfusion are matched. The major question is how long does this process take in humans?

H.W. Strauss, M.D.

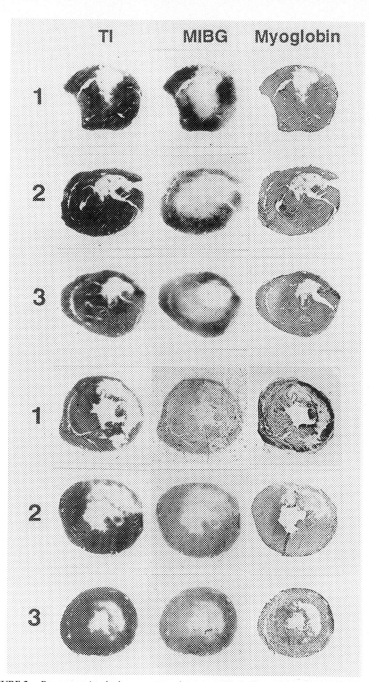

FIGURE 2.—Representative dual-tracer autoradiograms with thallium-201, iodine-125 metaiodobenzylguanidine (*MIBG*), and myoglobin immunostaining of hearts from 3 different rats with 30-minute coronary artery ligation. Myoglobin immunostaining and ^{201}Tl autoradiograms show identical defect regions representing myocardial infarction. Normal uptake of ^{201}Tl and [^{125}I]MIBG has almost disappeared from the infarcted region. **Upper panel,** 4 hours after reperfusion. **Lower panel,** 2 days after reperfusion. (Reprinted by permission of the Society of Nuclear Medicine, from Iwasaki T, Suzuki T, Tateno M, et al: Dual-tracer autoradiography with thallium-201 and iodine-125-metaiodobenzylguanidine in experimental myocardial infarction of rat. *J Nucl Med* 37:680–684, 1996.)

Influence of Downscatter in Simultaneously Acquired Thallium-201/ Technetium-99m-PYP SPECT

Ando H, Fukuyama T, Mitsuoka W, et al (Matsuyama Red Cross Hosp, Ehime, Japan)
J Nucl Med 37:781–785, 1996   10–34

Background.—There is growing interest in simultaneously acquired dual-isotope imaging as a means of shortening acquisition times and reducing errors caused by image misalignment. However, photon spillover from the other tracer is a potential source of problems with this technique. To evaluate the effects of technetium-99m downscatter on the thallium-201 images, an analysis of simultaneously acquired ^{201}Tl/^{99m}Tc-pyrophosphate dual-isotope SPECT in patients with acute myocardial infarction was done.

Methods.—Seventeen patients with acute myocardial infarction underwent dual-isotope ^{201}Tl/^{99m}Tc pyrophosphate SPECT. The ^{201}Tl studies were performed first, starting with a ^{201}Tl photopeak window after ^{201}Tl injection. These early ^{201}Tl images were followed by injection of ^{99m}Tc, with SPECT images acquired using dual-isotope windows (dual ^{201}Tl images). Finally, ^{201}Tl images were obtained 24 hours after injection of ^{99m}Tc. The 3 sets of ^{201}Tl images were analyzed to determine the thallium defect size and severity scores.

Results.—Images from all patients showed varying degrees of ^{99m}Tc accumulation. The early ^{201}Tl images and the 24-hour ^{201}Tl images had the same defect size and severity scores. However, in the dual ^{201}Tl images, the size scores were reduced by 36% and the severity scores by 53%.

Conclusions.—In simultaneously acquired dual-isotope ^{201}Tl/^{99m}Tc pyrophosphate imaging studies of patients with acute myocardial infarction, downscatter of ^{99m}Tc into ^{201}Tl is a potential source of problems. This ^{99m}Tc downscatter is sufficient to cause misinterpretations of both infarct size and myocardial viability. Several techniques to compensate for downscatter have been proposed, but these require validation.

▶ Downscatter from 20 mCi of pyrophosphate, even in the circumstance of minimal myocardial uptake, will make a big difference in the appearance of the resultant image. The situation is compounded because the investigators used an older 37-tube camera. Modern cameras generally have more efficient scatter rejection, making this kind of dual-tracer imaging more reliable. However, even newer instruments will have difficulty when sixfold more of the higher energy radionuclide is administered. These studies should be done with no more than a threefold difference, and preferably with less of the higher energy than the lower energy radionuclide.

H.W. Strauss, M.D.

Comparison and Reproducibility of Visual Echocardiographic and Quantitative Radionuclide Left Ventricular Ejection Fractions

van Royen N, Jaffe CC, Krumholz HM, et al (Yale Univ, New Haven, Conn)
Am J Cardiol 77:843–850, 1996   10–35

Introduction.—Equilibrium radionuclide angiography and echocardiography are commonly used to determine the left ventricular ejection fraction (LVEF) in patients with coronary artery disease. This measurement forms the basis for many important clinical decisions, and the 2 techniques are commonly regarded as interchangeable. The LVEF determinations made by 2-dimensional echocardiography and equilibrium radionuclide angiography were compared, including the reproducibility of both techniques and the clinical significance of any differences.

Methods.—The study included 73 patients who underwent equilibrium radionuclide angiography and echocardiography within a 4-day period. The patients, who had various indications, all were in clinically stable condition. Three echocardiographers and 3 nuclear cardiology technologists assessed LVEF in blinded fashion using both techniques. The readings were repeated after 1 week to assess reproducibility. In the repeat assess-

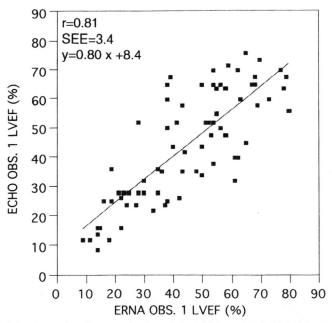

FIGURE 1.—Comparison between visually estimated left ventricular ejection fraction (*LVEF*) by echocardiographer #1 and quantitative assessment of LVEF by nuclear technologist #1. The mean difference is −0.6 ± 23.6% (2 standard deviations). *Abbreviations: ECHO*, 2-dimensional echocardiography; *ERNA*, equilibrium radionuclide angiography; *OBS*, observer. (Reprinted by permission of the publisher from van Royen N, Jaffe CC, Krumholz HM, et al: Comparison and reproducibility of visual echocardiographic and quantitative radionuclide left ventricular ejection fractions. *Am J Cardiol* 77:843-850, Copyright 1996 by Excerpta Medica, Inc.)

ments, a difference of 10% or greater ejection fraction units was considered to be of potential clinical significance.

Results.—Good correlation was found between the 2 techniques, $r =$ 0.81 (Fig 1). However, the limit of agreement in individual patients was 24%. Both intraobserver and interobserver reproducibility were somewhat better for the radionuclide study than for the echocardiographic study. The limits of agreement for radionuclide angiography were 2% to 4%, compared with 13% to 17% for echocardiography. Repeat analysis of the radionuclide studies did not disclose clinically relevant differences. In contrast, potentially important differences were found in 8% to 26% of cases on echocardiographic studies.

Conclusions.—Equilibrium radionuclide angiographic and echocardiographic determinations of LVEF show good agreement and provide clinically applicable information. However, radionuclide studies appear to be the better choice for patient management decisions requiring high reproducibility. When the goal is to find patients with severely depressed or definitely normal LVEF and to evaluate cardiac structure and function, 2-dimensional echocardiography may be preferred.

▶ Comparison of an objective to a subjective technique may not seem fair, but that is how the techniques are used in clinical care. The lack of reproducibility of the echo measurement raises serious concern about the value of this approach for serial measurements.

H.W. Strauss, M.D.

Iodine-123 Metaiodobenzylguanidine in the Assessment of Late Cardiac Effects From Cancer Therapy
Olmos RAV, ten Bokkel Huinink WW, Dewit LGH, et al (The Netherlands Cancer Inst, Amsterdam)
Eur J Nucl Med 23:453–458, 1996   10–36

Objective.—Survivors of cancer treatment are at risk of late adverse cardiac effects, particularly caused by anthracycline chemotherapy and radiotherapy involving the heart. Many patients have detectable but subclinical cardiac sequelae, which might place them at high risk if they were treated for recurrent cancer with potentially cardiotoxic treatments. Heart scintigraphic studies with iodine-123 metaiodobenzylguanidine (MIBG) were evaluated for their ability to identify patients with late cardiac effects after cancer therapy.

Methods.—The study included 18 patients with cancer, 11 of whom had received thoracic irradiation involving the heart a median of 60 months previously. In 5 patients, the radiotherapy was combined with anthracycline treatment. The 7 control patients had received neither anthracycline chemotherapy nor chest radiotherapy. All patients underwent ^{123}I MIBG heart scintigraphy to seek abnormalities of myocardial adrenergic neuron function, and the results were compared against the left ventricle ejection fraction (LVEF). Cardiac uptake of ^{123}I MIBG was expressed as a heart-to-mediastinum ratio on planar images after 4 hours, and myocardial ^{123}I MIBG washout was determined from planar images obtained at 15 minutes and 4 hours.

Results.—The median ^{123}I MIBG cardiac uptake was 1.56 patients exposed to potentially cardiotoxic treatments, compared with a value of 1.9 in the control patients. There also were significant differences between groups in myocardial ^{123}I MIBG washout and in LVEF, although these values overlapped between groups. In the patients receiving potentially cardiotoxic treatments, the cardiac abnormalities ranged from focal defects to diffuse reductions in myocardial uptake, as shown by planar images and additional SPECT images. The most severe abnormalities in the exposed group were noted in patients older than 60 years.

Conclusions.—Heart scintigraphic studies using ^{123}I MIBG can identify cancer treatment survivors with late cardiac sequelae. This nuclear medicine technique may be useful in risk assessment of patients who require retreatment with potentially cardiotoxic forms of therapy. It may be especially valuable in following adult patients with cancer who receive chest radiotherapy and in monitoring the long-term cardiac effects of cancer therapy in children.

▶ This is further evidence that cardiac irradiation and cardiotoxic chemotherapy cause changes in the heart. Accelerated atherosclerosis, possible abnormal endothelial function, and now abnormal adrenergic innervation have been described. It is important to bear in mind, however, that the goal is to treat the cancer as effectively as possible. This should be done to the limits of cardiac function.

H.W. Strauss, M.D.

Comparison of Technetium-99m Sestamibi Left Ventricular Wall Motion and Perfusion Studies With Thallium-201 Perfusion Imaging: In Search of the Combination of Variables With the Highest Accuracy in Predicting Coronary Artery Disease
Verzijlbergen JF, Zwinderman AH, Ascoop CAPL, et al (St Antonius Hosp, Nieuwegein, The Netherlands; Univ Hosp, Leiden, The Netherlands) *Eur J Nucl Med* 23:550–559, 1996   10–37

Background.—Myocardial perfusion and ventricular function measures are expected to provide useful information for detecting coronary artery disease (CAD). The current study determined the extent to which technetium-99m–labeled sestamibi wall motion yields information different from that provided by ^{99m}Tc-labeled sestamibi and thallium-201 perfusion, what information is useful in diagnosing CAD, and the most diagnostically accurate combination of variables.

Methods.—Sixty patients with suspected CAD were studied. Perfusion and wall motion scores obtained from visual and quantitative planar [201]Tl

TABLE 4.—Summary of the Sensitivity and Specificity for the Visual
and Quantitative Analyses

	Sensitivity	Specificity
^{201}Tl, visual	89%	79%
^{201}Tl, quantitative	70%	93%
^{99m}Tc-sestamibi, visual	89%	79%
^{99m}Tc-sestamibi, quantitative	89%	64%

(Courtesy of Verzijlbergen JF, Zwinderman AH, Ascoop CAPL, et al: Comparison of technetium-99m sestambi left ventricular wall motion and perfusion studies with thallium-201 perfusion imaging: In search of the combination of variables with the highest accuracy in predicting coronary artery disease. *Eur J Nucl Med* 23:550–559, 1996, Copyright Springer-Verlag.)

and ^{99m}Tc-labeled sestamibi scintigraphy were compared with angiographic findings in a polytomous logistic regression model. The diagnostic values were compared with one another.

Findings.—Thallium-201 stress and redistribution variables were correlated in comparative studies. Stepwise logistic regression analysis indicated that the combination of ^{201}Tl visual analysis of the stress images with quantitative redistribution images had the strongest diagnostic power, with a sensitivity of 93% and a specificity of 71%. All combinations of visual and quantitative analyses of the exercise and redistribution images had comparable diagnostic power. The diastolic stress image scores had the strongest diagnostic power of the ^{99m}Tc-labeled sestamibi variables, with a sensitivity of 91% and a specificity of 79%. Wall motion studies did not increase diagnostic power (Table 4).

Conclusions.—Technetium-99m–labeled sestamibi enables simultaneous measurement of myocardial perfusion and left ventricular function. However, there was no incremental value when the findings of combined perfusion and wall motion studies at rest and during exercise were compared with ^{201}Tl or ^{99m}Tc-labeled sestamibi perfusion studies alone.

▶ Once again, visual analysis by qualified readers performs well. It is surprising that the use of diastolic images with ^{99m}Tc-labeled sestamibi did not perform better. This may have been because of the difficulty in eliminating artifacts from attenuation (especially in the stomach after the patients ate). Now we need to see this study performed with gated SPECT imaging and attenuation correction.

H.W. Strauss, M.D.

Prediction of Functional Outcome After Myocardial Infarction Using BMIPP and Sestamibi Scintigraphy

Franken PR, Dendale P, De Geeter F, et al (Free Univ of Brussels, Belgium)
J Nucl Med 37:718–722, 1996   10–38

Background.—Radiolabeled fatty acids such as β-methyl iodophenyl pentadecanoic acid (BMIPP) may be useful in assessing reversible dysfunction in patients with subacute myocardial infarction. Previous studies have found differences between BMIPP uptake and perfusion, and regions showing greater reductions in BMIPP uptake than thallium-201 or sestamibi uptake at rest have been associated with successful reperfusion. The combination of BMIPP and sestamibi imaging was evaluated for its ability to predict long-term functional outcome after acute myocardial infarction.

Methods.—Eighteen patients with persistent regional wall motion abnormalities were studied 4–10 days after acute myocardial infarction. Each underwent BMIPP and sestamibi studies at rest as well as echocardiographic studies under low-dose dobutamine stimulation (Fig 1). The

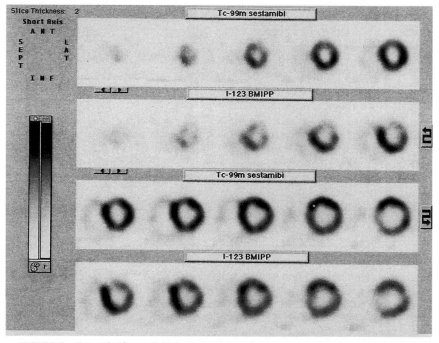

FIGURE 1.—Sestamibi (**first and third rows**) and β-methyl iodophenyl pentadecanoic acid (*BMIPP*) (**second and fourth rows**) left ventricular short-axis slices obtained 7–8 days after anterior myocardial infarction. There is mild to moderate reduction of sestamibi uptake in the apical and midventricular anterior segments. The BMIPP study shows similar defect intensity in the apex (matching) but more severe defects in the anterior and lateral walls (mismatching). (Reprinted with permission of the Society of Nuclear Medicine, from Franken PR, Dendale P, de Geeter F, et al: Prediction of functional outcome after myocardial infarction using BMIPP and sestamibi scintigraphy. *J Nucl Med* 37:718–722, 1996.)

functional outcomes were evaluated at 6 months by repeated rest echocardiographic studies.

Results.—Eighty-two percent of segments with mismatching between BMIPP and sestamibi studies showed improved wall motion at follow-up, compared with only 10% of segments with matched BMIPP and sestamibi defects. The combination of BMIPP and sestamibi imaging was 85% accurate in predicting the functional outcome of segments, compared with an accuracy of 77% with sestamibi alone. Eighty percent of segments showing contractile reserve had improved wall motion, whereas 63% of segments with negative results from dobutamine tests showed no improvement; dobutamine echocardiography thus had an accuracy of 69%. Combining the SPECT and echocardiography techniques produced positive and negative predictive values of 94%.

Conclusions.—A mismatch between BMIPP and sestamibi uptake after myocardial infarction is associated with improved long-term functional recovery after acute myocardial infarction. No improvement is seen in segments with matched BMIPP and sestamibi defects, suggesting the presence of only scar tissue. The combination of BMIPP and sestamibi SPECT also is more accurate than dobutamine echocardiography.

▶ Predicting the return of regional wall motion after an ischemic injury is important. The degree of perfusion impairment often is the standard used for this purpose. These authors demonstrate that adding information about the relationship of perfusion to fatty acid uptake increases the predictive value of this determination. In 82% of the areas of perfusion/fatty acid uptake mismatched wall motion improved at 6 months, whereas there was no improvement in 90% of segments in which the perfusion/fatty acid uptake was similarly decreased. Such a perfusion may be a useful approach to make this determination. A major question is whether anyone will pay for it.

H.W. Strauss, M.D.

Coronary Flow Reserve: Noninvasive Measurement in Humans With Breath-hold Velocity-encoded Cine MR Imaging
Sakuma H, Blake LM, Amidon TM, et al (Univ of California, San Francisco; GE Med Systems, Waukesha, Wis)
Radiology 198:745–750, 1996   10–39

Background.—The anatomical severity of coronary stenosis, as depicted by x-ray coronary angiography, does not necessarily reflect its functional significance. The small diameter of the coronary arteries has made it difficult to measure the blood flow velocity in those vessels. Using data acquired during a single breath-hold, fast velocity-encoded cine MRI has proven capable of providing a phasic flow-velocity time curve for the human coronary arteries. This technique was used to measure coronary vasodilator reserve in humans.

Methods.—Eight healthy adults were studied using a 1.5-tesla MRI unit. The velocity-encoded cine MR images were obtained during a single breath-hold in 25 seconds, using k-space segmentation and view-sharing reconstruction. The velocity encoding value was ± 1 m/sec; the repetition time, 16 milliseconds; and the echo time, 9 milliseconds. Two measurements of flow velocity in the left anterior descending artery were made both before and after IV administration of 0.56 mg of dipyridamole per kilogram.

Results.—The mean peak diastolic flow velocity in the left anterior descending artery increased from 15 seconds at baseline to 46 seconds after dipyridamole administration. This corresponded to an average coronary reserve of 3. Interstudy and reproducibility for peak diastolic velocity at baseline was 10% and interobserver reproducibility was 7% at baseline. Corresponding values were 7% and 3% after dipyridamole administration.

Conclusions.—Reproducible measurements of human coronary flow reserve can be obtained using the breath-hold velocity-encoded cine MRI technique described in this study. The accuracy of the flow velocity and volume measurements obtained by this technique must be evaluated further in animal studies using ultrasound flow probes.

▶ Velocity is not flow, but it is an interesting parameter. The surrogates for measuring perfusion are like a siren song, always alluring to the unwary. Determinations such as the blush on an arteriogram, the time activity curve of material through a tissue, the change in velocity from state A to state B, all have been advocated as indicators of perfusion. Although a relationship exists with each of these parameters, the relationship is not linear.

H.W. Strauss, M.D.

11 Correlative Imaging

Introduction

This chapter began just a few years ago as an experimental undertaking designed to discuss how and where our nuclear niche belongs in the integrated imaging patient workup. It is the least structured of all of the sections, but it tends to have more bone studies than anything else. This is probably because we do a lot of bone studies and the other modalities provide images that either integrate or compete. Similarly, we often have several brain papers, because both MRI and CT do a lot of brain work and we sometimes integrate or compete. My hope for this chapter is to provide you with ammunition to fight some of the integrated imaging wars that come your way and occasionally to provide you with a new nuclear niche to extend the work that you do. Frankly, I am not sure I am successful in either of these goals, and I have challenged you in the past to write me to let me know whether you think this section is useful to you at all. To date, no one has taken me up on this challenge. You know what they say about "no news," so we will keep on presenting these papers. However, if any of you have constructive criticism you would like to voice, don't be shy. I would like to hear it.

Alexander Gottschalk, M.D.

Serial MRI in Early Creutzfeldt-Jacob Disease With a Point Mutation of Prion Protein at Codon 180
Ishida S, Sugino M, Koizumi N, et al (Osaka Med College, Japan; Osaka Gen Hosp, Osaka City, Japan; Kyusyu Univ, Hukuoka City, Japan)
Neuroradiology 37:531–534, 1995   11–1

Background.—Creutzfeldt-Jakob disease (CJD) is a genetically transmitted neurodegenerative disease caused by a prion protein (PrP). Point mutations of the PrP gene have been identified at codons 102, 117, 129, 178, 198, and 200. A patient with CJD, in whom a new point mutation of the PrP gene was identified, was studied with serial MRI examinations.

Case Report.—Woman, 66, was admitted in September 1991 for progressive amnesia beginning 1 year earlier. She had muscle rigid-

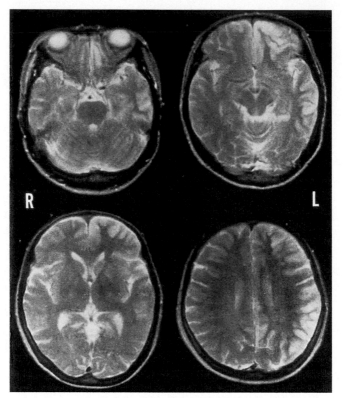

FIGURE 1.—Axial T2-weighted images (TR 2,000/TE 120) in June 1991 showed high signal in the left frontal, parietal, and temporal cortex. (Courtesy of Ishida S, Sugino M, Koizumi N, et al: Serial MRI in early Creutzfeldt-Jacob disease with a point mutation of prion protein at codon 180. *Neuroradiology* 37:531–534, 1995. Copyright Springer-Verlag.)

ity in her legs, exaggerated reflexes, aphasia, apraxia, disorientation, and memory disturbance. There were no periodic sharp waves on the electroencephalogram at any point throughout the clinical course. The MRI in June 1991 revealed increased signal in the cortex of the left frontal, parietal, and temporal lobes on T2-weighted images (Fig 1). Three months later the hyperintense cortical areas were larger and included the right frontal lobe. A technetium-99m–hexamethylpropyleneamine oxime study revealed left cerebral perfusion defects (Fig 3). The patient experienced progressive clinical deterioration, with akinesis, mutism, and myoclonic jerks occurring by October 1991. The MRI at that time revealed hyperintense spreading in the right cerebral cortex and into the basal ganglia bilaterally on T2-weighted images, and the T1-weighted images demonstrated frontal cortical atrophy. Examination of tissue obtained in an open brain biopsy of the left frontal lobe with the Western blot technique established the diagnosis of

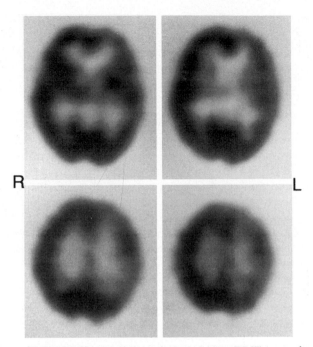

R   L

FIGURE 3.—Technetium-99m–hexamethylpropyleneamine oxime SPECT 1 year after onset demonstrated abnormal decrease in activity in the left cerebral hemisphere. (Courtesy of Ishida S. Sugino M. Koizumi N, et al: Serial MRI in early Creutzfeldt-Jacob disease with a point mutation of prion protein at codon 180. *Neuroradiology* 37:531–534, 1995. Copyright Springer-Verlag.)

CJD. Genetic analysis of DNA from peripheral blood leukocytes identified a G to A transition at codon 180.

Discussion.—The patient had both an atypical clinical course and atypical MRI findings. These variants may have been related to the finding of a variant mutation of the PrP gene.

▶ I am sure you guessed that in this year of the "mad cow" we would find something to put in the YEAR BOOK relating to Creutzfeldt-Jakob disease. Frankly, we're not sure what to make of this case report because—as the authors point out—the MRI findings are not uniform. Presumably the SPECT findings would be inconsistent as well.

A. Gottschalk, M.D.

Cerebral Demyelination Syndrome in a Patient Treated With 5-Fluorouracil and Levamisole: The Use of Thallium SPECT Imaging to Assist in Noninvasive Diagnosis. A Case Report

Savarese DM, Gordon J, Smith TW, et al (Univ of Massachusetts, Worcester)
Cancer 77:387–394, 1996   11–2

Background.—Patients with stage III adenocarcinoma of the colon are currently treated with 5-fluorouracil (5-FU) and levamisole. This treatment regimen is usually well tolerated, but there have been several reports of cerebral demyelination in patients treated with this combined therapy. This rare toxicity has a clinical picture suggesting multiple brain metastases. The imaging evaluation of a patient with this treatment-related syndrome was reported.

> *Case Report.*—Woman, 68, was admitted with left facial weakness, slurred speech, ataxia, and left arm and leg weakness. She had been treated for stage III adenocarcinoma of the sigmoid colon with adjuvant 5-FU/levamisole. Computed tomographic scanning was nondiagnostic. Symptoms improved when 5-FU/levamisole treatment was interrupted and worsened when treatment was reinstituted. An MRI scan with and without contrast showed several

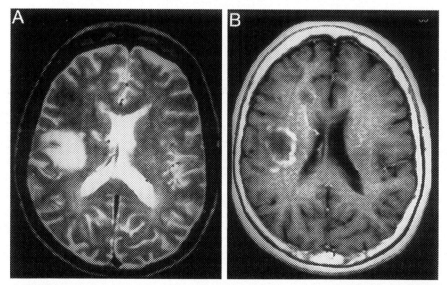

FIGURE 2.—Magnetic resonance image of the head at time of presentation. **A,** T2 (TR 2,500; TE 20). A focal area of abnormal T2 hyperintensity is seen at the corona radiata on the right. There are smaller scattered areas of punctate T2 hyperintensity. **B,** T1 (TR 600; TE 17) axial MR image with gadolinium reveals peripheral ring-type enhancement about the focus of abnormal T2 hyperintensity. Note the central area of T1 hypointensity, suggestive of focally increased tissue water content. (From Savarese DM, Gordon J, Smith TW, et al: Cerebral demyelination syndrome in a patient treated with 5-fluorouracil and levamisole: The use of thallium SPECT imaging to assist in noninvasive diagnosis. A case report. *Cancer* 77:387–394, 1996. Copyright © 1996 American Cancer Society. Reprinted by permission of Wiley-Liss, Inc., a division of John Wiley & Sons, Inc.)

bilateral infratentorial and supratentorial enhancing lesions and irregular ring-type enhancement of the right cerebral white matter (Fig 2). These features were atypical for brain metastasis. Indeed, there was no uptake with a radionuclide SPECT brain scan with thallium-201. Histologic analysis of a CT-guided stereotactic brain biopsy revealed demyelination with axonal sparing with no malignant cells. The patient was treated with dexamethasone, and her symptoms resolved. The MRI scans after treatment showed decreased but persistent areas of hyperintensity but no irregular ring enhancement.

Discussion.—Both 5-FU and levamisole have been implicated in this toxic syndrome, but there is increasing evidence of the pathogenetic role of levamisole, because patients rechallenged with each agent individually have had recurrences only with levamisole. The use of ^{201}Tl SPECT can distinguish noninvasively between malignant and nonmalignant disease, thus avoiding potentially devastating radiation treatment in patients with demyelinating disease.

▶ I am sorry we could not show you the thallium image because it was printed in color. However, believe me when I tell you that there was absolutely *no* uptake seen adjacent to the right lateral ventricle. Although metastasis is certainly a common cause of ring enhancement on MRI, particularly in a patient with a known primary such as this patient, this lesion is somewhat irregular in contour and not quite round. Consequently, the astute neuroradiologist would be leary of definitively calling this metastatic disease. If he knows what he is doing, he will consult you next—be ready with the thallium.

A. Gottschalk, M.D.

Case Report: Imaging of Central Nervous System Sarcoidosis With Gallium-67 Single Photon Emission Computed Tomography
Jarman PR, Whyte MKB, Glass DM, et al (Hammersmith Hosp, London)
Br J Radiol 69:192–194, 1996   11–3

Introduction.—Sarcoidosis is a granulomatous disease with multisystem involvement. Involvement of the nervous system is uncommon, reported in approximately 5% of the patients. It is difficult to establish a definitive diagnosis of neurosarcoidosis because of the difficulty of obtaining a biopsy specimen of nervous system tissue. Therefore, imaging and biopsy specimens obtained from other organs that demonstrate sarcoid granulomas usually establish the diagnosis. Gallium-67 scintigraphy has been relied on to identify sarcoidosis; however, SPECT may be more useful, providing improved spatial resolution. That technique was used in a patient with neurosarcoidosis.

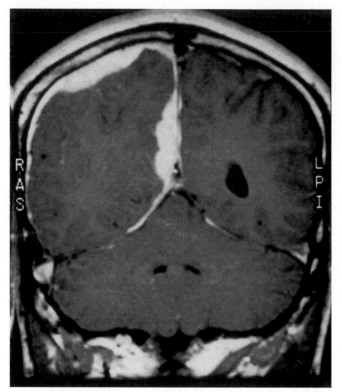

FIGURE 1.—Coronal MRI (T1-weighted spin echo) with gadolinium enhancement showing brightly enhancing, lobulated thickening of the falx and meninges over the right posterior cerebral hemisphere. (Courtesy of Jarman PR, Whyte MKB, Glass DM, et al: Case report: Imaging of central nervous system sarcoidosis with gallium-67 single photon emission computed tomography. *Br J Radiol* 69:192–194, 1996.)

Case Report.—Man, 28, had a 3-month history of brief episodes of altered consciousness. There was nodular shadowing and a bilateral loss of volume in the upper lobes on both a chest radiograph and CT. Excess lymphocytes, suggestive of sarcoidosis, were present in the bronchoalveolar lavage fluid, but results of the transbronchial biopsy were normal. Unenhanced CT of the brain demonstrated a mass in the right side of the chiasmatic cistern and a hypodense area in the right occipital cortex. Meningeal thickening appeared over the right posterior cerebral hemisphere extending along the falx cerebri into the midline on MRI (Fig 1). Whole-body planar scans with ^{67}Ga scintigraphy showed uptake at several points within the chest and an area of abnormal uptake in the right occipitoparietal area. Imaging with SPECT clarified the radionuclide activity in the brain, which was localized over the occipitoparietal cortex, extending into the brain along the posterior portion of the falx cerebri (Fig 4). A meningeal biopsy confirmed the presence of confluent granulomatous inflammation. This, along

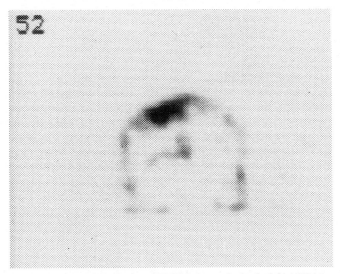

FIGURE 4.—Detail of coronal gallium-67 SPECT image at the level of the MRI image (Figure 1), showing meningeal lesions in a similar distribution. (Courtesy of Jarman PR, Whyte MKB, Glass DM, et al: Case report: Imaging of central nervous system sarcoidosis with gallium-67 single photon emission computed tomography. *Br J Radiol* 69:192–194, 1996.)

with the pulmonary abnormalities, established the diagnosis of neurosarcoidosis. The patient was treated with high-dose corticosteroids for 3 months and had no further episodes of altered consciousness.

Conclusion.—Gallium-67 SPECT imaging can improve localization of brain lesions in patients with CNS sarcoidosis.

▶ Frankly, it seems much more likely that the diagnosis here will be made with MRI. We have made a diagnosis like this in many cases of neurosarcoidosis without a lot of difficulty, particularly when gadolinium enhancement is used.

On the other hand, it may be that your patient has a fever of unknown origin and gets a whole-body nuclear medicine screen with [67]Ga. In that case, these findings should allow you to suggest the correct diagnosis.

A. Gottschalk, M.D.

MR and Positron Emission Tomography With Fludeoxyglucose F 18 in Gliomatosis Cerebri

Dexter MA, Parker GD, Besser M, et al (Royal Prince Alfred Hosp, Sydney, Australia)
AJNR 16:1507–1510, 1995   11–4

Background.—Cerebral angiography, pneumoencephalography, and CT have not been useful in identifying specific morphologic changes in patients with gliomatosis cerebri, even when the clinical changes were profound. It has been suggested that MRI could allow the definitive diagnosis and localization of gliomatosis cerebri. The findings with MRI and PET with FDG in the preoperative evaluation of a patient with unilateral painless third nerve palsy as the first sign of gliomatosis cerebri were described.

Case Report.—Girl, 16 years, first appeared with diplopia, which was found to be associated with a right third nerve palsy with pupillary sparing. There were no CT abnormalities. Magnetic resonance imaging studies showed focal areas of cortical thickening (with slightly increased intensity on T2-weighted images) in the lateral and mesial right frontal lobe and insula, but no underlying white matter abnormalities. Three months later, the MRI studies revealed increased gyral thickening in the right frontal and temporal lobes and right third nerve compression, but still no white matter abnormalities. Nine months later, the patient was admitted to the hospital with diplopia and left-sided weakness. She had bilateral third nerve palsies with pupillary sparing. The MRI studies showed further increased cortical thickening in the right frontal lobe and insula as well as hyperintensity in the left mesial frontal cortex, right thalamus, and right striatum, with no white matter abnormalities. An FDG PET study showed reduced uptake in the right temporal and both frontal lobes, with uptake lower in the right thalamus and striatum than on the left. Bilateral fourth nerve palsies, a right sixth nerve palsy, and drowsiness quickly developed. The patient was treated surgically with the excision of the anterior 3 cm of the right temporal lobe, which resulted in marked symptomatic improvement. The histologic evaluation revealed the characteristic signs of gliomatosis cerebri.

Discussion.—Multiple cranial nerve palsies and hemiparesis indicate brain stem involvement, which was not detected with either MRI or FDG PET studies. However, both studies demonstrated the extent and progression of the disease process and were useful in planning surgical biopsy.

▶ I cannot decide whether this is a tour-de-force or a tour-de-farce. I say that because this patient underwent elegant workup with MR and FDG PET and yet, as the authors point out, the lesion causing the patient's symptoms was not detected with either study. I think the trick in making this diagnosis is to find the diffuse activity seen on the MR and the hypometabolism seen on the PET suggesting that although this is extensive disease, it is low-grade disease. Hopefully this will trigger the right diagnostic response in your own cerebrum. I am sorry that the PET study was in color so we could not print the images.

A. Gottschalk, M.D.

Osteonecrosis of the Medial Part of the Tibial Plateau
Ecker ML, Lotke PA (Univ of Pennsylvania, Philadelphia)
J Bone Joint Surg (Am) 77A:596–601, 1995   11–5

Background.—Usually, the initial plain roentgenogram does not detect osteonecrosis of the medial femoral condyle, although increased uptake is seen on the radionuclide bone scan and the T1-weighted MRI shows a subchondral area of hypointensity instead of the normal hyperintense signal from the fat in the marrow. However, osteonecrosis of the knee has been seen on radionuclide scintiscans but not on MRI. Plain roentgenograms demonstrated tibial osteonecrosis in a large number of affected patients.

Methods.—In a 14-year period, 16 knees in 15 elderly patients with acute knee pain were evaluated with plain roentgenograms, technetium radionuclide bone scans, and MRI. Because of symptom progression, 9 knees were treated with a total knee arthroplasty and 3 were treated with a unicompartmental replacement. Surgery was also recommended but refused for 2 additional knees. The symptoms resolved spontaneously in the last 2 knees.

Results.—The initial plain roentgenograms of 9 of the 16 knees demonstrated a radiolucent area at the site of tenderness. Of the remaining 7 knees, radionuclide bone scans revealed focal technetium uptake at the site of tenderness in 4, and MR images showed focal areas of hypointensity at the site of tenderness in the other 3. Surgery resulted in satisfactory outcome in all 12 knees. Histologic findings indicated late-stage osteonecrosis of the tibial plateau. Later operations in 3 knees revealed a degenerative tear in the medial meniscus, which corresponded with the areas of hypointensity on MRI but did not show up on the initial plain roentgenograms.

Conclusions.—The characteristic roentgenographic, radionuclide, and MRI findings of tibial osteonecrosis should be sought in patients with acute knee pain. When these signs appear, arthroscopic débridement is contraindicated, even in patients with a degenerative tear in the meniscus, which is common in the elderly.

▶ These authors make an excellent point that all nuclear physicians should understand. Impressive uptake on the medial side of the tibial plateau on the bone scan must raise a serious question of osteonecrosis in the elderly patient. In the first place, the routine MRI study of the knee will almost always show serious meniscal pathologic changes. Most commonly these menisci are macerated in this age group. And, as the authors point out, the MRI examination may not show the underlying osteonecrosis. Consequently, the diagnosis rests on appropriate clinical findings and the positive findings on a radionuclide bone scan. In short, the ball is in our court—let's not drop it.

A. Gottschalk, M.D.

Tibial Stress Reaction in Runners: Correlation of Clinical Symptoms and Scintigraphy With a New Magnetic Resonance Imaging Grading System
Fredericson M, Bergman AG, Hoffman KL, et al (Stanford Univ, Calif)
Am J Sports Med 23:472–481, 1995   11–6

Objective.—Stress fractures are a common form of sports medicine injury that may be difficult to diagnose and manage. Traditionally, runners with medial tibial pain have been regarded as having either a shinsplint syndrome or a stress fracture. However, only about half of symptomatic patients will ever show radiographic evidence of a stress reaction. Magnetic resonance imaging may be able to document a progression of injury, from periosteal edema through progressive marrow involvement, and finally to frank cortical stress fracture. An MRI-based grading system for the evaluation of tibial stress injuries in runners was evaluated, including an attempt to identify clinical factors indicating more severe grades of stress injury.

Methods.—The analysis included 18 symptomatic legs in 14 runners. All underwent clinical examination, bone scans, and MRI, all of which were performed within 10 days. The MRI findings were graded from 0 to 4: grade 0 indicated a normal examination; grade 1, mild to moderate periosteal edema on T2-weighted images only; grade 2, more severe periosteal edema and bone marrow edema on T2-weighted images only (Fig 2); grade 3, moderate to severe periosteal and marrow edema on T1- and T2-weighted images; and grade 4, low-signal fracture line on all sequences, along with severe marrow edema on T1- and T2-weighted images. The MRI results were compared with the clinical and bone scan findings.

Results.—The MRI result was grade 0 in 11% of legs, grade 1 in 11%, grade 2 in 17%, grade 3 in 56%, and grade IV in 6%. Fourteen of the 18 legs had similar results on bone scanning; 2 had a more severe injury detected on MRI, and 2 had normal MRI findings but a grade 1 injury on bone scanning. According to MRI, the location of injury was the proximal tibia in 7 cases, the midtibia in 6, and the distal tibia in 3. All of the injuries were found along the compressive side of the tibia, on the posteromedial border, which is subject to compressive forces during running. Eighty-eight percent of legs showed periosteal involvement. In most cases, the periosteal

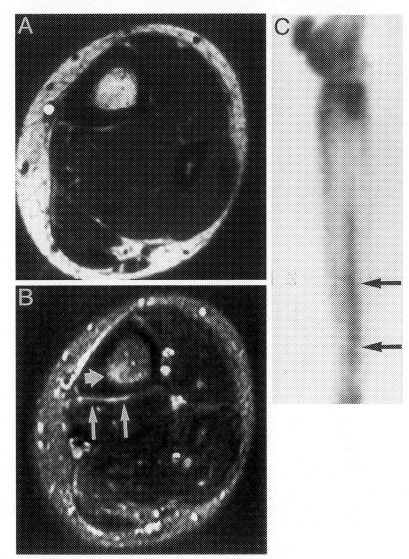

FIGURE 2.—Grade 2 MRI findings in the left lower leg in an 18-year-old female varsity runner. Axial T1-weighted MR image (**A**) shows no detectable abnormality, but the T2-weighted image (**B**) shows moderate periosteal edema (*long arrows*) along the posterior and medial aspect of the tibia, and there is marrow edema (*short arrow*) in the adjacent part of the tibia. The bone scintigraphy (**C**) shows increased activity along the distal half of the tibial diaphysis (*arrows*). (Courtesy of Fredericson M, Bergman AG, Hoffman KL, et al: Tibial stress reaction in runners: Correlation of clinical symptoms and scintigraphy with a new magnetic resonance imaging grading system. *Am J Sports Med* 23:472–481, 1995.)

edema involved the bony insertions of the tibialis posterior, the flexor digitorum longus, and soleus muscles.

Conclusions.—Magnetic resonance imaging helps to define the location and extent of tibial stress reaction in runners. Physical findings such as localized tibial tenderness and pain on direct percussion over the involved area are linked with more involved marrow and cortical abnormalities. Tenderness to indirect percussion is a very specific indicator of grade 3 or 4 injury. There is good correlation between the results of bone scanning and MRI. Periosteal edema appears to represent the initial injury on a spectrum that can progress to a more serious bone injury. The article includes illustrations of the newly developed MRI grading system for runners with medial tibial pain.

▶ The thing that makes these studies work is the use of the fat-suppressed, fast T2-weighted MR images—an excellent technique for seeing small amounts of edema in the soft tissues or bone marrow. Similar results can be obtained by using fast T2-weighted inversion recovery images as well. Both of these sequences are relatively new, and both are very sensitive for fluid and particularly useful in patients like the ones studied here. In fact, I wonder whether this technique is too sensitive. This study would have been better had a series of asymptomatic runners been used as a control to be sure the lower grades of edema were not discovered in the controls on these ultra-sensitive MRI studies.

Even if this turns out not to be the case, we think there is a good argument—overlooked in this article—for still using the bone scan to look at the legs of these runners. I call it the "double trouble" sign (a term I learned from a former colleague, Jack Lawson, a bone radiologist at Yale). Many times, when we see shinsplints in one leg, we find an occult stress fracture on the other side from the gait disturbance the pain has caused. Virtually all of the runners—the better the caliber, the more likely this is to happen—will run "through the pain" for a while before they even go see the trainer or sports physician. Consequently, they run with an altered gait, which probably causes the "double trouble" (in my experience usually a stress fracture in the metatarsal). Lesion number 2 is clinically occult because the pain of the second lesion is masked by the more severe pain in the opposite shinsplint leg. The bone scan, by looking at all of both legs (at least), finds both lesions. The MRI will not do that because it will be a directed scan looking at the lower extremity in question; even if it gets both legs (which it often will), it is unlikely to look at the foot, where the second trouble area is most likely to be.

A. Gottschalk, M.D.

The "Gray Cortex": An Early Sign of Stress Fracture
Mulligan ME (Univ of Maryland, Baltimore)
Skeletal Radiol 24:201–203, 1995   11–7

Background.—Recognizing stress injuries early can prevent more serious injury and hasten rehabilitation. However, it is often difficult to establish an early plain film radiologic diagnosis of stress injury, leading to the use of more expensive imaging technologies. However, a focal graying

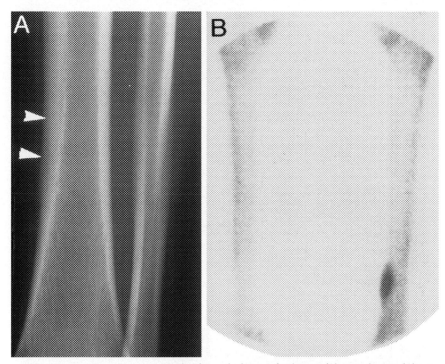

FIGURE 3.—Case 3. **A**, conventional radiograph shows a focal area of decreased cortical density ("gray cortex" sign). **B**, technetium-99m bone scan (done the same day as **A**) shows a corresponding focal, unilateral area of increased uptake oriented vertically along the medial cortex of the tibia. (Courtesy of Mulligan ME: The "gray cortex": An early sign of stress fracture. *Skeletal Radiol* 24:201–203, 1995.)

of the cortex has been described as an early radiographic sign of stress injury. This sign appeared in 3 patients with stress injury.

Patients.—Three patients, aged 30–32 years, were seen with lower-extremity pain. Two of the patients ran 2–5 miles per day and the third played lacrosse. All the patients had focal tenderness, 2 at the medial aspect of the distal tibia and 1 in the proximal tibia. In each patient, the initial radiographic studies showed focal areas of cortex that were slightly more gray than adjacent areas (Fig 3). The difference was subtle enough to be missed in the original interpretation in 1 patient. The diagnosis of stress injury was confirmed with technetium-99m bone scan and/or CT. Conservative treatment resulted in progressive healing (Fig 1).

Discussion.—Although the more typical radiographic sign of stress injury is a linear horizontal area of increased density, this usually occurs late. The graying of the cortical bone is an early radiographic sign of stress injury. This finding along with an appropriate clinical history should alert the clinician to suspect stress injury. The distal tibia, although recognized as a common site for insufficiency fractures in patients with rheumatoid arthritis or after ankle fractures, may also be a more common site for fatigue fracture than has previously been recognized.

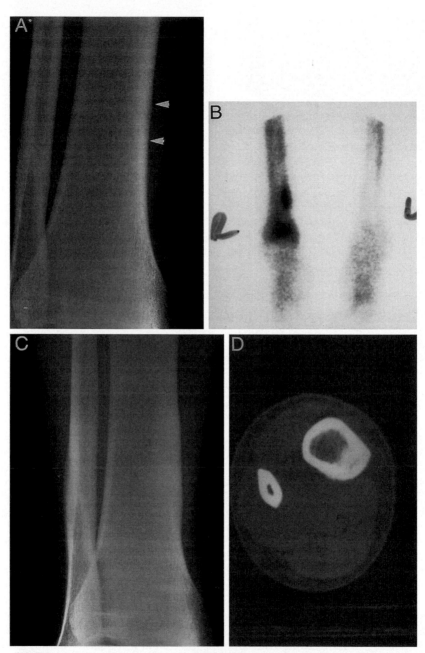

FIGURE 1.—A, conventional radiograph shows subtle areas of decreased cortical density ("gray cortex" sign) in the medial aspect of the distal tibia (*arrowheads*). **B,** technetium-99m bone scan (3 weeks after **A**) shows focal, unilateral, vertically oriented area of increased uptake along the medial cortex of the tibia. **C,** axial CT section (4 months after **A**) shows endosteal and periosteal new bone formation with a linear fracture line posteromedially. **D,** follow-up radiograph (9 months after **A**) shows focal remodeling of distal tibial medial cortex. (Courtesy of Mulligan ME: The "gray cortex": An early sign of stress fracture. *Skeletal Radiol* 24:201–203, 1995.)

▶ Hopefully, you or your skeletal radiologist will be smart enough to recognize the plain film findings, but it is likely that the bone scan may be the first characteristic test obtained. I want to be sure that you know what all the other correlative modalities will show.

This author gives credit to the late Lee Theros for the plain film "gray cortex sign." Lee, an old friend, died in the interim between the time this paper was written and it was published. You might be interested to know that he was the first person to popularize the radioisotopic finding that radiation therapy causes a portal-shaped defect on either the colloid or hepatocellular liver scan when doses in the range of 2,300 to 2,800 cGy have been delivered.

A. Gottschalk, M.D.

Quantification of Inflammation in the Wrist With Gadolinium-enhanced MR Imaging and PET With 2-[F-18]-Fluoro-2-Deoxy-D-Glucose
Palmer WE, Rosenthal DI, Schoenberg OI, et al (Harvard Med School, Boston; New England Deaconess Hosp, Boston; Harvard Univ, Cambridge, Mass)
Radiology 196:647–655, 1995   11–8

Objective.—Patients with inflammatory arthritis were examined with MRI and PET to assess the ability of these imaging methods to quantify joint inflammation and response to therapy.

Patients and Methods.—Twelve patients (11 women and 1 man) took part in the study. Nine had rheumatoid arthritis and 3 had psoriatic arthritis; all had synovitis of the wrist in addition to active systemic disease. A baseline examination was performed after a 1- to 2-week washout period during which nonsteroidal anti-inflammatory drugs were withheld. Two weeks later, patients were assessed after treatment with either piroxicam, 20 mg/day, or prednisone, 10 mg/day. The third assessment was performed after 12–14 weeks of methotrexate therapy (5–10 mg/week). Each assessment period included clinical evaluation and gadolinium-enhanced MRI and 2 FDG PET of the wrist. The volume of enhancing pannus (VEP) was measured by MRI and uptake of FDG by PET.

Results.—A comparison of PET and MR images showed the regions of greatest FDG uptake on PET images to correspond in location to the presence of enhancing pannus on MR images. Combined data from the 3 assessments showed strong linear relationships between VEP and both regional and total FDG uptake. There was a strong association between VEP and FDG uptake and clinical findings in the wrists with active synovitis; the association between VEP and FDG uptake and treatment outcome was not significant.

Conclusion.—Contrast-enhanced MRI and FDG PET can be useful in the quantification of joint inflammation and in monitoring and comparing the efficacy of anti-inflammatory drugs. There was a close correlation between treatment-related changes in the volume and metabolic activity of pannus.

▶ This is an elegant study using elegant MRI and elegant tracer technique. However, if you think about it a little bit, the MRI study simply reflects the distribution of the gadolinium-enhanced image, and gadolinium is comparable to labeled DTPA. It makes you wonder whether you could get the same results by giving the patient technetium-99m DTPA, using a probe to count each wrist, and creating a diagnostic ratio. It would be much cheaper, much less elegant, but the physiology is the same. If any of you out there decide to try it, please let us know how it works.

A. Gottschalk, M.D.

Hyperphosphataemic Tumoral Calcinosis in Bedouin Arabs: Clinical and Radiological Features
McGuinness FE (King Khalid Natl Guard Hosp, Jeddah, Saudi Arabia)
Clin Radiol 50:259–264, 1995   11–9

Introduction.—Recent studies suggest that tumoral calcinosis has a genetic origin associated with hyperphosphatemia and elevated serum 1,25-dihydroxy vitamin D levels. The 4 cases presented here are the first to be reported among Bedouin Arabs.

> *Case Report.*—Boy, 13 years, was seen with a large calcified
> right gluteal mass that had ulcerated the overlying skin (Fig 2).

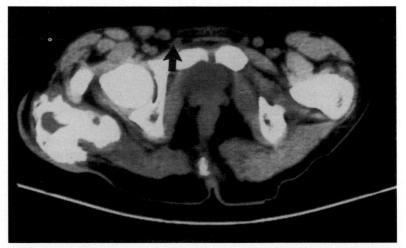

FIGURE 2.—Axial CT through the floor of the pelvis. A right-sided mass of tumoral calcinosis replaces most of the gluteal muscle and subcutaneous tissues. Calcification of the right femoral artery is present (*broad arrow*). (Courtesy of McGuinness FE: Hyperphosphataemic tumoral calcinosis in Bedouin Arabs: Clinical and radiological features. *Clin Radiol* 50:259–264, 1995.)

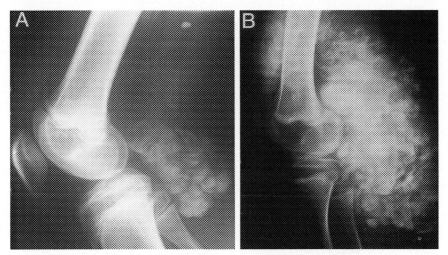

FIGURE 6.—Plain radiographs of the right knee at (A) age 15 and (B) age 16 years, showing a rapidly developing mass of tumoral calcinosis on the posterior aspect of the knee (later involving the suprapatella region) (B). (Courtesy of McGuinness FE: Hyperphosphataemic tumoral calcinosis in Bedouin Arabs: Clinical and radiological features. *Clin Radiol* 50:259–264, 1995.)

Surgical scars suggested that lesions of tumoral calcinosis had previously been excised from both feet. The patient had hyperphosphatemia. Histologic examination of the excised gluteal mass confirmed tumoral calcinosis. A CT scan showed vascular calcification in the femoral artery. The patient was seen on a number of occasions between the ages of 13 and 17. During this period, plain radiographs showed a rapidly developing mass of tumoral calcinosis in the right knee (Fig 6), and, more recently, another mass in the right popliteal fossa was seen with technetium bone scintigraphy (Fig 12).

Discussion.—Two of the other patients were brothers of the boy described here and the fourth patient was their female first cousin. Involvement of the knee is uncommon in tumoral calcinosis, and a mass on the flexor aspect of the knee, as in this case, has not previously been reported. Episodes of calcific myelitis in 2 of the 4 cases appeared clinically to be acute osteomyelitis. Plain films in all 4 patients demonstrated layering of calcium in the tumoral calcinosis lesions; CT demonstrated the sedimentation sign in 3 patients and extensive vascular calcifications in 2. Although a low-calcium diet is sometimes helpful in tumoral calcinosis, 2 of the 4 patients failed to respond to such a regimen. Hyperphosphatemia with normal renal function was present in all 4 cases. The arterial calcification observed in 2 patients has not previously been described.

▶ I have seen a few cases of this entity, and the radionuclide bone scan always made me think of osteosarcoma because of the extensive apparent uptake inside and outside the bone. However, these are wonderful cases to

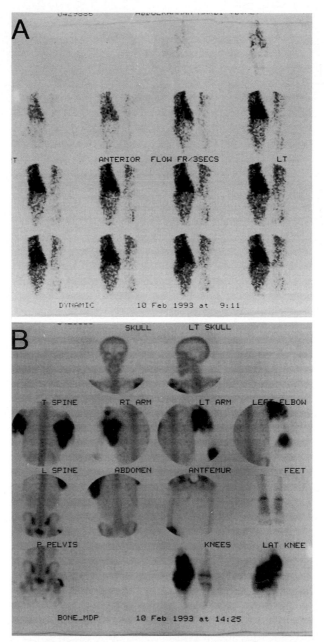

FIGURE 12.—A and B, during a second episode of calcific myelitis. Technetium bone scintigraphy in the dynamic and static phases. The dynamic images indicate that the lesion is confined to the lower femoral metaphysis. The patient was clinically thought to have septic arthritis of the knee. Static scans confirm increased uptake in the lower femoral metaphysis and the knee joint is not affected. Large tumoral calcinosis masses behind the knee and around both shoulders show increased uptake of the isotope. (Courtesy of McGuinness FE: Hyperphosphataemic tumoral calcinosis in Bedouin Arabs: Clinical and radiological features. *Clin Radiol* 50:259–264, 1995.)

correlate with a CT because you should see a fluid-fluid calcium level (which these authors refer to as the sedimentation sign), which is a diagnostic dead giveaway. Some of you out there with super SPECT units might even be able to show this on a high-resolution SPECT slice through the lesion. If you do this, send me the reprint and we will put it in the YEAR BOOK.

A. Gottschalk, M.D.

Assessment of Skull Base Involvement in Nasopharyngeal Carcinoma: Comparisons of Single-photon Emission Tomography With Planar Bone Scintigraphy and X-ray Computed Tomography
Lee C-H, Wang P-W, Chen H-Y, et al (Chang Gung Mem Hosp, Kaohsiung, Taiwan, Republic of China; Chang Gung Med College, Kaohsiung, Taiwan, Republic of China)
Eur J Nucl Med 22:514–520, 1995   11–10

Background.—The overlapping bony structures make evaluation of the skull base with planar bone scintigraphy difficult in patients with nasopharyngeal carcinoma (NPC). Because skull base and intracranial involvement may have prognostic significance in these patients, imaging evaluation is important. The usefulness of SPECT for this purpose was evaluated.

Methods.—Two hundred patients with biopsy-proven NPC were evaluated with planar bone scintigraphy, CT, and SPECT bone scintigraphy of the skull within 1 week. To establish normal skull appearance, SPECT images were also obtained of 5 patients with no head and neck disease.

Results.—Skull base lesions were identified in 141 patients with SPECT (Figs 2 and 4). Of these 141 patients, the lesions were missed in 34 (24%) with planar bone scintigraphy and in 69 (49%) with CT examination (Table 1). No lesions were discovered with CT or planar bone scintigraphy in patients with negative results on SPECT. Of the 107 patients with lesions detected with planar scintigraphy, all lesions were also detected with SPECT but 39% were missed by CT (Table 3). Of the 72 patients with lesions detected with CT, all lesions were detected with SPECT but 10% were missed with planar scintigraphy (Table 2). Thirty-five patients had cranial nerve palsy. Skull base lesions were detected in all of these patients with SPECT, in 27 patients with CT, and in 31 patients with planar bone scintigraphy.

Conclusions.—Single-photon emission CT is more sensitive and specific than either CT or planar bone scintigraphy in the diagnosis of skull base involvement in patients with NPC. The technique provides improved localization and information about the extent of disease.

▶ As Figures 2 and 4 show, SPECT certainly makes the diagnosis simple in these cases. However, one could argue that the gold standard might well be MRI, not CT. These results are still quite impressive except for one thing. There is no proof that there is actual bone involvement. Because all these patients received only radiation therapy or chemotherapy or both, we never

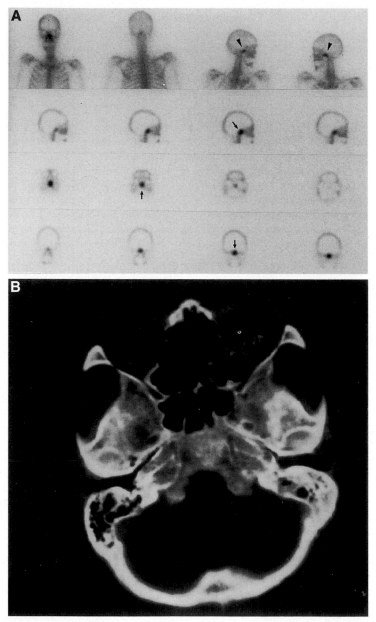

FIGURE 2.—An example of positive planar bone scintigraphy and SPECT, but negative CT study. **A,** the planar bone scan and SPECT showed similar findings. The planar bone scan **top row** revealed symmetrically intense uptake in the skull base, corresponding to the clivus *arrowheads*. The SPECT images (**row 2–4**) did not reveal any additional site (*arrows*) and the CT scan (**B**) revealed no bony destruction. (Courtesy of Lee C-H, Wang P-W, Chen H-Y, et al: Assessment of skull base involvement in nasopharyngeal carcinoma: Comparisons of single-photon emission tomography with planar bone scintigraphy and x-ray computed tomography. *Eur J Nucl Med* 22:514–520, 1995. Copyright Springer-Verlag.)

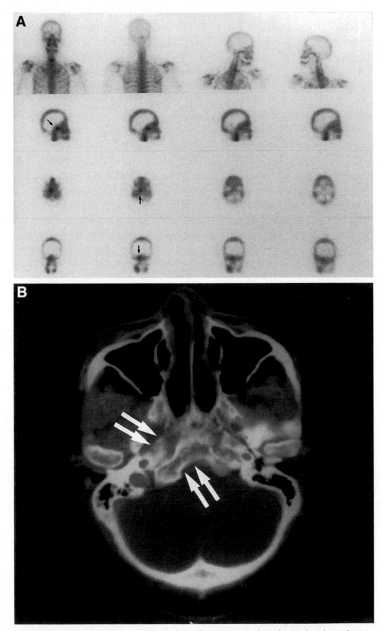

FIGURE 4.—An example of lesions detected by the SPECT study only. **A,** the planar bone scan (**top row**) showed normal uptake but the SPECT images (**rows 2–4**) showed increased uptake at the right portion of sphenoid bone (*arrows*). **B,** the CT scan revealed a similar location of the lesions to that seen on the SPECT study (*double arrows*). (Courtesy of Lee C-H, Wang P-W, Chen H-Y, et al: Assessment of skull base involvement in nasopharyngeal carcinoma: Comparisons of single-photon emission tomography with planar bone scintigraphy and x-ray computed tomography. *Eur J Nucl Med* 22:514–520, 1995. Copyright Springer-Verlag.)

TABLE 1.—Comparison of SPECT With Planar Bone Scintigraphy

SPECT	Planar	No. of examined patients	No. with cranial nerve involvement
+	+	34	2
+*	+	73	29
+	−	34	4
−	−	59	0

* Better localization and definition.
Note: *plus sign*, positive; *minus sign*, negative.
(Courtesy of Lee C-H, Wang P-W, Chen H-Y, et al: Assessment of skull base involvement in nasopharyngeal carcinoma: Comparisons of single-photon emission tomography with planar bone scintigraphy and x-ray computed tomography. *Eur J Nucl Med* 22:514–520, 1995. Copyright Springer-Verlag.)

TABLE 3.—Comparison of Planar Bone Scintigraphy With CT

Planar	CT	No. of examined patients	No. with cranial nerve involvement
+	+	65	23
+	−	42	8
−	−	86	0
−	+	7	4

Note: *plus sign*, positive; *minus sign*, negative.
(Courtesy of Lee C-H, Wang P-W, Chen H-Y, et al: Assessment of skull base involvement in nasopharyngeal carcinoma: Comparisons of single-photon emission tomography with planar bone scintigraphy and x-ray computed tomography. *Eur J Nucl Med* 22:514–520, 1995. Copyright Springer-Verlag.)

TABLE 2.—Comparison of SPECT With CT

SPECT	CT	No. of examined patients	No. with cranial nerve involvement
+	+	72	27
+	−	69	8
−	−	59	0

Note: *plus sign*, positive; *minus sign*, negative.
(Courtesy of Lee C-H, Wang P-W, Chen H-Y, et al: Assessment of skull base involvement in nasopharyngeal carcinoma: Comparisons of single-photon emission tomography with planar bone scintigraphy and x-ray computed tomography. *Eur J Nucl Med* 22:514–520, 1995. Copyright Springer-Verlag.)

have complete surgical or pathologic correlation. Therefore, I am not sure we can prove bone involvement as distinct from regional soft-tissue vascular irritation. Nevertheless, the point remains that SPECT bone scintigraphy provides a "hot" target, whereas CT provides bony destruction—a negative assessment. This makes the radionuclide evaluation much easier.

A. Gottschalk, M.D.

Chondroblastoma of the Patella Presenting as Knee Pain in an Adolescent
Wolfe MW, Halvorson TL, Bennett JT, et al (Tulane Univ, New Orleans, La)
Am J Orthop 24:61–64, 1995   11–11

Background.—Chondroblastoma is a tumor arising from cartilage, typically in a long-bone epiphysis. These are usually nonaggressive tumors, with rare reports of metastasis of benign tumors or locally large, aggressive tumors. A rare case of chondroblastoma of the patella was seen in a patient who had an aneurysmal bone cyst and pathologic fracture at the time of diagnosis.

Case Report.—Girl, 13 years, complained of a 5-week history of pain and swelling in her left knee. She had a stable knee joint with full range of motion. There was tenderness to touch and effusion at the anterior aspect of the patella. She had no abnormalities on laboratory examinations. Roentgenographic studies revealed a lesion of the left patella with a possible pathologic fracture of the posterolateral cortex. This area had increased uptake on a technetium bone scan. Surgical exploration revealed significant synovitis with fibrocartilage over the fracture site. The osteolytic lesion was excised through an anterior patellar window. Pathologic analysis identified chondroblastoma with secondary aneurysmal changes. Follow-up roentgenographs at 7 months showed signs of persistent or recurrent disease. The chondroblastoma was resected and regrafted. Ten months after excision, there was no evidence of recur-

TABLE.—Differential Diagnosis of Osteolytic Lesions of the Patella

Nonneoplastic	Benign	Malignant
Dorsal defect	Chondroblastoma	Lymphoma
Hyperparathyroidism	Giant-cell tumor	Hemangioendothelioma
Osteomyelitis	Simple bone cyst	Metastasis
Osteochondritis dissecans	Hemangioma	
Rheumatoid cyst	Osteochondroma	
Paget's disease	Lipoma	
	Osteoblastoma	

(From Wolfe MW, Halvorson TL, Bennett JT, et al: Chondroblastoma of the patella presenting as knee pain in an adolescent. *Am J Orthop* 24:61–64, 1995. Adapted with permission from *American Journal of Orthopedics*.)

rence. The patient was pain-free and had full range of motion and normal ambulation.

Discussion.—With 35 previously published case reports of chondroblastoma of the patella, this site should be considered common for the epiphyseal lesion. However, radiographic evidence of osteolytic lesions of the patella can suggest differential diagnosis of numerous nonneoplastic, benign, and malignant lesions (Table). Although chondroblastoma usually grows in a metaphyseal direction, in conjunction with a secondary aneurysmal bone cyst, it is more likely to invade the joint space and cause pathologic fracture. It is best managed with curettage and bone grafting. Preservation of the patella is desirable but may not be possible with very large lesions or extensive patellar destruction.

▶ I doubt you will ever see a case like this, but the table presents a useful gamut of diagnostic lesions to use if you ever come across a hole in the kneecap.

A. Gottschalk, M.D.

Legg-Calvé-Perthes Disease: Comparison of Conventional Radiography, MR Imaging, Bone Scintigraphy and Arthrography
Kaniklides C, Lönnerholm T, Moberg A, et al (Univ Hosp, Uppsala, Sweden)
Acta Radiol 36:434–439, 1995   11–12

Background.—In patients with Legg-Calvé-Perthes disease (LCPD), the most important prognostic factors are the extent to which the femoral head is involved and the presence of lateral subluxation of the hip. These factors cannot be assessed by conventional radiographs, so additional studies such as arthrography, bone scintigraphy, and MRI are often needed. These 4 radiologic studies—conventional radiography, arthrography, bone scintigraphy, and MRI—were compared for their ability to evaluate the size of the necrosis, the degree of lateral subluxation, and the disease stage in patients with LCPD.

Methods.—The prospective study included 24 hips of 22 patients with LCPD. All hips were evaluated by all 4 studies within a 1-month period at the time of diagnosis. Conventional radiography included anteroposterior and Lauenstein projections of both hips. The MRI scans included coronal views of both hips and sagittal views of the affected hip. The bone scintigrams, also performed in anteroposterior and Lauenstein projections, were obtained 2 hours after injection of hydroxydiphosphonate, and bilateral arthrography was performed with the use of general anesthesia. Three radiologists evaluated each of the imaging studies independently.

Results.—The best technique for evaluating the extent of involvement of the femoral head—better than conventional radiography or bone scintigraphy—was MRI. However, arthrography was at least as good as MRI in depicting the shape of the articular surfaces and in determining whether lateral subluxation was present. The conventional radiographs were not very sensitive in determining the degree of lateral subluxation and the extent of femoral head necrosis. Valuable anatomical and pathophysiologic information about the extent and location of femoral head involvement, and about the degree of lateral subluxation, was provided by MRI. Magnetic resonance imaging was also better than bone scintigraphy at showing revascularization.

Conclusions.—Conventional radiography remains an important technique for the diagnosis of LCPD. Magnetic resonance imaging can establish or exclude this diagnosis, as well as detect revascularization or loss of containment and provide important information about the extent and location of necrosis. For patients with advanced deformity, significant lateral subluxation, or extremely restricted abduction, dynamic arthrography may be needed to tell whether containment of the femoral head is surgically achievable.

▶ Unfortunately, I suspect these authors are correct. However, it is worth pointing out to you that they included no bone scintigraphy images in this article. The doses used (3–4mCi) seem light for some of the older children, and I have no clue how many counts were obtained, even though they do tell us they used pinhole images. Furthermore, at the University of Uppsala, nuclear medicine is not done in the same department as diagnostic radiology, which may explain why there is so little detail here about the nuclear images. In short, in this series, it is possible that the radionuclide studies may not be getting a fair shake.

A. Gottschalk, M.D.

The Role of 131 Iodine-Metaiodobenzylguanidine Scanning in the Correlative Imaging of Patients With Neuroblastoma
Andrich MP, Shalaby-Rana E, Movassaghi N, et al (Children's Natl Med Ctr, Washington, DC; George Washington Univ, Washington, DC)
Pediatrics 97:246–250, 1996   11–13

Introduction.—Metaiodobenzylguanidine (MIBG) labeled with radioactive iodine has been used for over a decade in the imaging of patients with neuroblastoma (NB). Uptake of MIBG indicates the presence of viable tumor cells and can identify primary and metastatic sites of NB. Serial MIBG scans of 27 pediatric patients were reviewed retrospectively to determine the impact of scanning results on staging, treatment, and prognosis.

Methods.—All patients had histologically proven or suspected NB; at diagnosis, 1 had a ganglioneuroblastoma (GNB) and 1 had a ganglioneuroma (GN). The mean age of the group was 2.9 years. Among those with NB, 3 were classified as stage 1, 7 as stage 3, 12 as stage 4, and 3 as stage 4S. Results of 103 MIBG scans, performed at initial diagnosis and at

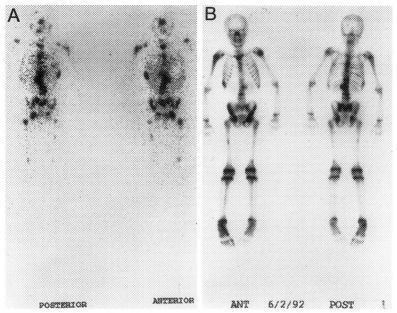

FIGURE 2.—Boy, 73 months, with stage 4 neuroblastoma and multiple bone metastases seen on both the metaiodobenzylguanidine scan (**A**) and bone scan (**B**). The studies were obtained after resection of a right retroperitoneal primary tumor. (Courtesy of Andrich MP, Shalaby-Rana E, Movassaghi N, et al: The role of 131 iodine-metaiodobenzylguanidine scanning in the correlative imaging of patients with neuroblastoma. Reproduced by permission of *Pediatrics* Vol 97, pp 246–250, Copyright 1996.)

varying intervals during and after therapy, were compared with the results of 105 bone scans and 239 CT scans.

Results.—Six patients underwent resection of NB before the first MIBG scans. At the time of initial MIBG scanning, primary tumors were present and visualized on CT scans of the remaining 19 patients. Fifteen of these tumors showed uptake of MIBG, for a sensitivity of 79%. The GN demonstrated uptake of MIBG but the GNB did not. In 11 children with stage 4 NB, metastases to bone were visualized on both the initial MIBG and bone scans (Fig 2). Multiple bone lesions were present in all 11 cases, and both scans showed metastases in the same general areas. The MIBG studies did not change staging by identifying additional lesions not seen on bone and CT scans. Eight children with stage 4 disease had relapses after completion of therapy. All areas of disease were visualized at relapse with CT and bone scans, but MIBG scans showed positive results in only 4 of 8 cases.

Conclusion.—The staging and treatment of these children with neural crest tumors was not altered by results of MIBG imaging. Some patients with initially positive MIBG results had serial studies that normalized during treatment, but these negative findings were not indicative of a favorable response. Routine use of serial MIBG scanning is not recommended for patients with NB because its impact on clinical decisions does not justify the cost, inconvenience, and radiation exposure.

▶ In contrast to Abstract 11–12, I know that this group does outstanding pediatric nuclear work. As a consequence, we look at these discouraging results and recognize that, as the late Howard Cosell used to say, they "told it like it is." This is a bad and discouraging disease, and MIBG just does not seem to help.

A. Gottschalk, M.D.

Persistent/Recurrent Hyperparathyroidism: A Comparison of Sestamibi Scintigraphy, MRI, and Ultrasonography
Numerow LM, Morita ET, Clark OH, et al (Univ of California, San Francisco)
J Magn Reson Imaging 5:702–708, 1995   11–14

Introduction.—Preoperative imaging is useful in patients with persistent or recurrent hyperparathyroidism, because localizing studies can improve the success rate of reoperation and decrease postoperative morbidity. Twenty-three patients with remaining abnormal parathyroid glands after previous surgical exploration took part in a study designed to compare the accuracy, sensitivity, and positive predictive value of MRI, technetium-99m sestamibi (MIBI) scintigraphy, and ultrasonography (US) in this setting.

Methods.—The patients had a mean age of 56 years and an average of 1.6 previous surgical explorations for hyperparathyroidism. At MRI, any nodular structure visualized in a region expected for normal and ectopic parathyroid glands was considered a positive finding. Abnormal parathyroid tissue was identified at MIBI scintigraphy as a dominant focus of increased activity in the neck or mediastinum that was identified on both early and delayed images. An abnormal finding at US was a relatively hypoechoic mass adjacent to, within, or inferior to the thyroid gland. Accuracy of imaging findings and of various combinations of tests were determined by comparison with operative reports.

Results.—Twenty-five abnormal glands were found at surgery, including 18 parathyroid adenomas and 7 hyperplastic glands. Sensitivities and accuracies were, respectively, 88% and 84% for MRI, 80% and 80% for MIBI, and 58% and 44% for US. The combination of MRI and MIBI yielded an accuracy of 92%, but combining either MRI or MIBI with US did not improve the accuracy of either test alone. When parathyroid adenomas were analyzed separately, sensitivities and accuracies were respectively, 89% and 89% for MRI, 94% and 94% for MIBI, and 58% and 39% for US; for parathyroid hyperplasia, corresponding values were, respectively, 83% and 71% for MRI, 43% and 43% for MIBI, and 57% and 57% for US. Both MRI and MIBI were significantly more sensitive and accurate than US, but the difference between MRI and MIBI was not statistically significant.

Conclusion.—In patients with persistent or recurrent hyperparathyroidism, MRI and MIBI were of equal value in localizing abnormal parathyroid glands and significantly better than US. Combining MRI and MIBI may yield the most accurate results.

▶ This is a large series discussing a very tough problem. I am pleased that the authors point out that this is a highly selected patient population and therefore sensitivity (i.e., true negatives) was not established because it would not be meaningful. Ordinarily, in this "managed care" world of ours, somebody suggesting that 2 tests in combination are a good idea is likely to be impaled on a cost-conscious spear. However, these patients are probably exceptions. They have been operated on before and they have a very difficult surgical problem. I think it is reasonable to do both MRI and sestamibi studies on this patient group. As the authors note, save money by not doing the US.

It is also important to point out that the authors did not hesitate to use good technetium pinhole thyroid views to be confident they knew precisely where the thyroid was, as many of these recurrent adenomas occur in immediate proximity to the thyroid gland. In short, they pulled out all the nuclear stops: a very good idea.

A. Gottschalk, M.D.

Role of Technetium-99m Pertechnetate Scintigraphy in the Management of Extra Abdominal Fibromatosis
Terui S, Terauchi T, Abe H, et al (Natl Cancer Ctr Hosp, Tokyo)
Skeletal Radiol 24:331–336, 1995   11–15

Introduction.—No imaging procedure has proven adequate for the study of extra-abdominal fibromatosis, a benign but locally aggressive tumor. A review of 11 patients with this tumor assessed the effectiveness of scintigraphy using technetium-99m pertechnetate as a scanning technique.

Methods.—The patients, 3 males and 8 females with an average age of 27 years, were seen during an 8-year period (1985–1993). In 10 cases, the tumor had recurred locally after 1 or more surgical treatments. Histologic diagnoses were determined from surgical and/or biopsy specimens stained with hematoxylin and eosin. The tumors were classified according to vascularity and cellularity. Scintigraphic images were recorded twice: an early scintigram was obtained 5–10 minutes after IV injection of 10 mCi (370 MBq) of ^{99m}Tc pertechnetate and a delayed scintigram 2–3 hours later.

Results.—Twenty tumors varying in size from 0.8 to 2.5 cm were identified from the initial scintigrams. All 20 presented clear images and appeared as hot spots on the ^{99m}Tc scintigram. Uptake of the scanning agent by the extra-abdominal fibromatosis was registered in both early and delayed studies. Two patterns of ^{99m}Tc distribution were observed. In 7 cases, there was even uptake and equivalent accumulation in early and delayed scintigrams. Early scintigrams in 4 patients showed uneven uptake, whereas delayed scintigrams revealed accumulations that extended

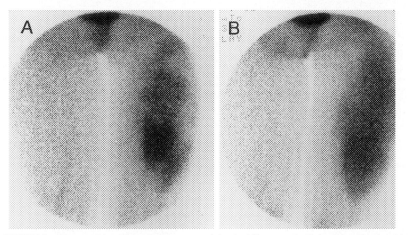

FIGURE 2.—Woman, 24, with a recurrent extra-abdominal fibromatosis of the right posterior thigh. **A**, early scintigram of the posterior of the right thigh demonstrates huge nodular accumulations consistent with the clinical findings. The margins of the tumors are well defined. **B**, delayed scintigram taken 3 hours after (**A**). The accumulation is diffusely extending to the surrounding tissue, and its uptake becomes evenly spread. However, the margin is still well defined. (Courtesy of Terui S, Terauchi T, Abe H, et al: Role of technetium-99m pertechnetate scintigraphy in the management of extra-abdominal fibromatosis. *Skeletal Radiol* 24:331–336, 1995.)

diffusely to the outer side (Fig 2). In both primary and recurrent cases of extra-abdominal fibromatosis, the ^{99m}Tc scintigram had a sensitivity and specificity of 100%.

Conclusion.—Extra-abdominal fibromatosis is a rare tumor with a high rate of recurrence after surgery. With ^{99m}Tc scintigraphy, the extent of the tumor can be determined and the whole patient surveyed. Strong uptake of the early scintigram appears to correspond to both the tumor's rich cellularity and vascularity, and the fused and extended uptake of the delayed image corresponds to the tumor cells embedded with the collagen fibers.

▶ I have come across this technique from time to time and wanted to call this article to your attention in case you ever see something like this on a Meckel scan, or any other nonspecific use of pertechnetate that comes your way. I am sorry the authors do not have some correlative technetium bone scans to show us; I would bet they would be positive, too.

A. Gottschalk, M.D.

12 Radiopharmaceuticals

Introduction

The future utility of nuclear medicine requires the development of exciting new radiopharmaceuticals. This year we see several interesting agents described for receptor imaging, such as high specific activity nicotine for determining the occupancy and distribution of cholinergic receptors, determination of metabolism, myocardial perfusion with technetium-labeled Q12, direct imaging of angiotensin II receptors, and animal studies verifying the imaging potential of a direct hypoxia marker. One of the most intriguing articles does not describe a new radionuclide, but rather tells about the discovery of technetium. This well-written and well-referenced article has intriguing implications. It took people with diverse interests, working on different continents, who had related but different goals, to discover this agent. The discovery of technetium stands as an important milestone for our specialty. It is also a tribute to the international collaboration and cooperation that makes science a great calling.

H. William Strauss, M.D.

Technetium, the Missing Element
de Jonge FAA, Pauwels EKJ (KCL Found, Leeuwarden, The Netherlands; Leiden Univ Hosp, The Netherlands)
Eur J Nucl Med 23:336–344, 1996   12–1

Introduction.—When the first periodic tables were created, the existence of a new element with an atomic weight of 100, called eka-manganese, was predicted. The history of the discovery of what was eventually called technetium was reviewed.

Early Discoveries of Nuclear Physics.—The discovery of subatomic particles led to the discovery of artificial radioactivity and the development of machines that could produce these radionuclides. The cyclotron, developed by Ernest Orlando Lawrence, was able to induce radioactivity by bombarding carbon with deuterons. Emilio Segre, a physicist in Palermo, visited Lawrence in 1936, saw the cyclotron, and noticed the radioactive metal scrap that could be his radioactive source.

The Discovery of Element 43.—Lawrence responded to Segre's request for radioactive metal scrap by mailing salvaged copper and molybdenum strips. By 1937, Segre and Carlo Perrier discovered element 43 in this scrap metal by proving that the radioactivity was not produced by radioisotopes of other known elements. Thus, the first artificially produced element was discovered. Later, Segre discovered its isomeric properties. Perrier and Segre proposed the name technetium in 1947.

Technetium in Nature.—Natural technetium was first discovered in the X-ray spectra of certain stars. Technetium isotopes were then discovered as products of spontaneous fission of uranium-238. Natural technetium was first isolated from Belgian Congo pitchblende. Although natural technetium exists, it does not exist in enough abundance to supply medical or industrial users.

Conclusion.—Therefore, it is necessary to produce technetium artificially in nuclear reactors. The greatest current source of technetium is molybdenum-99, produced either as a direct fission product or from neutron activation of natural molybdenum or targets enriched with ^{98}Mo.

▶ This is an excellent review of the history of technetium. Among other things, it shows the importance of personal collaboration between investigators, who are geographically separated, to major scientific advances. In addition to teaching us our history, the article is fun to read.

H.W. Strauss, M.D.

Iodine-123 *N*-Methyl-4-Iododexetimide: A New Radioligand for Single-photon Emission Tomographic Imaging of Myocardial Muscarinic Receptors
Hicks RJ, Kassiou M, Eu P, et al (Heidelberg Hosp, Melbourne, VIC, Australia; Australian Nuclear Science and Technology Organisation, Sydney, NSW, Australia)
Eur J Nucl Med 22:339–345, 1995   12–2

Introduction.—The mediation of parasympathetic effects on the heart by muscarinic cholinergic receptors (mAChR) leads to a slowing in the rate and a decrease in the force of contraction. In an animal model, decreased muscarinic receptor density was described in cardiac failure. A new radiopharmaceutical, [iodine-123]N-methyl-4-iododexetimide, was evaluated for its potential as an imaging agent for muscarinic receptor distribution in the heart.

Methods.—Initial biodistribution studies of the radiopharmaceutical were performed in male Wistar rats. To assess receptor-specific myocardial uptake with co-administration of radiotracer and the nonradioactive receptor antagonist, the ability of the muscarinic receptor antagonist methylquinuclidinyl benzylate (MQNB 1 mg/kg) to displace [^{123}I]N-methyl-4-iododexetimide was investigated in 5 animals. Imaging studies were then performed in rabbits and, primarily, in dogs.

Results.—The biodistribution studies showed high cardiac uptake (2.4%ID/g) 10 minutes after injection, with a ratio of heart to lung activity of 5:1. Also demonstrated in these studies were the specificity and stereoselectivity of cardiac binding. Two studies in a single rabbit showed definite cardiac uptake and other findings concordant with rat biodistribution data. In the dogs, dynamic images studies revealed rapid and high myocardial uptake and low lung binding, with stable heart to lung activity ratios of greater than 2.5:1 between 10 and 30 minutes. When an excess of the unlabeled muscarinic antagonist was administered, myocardial activity was rapidly displaced to background levels. This finding (Fig 3)

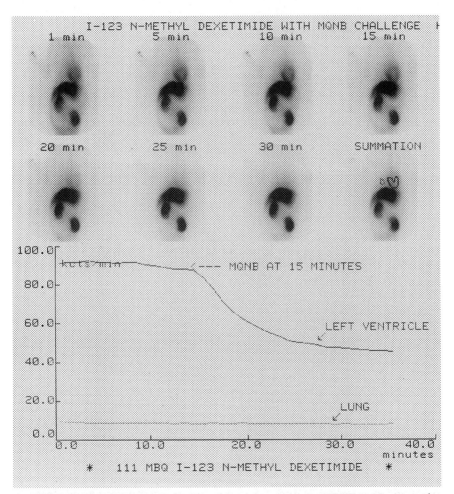

FIGURE 3.—The administration of a muscarinic receptor antagonist (*MQNB*) at 15 minutes after injection of [iodine-123]N-methyl-4-iododexetimide into the greyhound revealed rapid and qualitatively complete displacement of activity from the heart, suggesting high specific binding to muscarinic receptors. (Courtesy of Hicks RJ, Kassiou M, Eu P, et al: Iodine-123 N-methyl-4-iododexetimide: A new radioligand for single-photon emission tomographic imaging of myocardial muscarinic receptors. *Eur J Nucl Med* 22:339–345, 1995. Copyright Springer-Verlag.)

suggested high specific binding to muscarinic receptors. Single-photon emission tomographic (SPET) imaging revealed excellent cardiac definition, with a myocardial to lung activity ratio of greater than 10:1 at the midventricular level.

Conclusion.—Previous efforts to develop a SPET agent that could evaluate the parasympathetic innervation of the heart have yielded disappointing results. The radiopharmaceutical evaluated here—[^{123}I]*N*-methyl-4-iododexetimide—shows promise in this setting and may aid in the evaluation of cardiac diseases (such as heart failure and diabetic heart disease) associated with changes in muscarinic receptor function.

► The biodistribution of [^{123}I]*N*-methyl-4-iododexetimide was determined in rats, and imaging studies were performed in 4 dogs and a rabbit. Within 10 minutes of injection, myocardial uptake was 2.4% of the dose/g, fivefold greater than that of the lung and about 20-fold greater than that of the blood. The kidney concentrated 20% of the dose/g. The uptake was specific for the *d* stereoisomer, because the *l* isomer had 0.14% in the myocardium.

This paper presents an interesting opportunity for identifying sites of potential arrhythmogenesis. One theory identified local excess of either sympathetic or parasympathetic activity as the source of arrhythmia. Although [^{131}I]metaiodobenzylguanidine offered an opportunity to see the sympathetic activity, there was no agent with high myocardial uptake to see the parasympathetic activity. It appears that Hicks et al. have now solved this problem.

H.W. Strauss, M.D.

Biokinetics and Dosimetry Analysis in Healthy Volunteers for a Two-injection (Rest-Stress) Protocol of the Myocardial Perfusion Imaging Agent Technetium 99m–labeled Q3
Rohe RC, Thomas SR, Stabin MG, et al (Univ of Cincinnati, Ohio; Oak Ridge Inst, Tenn; Mallinckrodt Med Inc, St Louis)
J Nucl Cardiol 2:395–404, 1995   12–3

Introduction.—Newer myocardial imaging agents have been developed to improve myocardial uptake compared with background activity in the liver. One of these agents is trans (N,N'-ethylene bis(acetylacetoneimine)) bis(tris(3-methoxy-1-propyl) phosphine) technetium-99m (III) ^{99m}Tc-Q3), which has shown diagnostic accuracy equal to that of thallium-201 in a shorter protocol. Biokinetic studies and a dosimetry analysis of ^{99m}Tc(III) were conducted.

Methods.—Six healthy volunteers received 2 injections of ^{99m}Tc(III) on the same day. The first injection, 241 MBq, was followed 15 minutes later by myocardial SPECT and 1.5 hours later by a whole-body scan. A treadmill test was then performed with an average stress injection of 744 MBq, given 2.4 hours after the rest injection. Myocardial SPECT and whole-body scans were performed at intervals of from 1.5 to 21.0 hours after stress injection. Conjugate counting methods were used to calculate absolute organ activities. Dosimetry analysis was performed by simplifying the data from both injections to a 1-injection equivalent data set.

Results.—At 1.5 hours after both injections, decay correct average percentage uptake values for the myocardium were 1.4%, with an average biological half-time of 26.4 hours. At 1.5 hours after the stress injection, the gallbladder had the highest organ uptake value at 5.5%, followed by the liver at 4.1% (Fig 4). About 6.5 hours after the stress injection, and

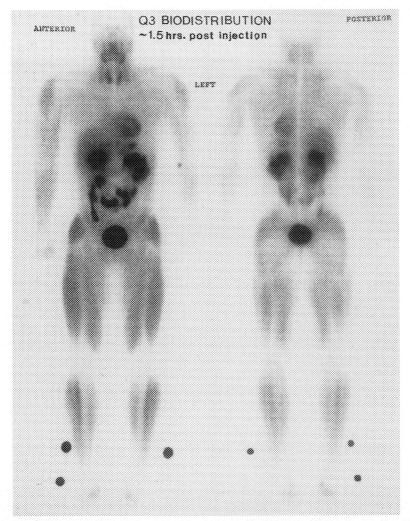

FIGURE 4.—Whole-body images obtained in a volunteer approximately 1.5 hours postress injection of technetium-99m–Q3. Scan acquisition time was 25 minutes. Myocardium, gallbladder, liver, kidneys, urinary bladder, and some intestine activity are seen clearly. (Courtesy of Rohe RC, Thomas SR, Stabin MG, et al: Biokinetics and dosimetry analysis in healthy volunteers for a two-injection (rest-stress) protocol of the myocardial perfusion imaging agent technetium 99m–labeled Q3. *J Nucl Cardiol* 2:395–404, 1995.)

before any fecal elimination of the imaging agent, the mean sum of all gastrointestinal tract components was 18.8%. Urine clearance in a 24-hour urine specimen was 17.1%. The dose to the gallbladder wall was 0.024 mGy/MBq, whereas that to the upper large intestine wall was 0.023 mGy/MBq.

Conclusions.—The estimated effective dose equivalent of ^{99m}Tc (III) is 0.01 mSv/MBq. For an administration of 1,110 MBq, or 30 mCi, this is less than half of that with a standard ^{201}Tl imaging protocol and similar to those reported for ^{99m}Tc-labeled sestamibi or tetrofosmin. The myocardial uptake of ^{99m}Tc(III) is similar to that of the latter 2 agents.

▶ It will be nice to have more radiopharmaceuticals to choose from for perfusion imaging. Although the technetium-labeled agents may have some similarities, they will not be identical, and each may have a clinical situation in which it is preferred. The low myocardial uptake of this agent, however, leaves us with the specter of decreased sensitivity for detection of subtle coronary disease.

H.W. Strauss, M.D.

Unexpected Keys in Cell Biochemistry Imaging: Some Lessons From Technetium-99m-Sestamibi
Mariani G (Univ of Genoa, Italy)
J Nucl Med 37:536–538, 1996   12–4

Objective.—Although it was designed as a myocardial perfusion imaging agent, technetium-99m–sestamibi (MIBI) has proven useful in examining the cellular function of other tissues. Patterns of uptake by different types of cells, such as tumor cells and cardiac myocytes, have been observed and may reflect differences in the intracellular density of storage organelles. Although the mechanisms of MIBI diffusion and transport from the extracellular to the intracellular space are not well understood, the mechanisms of its intracellular distribution and its exit from cells have been studied. The active storage of MIBI in a subcellular compartment, i.e., the mitochondria, forms the basis for its flow-dependent imaging characteristics. However, some important questions remain. Insights from research using MIBI for cell biochemistry imaging were discussed.

Sestamibi in Cell Biochemistry Imaging.—In vitro cell culture studies have not aided our understanding of the varying washout rates of MIBI from different types of cells. Lipophilicity, which is one of the properties that helps transport MIBI across cell membranes, has also limited its clinical applications in tumor imaging. However, there may be some time-windows useful for MIBI imaging of abdominal tumors. Studies assessing the use of MIBI to evaluate tumor response to therapy have given disappointing results. Research does show that MIBI is actively extruded out of tumor cells by the permeability glycoprotein (P-gp) pump, as are the cytotoxic agents involved in tumor multidrug resistance. Also, active extrusion of MIBI from tumor cells is directly correlated with expression of the multidrug-resistance gene, in vitro studies have found. Thus, MIBI scintigraphy could become useful as a prognostic indicator of the level of P-gp expression in tumors, opening the way to pharmacologic manipulations to increase tumor responsiveness to cytotoxic chemotherapy. Some of these concepts are already finding their way into clinical practice.

Summary.—Technetium-99m–sestamibi and other new radiopharmaceuticals are proving useful for in vivo evaluation of complex cell functions. The precise mechanisms by which these agents accumulate in and wash out of tissues remain to be determined. Once these interactions are better described, they may lead to a better understanding of tumor biology and perhaps to new cancer treatments.

▶ This is a thoughtful, well-referenced review of some unexplained facts about the kinetics of sestamibi in tissues. Why are there differences in the clearance of MIBI from different tissues? Is the release of MIBI from tissue a purely passive process? These questions need to be asked so we can begin to explore the answers.

H.W. Strauss, M.D.

Preclinical Animal Studies With Radioiododeoxyuridine
Kassis AI, Adelstein SJ (Harvard Med School, Boston)
J Nucl Med 37:10S–12S, 1996   12–5

Background.—A therapeutic/diagnostic agent is sometimes used to facilitate targeting to tumors. The ideal agent can be freely diffused throughout the target tissues, is selectively taken up only by tumor cells, can be quickly converted into a nontoxic form or excreted if it diffuses out of the target area, and is not biologically altered by repeat or prolonged injection. The efficacy of 5-iodo-2'-deoxyuridine (IUdR), radiolabeled with the Auger electron emitters iodine-123 or iodine-125, as a therapeutic and/or diagnostic agent was evaluated in various animal tumor models.

Methods.—Iodine-125–labeled IUdR was administered by intraperitoneal injection into mice with ovarian cancer. The tumor/nontumor ratios were determined with biodistribution studies, and tumor cell survival was compared with 3 doses of IUdR. In addition, the biodistribution patterns were studied in rats with bladder tumors treated with the intravesical administration of [^{125}I] IUdR. Brain tumors were induced in rats with injection of gliosarcoma cells in the right caudate nucleus. The same areas were later injected with [^{123}I]IUdR and [^{125}I] IUdR. Both tumor cells and radiopharmaceutical were delivered intrathecally in rats; biodistribution and survival were evaluated after treatment.

Results.—In the murine ovarian tumor model, intraperitoneal injection of [^{125}I] IUdR resulted in excellent tumor/nontumor ratios and decreased tumor cell survival. Excellent tumor/nontumor ratios were also found in the diagnostic administration of radiolabeled IUdR in rats with bladder tumors, brain tumors, and intrathecal tumors. Survival in the rats with brain tumors was not affected by nonradioactive [^{127}I] IUdR, but it was significantly prolonged by treatment with [^{125}I] IUdR, which also prolonged survival in rats with intrathecal tumors.

Conclusions.—The agent, IUdR, radiolabeled with ^{123}I or ^{125}I, shows promise in the scintigraphic diagnosis or treatment of tumors that are accessible to direct radiopharmaceutical administration, including ovarian, bladder, CNS, breast, prostate, and hepatic cancers.

▶ Radionuclide therapy is likely to play a role in selected tumors. Radiolabeled IUdR has shown remarkable tumoricidal ability in selected animal studies. This paper summarizes the results of these preclinical studies and identifies the problems with future development of this agent.

H.W. Strauss, M.D.

Labelling of Leucocytes With Technetium-99m Exametazime Causes In Vitro Upregulation of Granulocyte CD11b Without Correlation to Tissue Uptake In Vivo

Almer S, Ljunghusen O, Lundahl J (Linköping Univ, Sweden; Univ Hosp, Linköping, Sweden; Karolinska Hosp, Stockholm)
Eur J Nucl Med 23:669–674, 1996   12–6

Objective.—In inflammatory bowel disease, leukocytes migrate to sites of inflammation. Interactions between leukocyte CD11b and endothelial intercellular adhesion molecule 1 are integral to this extravasation process. Labeling of leukocytes with technetium-99m exametazime has been shown to cause upregulation of the cellular activation marker, CD11b, on granulocytes. A study was conducted to investigate whether labeling affects the expression of CD11b and to determine whether CD11b expression correlates with tracer uptake in the bowel, lungs, or reticuloendothelial system of patients with inflammatory bowel disease.

Methods.—Expression of CD11b on granulocytes was studied in 15 patients with Crohn's disease and 10 patients with ulcerative colitis (10 women) aged 17–63 years. Monocyte expression was investigated in 20 of

TABLE 1.—Expression of Adhesion Molecule CD11b on Granulocytes and Monocytes From 25 Patients With Inflammatory Bowel Disease Before and After Labeling With Technetium-99m Exametazime

	Unlabeled cells	Labeled cells
Granulocytes ($n=250$)	11.4 (8.0–17.2)0	16.3 (12.4–25.0)*
Monocytes ($n=20$)	28.3 (21.0–33.2)	21.7 (19.5–29.7)†

Note: Values are expressed as medians (interquartile range) of the mean fluorescence intensity.
* $P < 0.01$ vs. unlabeled cells by Wilcoxon signed rank test.
† $P > 0.05$ (NS) vs. unlabeled cells by Wilcoxon signed rank test.
(Courtesy of Almer S, Ljunghusen O, Lundahl J: Labelling of leucocytes with technetium-99m exametazime causes in vitro upregulation of granulocyte CD11b without correlation to tissue uptake in vivo *Eur J Nucl Med* 23:669–674, 1996. Copyright Springer-Verlag.)

these patients. Results were compared with those of 11 healthy controls. Patients' leukocytes were labeled and reinjected and imaging studies were performed. Leukocytes were reisolated from blood samples, and receptor mobilization and immunostaining were performed. Samples were analyzed by flow cytometry.

Results.—After labeling, there was a small but significant increase of CD11b expression on granulocytes but not on monocytes (Table 1). Expression was higher in patients treated with prednisolone than in untreated patients. Expression of CD11b on unlabeled granulocytes and monocytes was significantly correlated. The increase in CD11b expression on granulocytes was lower than, and not correlated with, either expression that mobilized spontaneously at 37°C or expression induced by N-formyl-methionyl-phenylalanine. After reinjection of labeled cells, expression of CD11b on unlabeled granulocytes correlated with uptake in bowel and lung at 45 minutes but not at 4 hours. There was no correlation between CD11b expression on labeled cells and tracer uptake in lungs or bowel. Patients with ulcerative colitis had significantly higher bowel uptake between 45 minutes and 4 hours than did patients with Crohn's disease.

Conclusion.—The increase in CD11b expression on granulocytes is not associated with a concomitant increase in tracer uptake in bowel and lungs.

▶ The investigators' protocol of sampling blood before injection of radiolabeled leukocytes and again after injection of radiolabeled leukocytes is particularly interesting. There is a slight increase in the expression of the CD11b adhesion molecule on the granulocytes but not on the monocytes. However, the standard deviation of the measurements is extremely large. This result is particularly interesting, because the investigators drew a total volume of 102 mL of venous blood in a patient whose total blood volume would be approximately 5L, for 1/50th of the total blood volume. After reinjection of the labeled cells, the dilution factor should have varied this response. These data raise the question about whether other substances in the injected mixture may be responsible for this apparent upregulation of the adhesion molecule.

H.W. Strauss, M.D.

Pharmacokinetics and Biodistribution of Samarium-153-labelled OC125 Antibody Coupled to CITCDTPA in a Xenograft Model of Ovarian Cancer
Kraeber-Bodéré F, Mishra A, Thédrez P, et al (INSERM Research Unit 211, Nantes, France; Nara Med Univ, Japan)
Eur J Nucl Med 23:560–567, 1996   12–7

Purpose.—Samarium-153 has been proposed for use in radioimmunotherapy of ovarian cancer. However, the instability of antibody labeling leads to high uptake concentrations of ^{153}Sm in liver and bone, thus limiting its use in radioimmunotherapy. To compare the pharmacokinetics and biodistribution of ¹⁵³Sm-labeled monoclonal antibody, in whole IgG or F(ab')₂ fragment form, with either diethylene triamine pentaacetic acid (DTPA) or the new ligand 6-*p*-isothiocyanatobenzyl diethylene triamine pentaacetic acid (CITCDTPA) (Fig 1), a study was done in mice.

Methods and Results.—Experiments were performed in nude mice grafted with ovarian adenocarcinoma cells expressing the CA 125 antigen. The immunoconjugates had a specific activity of 18.5–55.5 MBq/mg with immunoreactivity of greater than 65%. Stability studies of ¹⁵³Sm-DTPA-OC125 F(ab')₂ showed that half of the metal remained bound to antibody. These antibodies had a retention half-life of 25 hours and blood clearance of 0.72 mL/hr. In biodistribution studies, tumor uptake at 24 hours was about 5% of injected activity/per gram (%ID/g), with a tumor-to-liver ratio of 0.23 and a tumor-to-bone ratio of 1.54.

In comparison, ¹⁵³Sm-CITCDTPA-OC125 F(ab')₂ had greater serum stability, with 87% of the metal bound to antibody. This preparation had a retention half-life of 22 hours and blood clearance of 2.23 mL/hr. Tumor uptake at 24 hours was 8% of injected dose, with a tumor-to-liver ratio of 1.17 and a tumor-to-bone ratio of 7.08. Renal retention was elevated with ¹⁵³Sm-CITCDTPA-OC125 F(ab')₂, with 30%ID/g at 24 hours. With whole IgG antibodies, both renal and tumor uptake were about 1%ID/g at 24 hours. The whole form showed greater liver uptake and slower blood clearance. The pharmacokinetics and biodistribution of ¹⁵³Sm-CITCDTPA made it more favorable for use in radioimmunotherapy than ¹⁵³Sm-DTPA. A quantitative comparison with conventional autoradiography showed that the imaging plate system produced values comparable to those of the biodistribution study for all tissues.

Conclusions.—In ¹⁵³Sm labeling of monoclonal antibodies for radioimmunotherapy, the new ligand CITCDTPA has qualities that make it more favorable than DTPA. It may even permit a study of radioimmunotherapy in an intraperitoneally xenografted animal model. Using macrocyclic ligands may be helpful in addressing problems with the labeling stability of

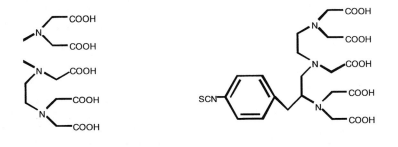

DTPA   CITC DTPA

FIGURE 1.—Structure of the chelating agents. (Courtesy of Kraeber-Bodéré F, Mishra A, Thédrez P, et al: Pharmacokinetics and biodistribution of samarium-153-labelled OC125 antibody coupled to CIT-CDTPA in a xenograft model of ovarian cancer. *Eur J Nucl Med* 23:560–567, 1996. Copyright Springer-Verlag.)

^{153}Sm and the tumor-to-normal tissue ratios. The imaging plate system has a key role to play in studying the biodistribution of radiolabeled antibodies.

▶ Another chelate with improved properties. The affinity of the chelate for the metal is improved by binding the chelate to the protein through the backbone instead of 1 of the chelate arms. It is impressive how important an additional arm can be.

H.W. Strauss, M.D.

Detection and Quantification of Protein-losing Enteropathy With Indium-111 Transferrin
de Kaski MC, Peters AM, Bradley D, et al (Hammersmith Hosp, London)
Eur J Nucl Med 23:530–533, 1996   12–8

Background.—Patients with protein-losing enteropathy have excessive loss of plasma protein into the gut. The clinical management of hypoalbuminemia depends on localization and quantification of the protein loss. With indium-111 transferrin, it may be possible to use a single test for both localization and quantification. Twenty-three patients with hypoalbuminemia were studied using ^{111}In chloride to localize and quantify protein loss.

Methods.—All patients had clinically suspected gastrointestinal protein loss after exclusion of urinary protein loss. A total of 25 ^{111}In transferrin studies were performed. The tracer was prepared by incubating autologous cell-free plasma with ^{111}In chloride for 15 minutes. An uncollimated gamma camera was used to measure whole-body counts at 3 hours and 5 or 6 days after injection of ^{111}In transferrin.

Results.—A gastrointestinal site of protein loss was revealed in 15 of the 25 studies. Thirteen of these studies showed ^{111}In excretion of 16% to 34%, compared with a normal value of less than 10%. Of the 10 ^{111}In imaging studies with negative results, 9 were in patients with normal whole-body ^{111}In excretion; the other patient, with ^{111}In excretion of 22%, had carcinoid syndrome. The mean ^{111}In excretion was 21% in patients with positive imaging studies vs. 7.5% in those with negative imaging studies.

Conclusions.—Gamma camera imaging with ^{111}In transferrin provides a single technique for localizing and quantifying protein loss in patients with protein-losing enteropathy. The technique is simple and convenient, requiring no special patient preparation or stool collection.

▶ Very nice technique. Although the imaging technique failed to identify 1 patient with protein-losing enteropathy, it was successful in most patients. These patients are rare, but it is often important to know the site of protein loss to facilitate therapy.

H.W. Strauss, M.D.

Technetium-99m Dextran: A Promising New Protein-losing Enteropathy Imaging Agent

Bhatnagar A, Singh AK, Lahoti D, et al (Inst of Nuclear Medicine and Allied Sciences, Delhi, India; Ram Manohar Lohia Hosp, New Delhi, India)
Eur J Nucl Med 23:575–578, 1996   12–9

Purpose.—Although technetium-99m human serum albumin is commonly used in imaging studies for protein-losing enteropathy (PLE), there have been few reported series of PLE diagnosed by this technique, raising questions about its sensitivity. Technetium-99m dextran was used for the diagnosis of 2 cases of PLE. This tracer was evaluated for its ability to diagnose PLE in a larger number of patients.

Methods.—Scintigraphy was performed after IV injection of ^{99m}Tc dextran in 22 patients with conditions commonly associated with PLE and 12 healthy controls. Nineteen of the patients had exudative gastrointestinal disease. The scans were evaluated to determine the source and amount of the leakage.

Results.—The radiotracer accumulated in significant amounts in the intestines of all 22 patients within 3–4 hours after injection. One patient with ulcerative colitis in remission had unsuspected tracer activity in the right iliac region but no significant large intestinal exudation. Significant tracer exudation, mainly at the site of involvement, was seen in all patients with active ulcerative colitis. Significant large intestinal exudation also occurred in all patients with enterocolitis, whereas patients with intestinal worms showed focal abnormalities. One third of the normal controls showed some minimal accumulation of the tracer late in the study. These findings could have been physiologic, related to food habits, or caused by unsuspected intestinal worms.

Conclusions.—Technetium-99m dextran appears to be a promising radiopharmaceutical agent for the diagnostic imaging of PLE. It seems to have better sensitivity than ^{99m}Tc HSA, with no adverse reactions. Some false positive results occurred in normal controls.

▶ A very good use for a radiopharmaceutical that has been around for more than a decade.

H.W. Strauss, M.D.

In Vivo Labeling of Angiotensin II Receptors With a Carbon-11-labeled Selective Nonpeptide Antagonist

Kim SE, Scheffel U, Szabo Z, et al (Johns Hopkins Med Insts, Baltimore, Md; Merck Research Labs, West Point, Pa)
J Nucl Med 37:307–311, 1996   12–10

Background.—Angiotensin II (ANG II) is an octapeptide that is the biologically active component of the renin-angiotensin system. It is responsible for initiating several different physiologic effects via binding to high-

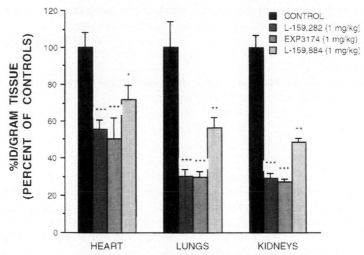

FIGURE 3.—Inhibition of [carbon-11]L-159,884 in vivo binding by L-159,282, EXP3174, and L-159,884 in heart, lungs, and kidneys. Data are means (± 1 standard deviation) of injected activity per gram expressed as percentages of controls. $n = 4$ for each drug. $*P < 0.05$; $**P < 0.01$; $***P < 0.001$. (Reprinted by permission of the Society of Nuclear Medicine, from Kim SE, Scheffel U, Szabo Z, et al: In vivo labeling of angiotensin II receptors with a carbon-11-labeled selective nonpeptide antagonist. *J Nucl Med* 37:307–311, 1996.)

affinity receptors. [Carbon-11]L-159,884, an AT1 subtype selective non-peptide antagonist, is reported as a promising radiotracer for in vivo study of ANG II receptors in PET.

Methods.—The binding, distribution, and kinetic characteristics of [^{11}C]L-159,884 PET studies were studied in mice. The tracer was prepared by alkylation of the nor precursor with [^{11}C]methyliodide. Additional studies were done to evaluate the effects of the AT2-selective ANGII antagonist PD-123319 and of α- and β-adrenergic drugs on the binding of [^{11}C]L-159,884.

Results.—Giving AT1 antagonists produced dose-dependent inhibition of renal binding of [^{11}C]L-159,884, consistent with the high density of AT1 receptors in the kidney. Pulmonary and cardiac binding was inhibited as well (Fig 3). Binding of [^{11}C]L-159,884 to AT1 receptors was unaffected by α- or β-adrenergic drugs. The tracer was rapidly taken up by the liver, kidneys, lungs, and heart, kinetic studies found. More than 20% of the total radioactivity was excreted via the intestine; urinary excretion accounted for less than 8%.

Conclusions.—Binding of the AT1 subtype selective nonpeptide antagonist in the mouse kidneys, lungs, and heart occurred. It is possible that [^{11}C]L-159,884 could be a useful radiotracer for study of ANG II receptors by PET.

▶ Is this the beginning of a new era in the evaluation of hypertension and heart failure? The angiotensin system plays a pivotal role in heart failure and possibly in cardiac remodeling after myocardial infarction. Defining the distribution of angiotensin II receptors, and their occupancy in these diseases, may mark the dawn of a new era in radionuclide imaging.

H.W. Strauss, M.D.

Radioiodination of Nicotine With Specific Activity High Enough for Mapping Nicotinic Acetylcholine Receptors
Kämpfer I, Sorger D, Schliebs R, et al (Univ of Leipzig, Germany; Paul Flechsig Inst of Brain Research, Leipzig, Germany)
Eur J Nucl Med 23:157–162, 1996   12–11

Background.—Recent reports have described the development of radioligands for nicotinic receptors in the brain. However, the radioligands synthesized so far have not been specific enough for in vivo nicotinic receptor-binding studies. A new radiochemical method of synthesizing 5-[^{123}I/^{125}I/^{131}I]-DL-nicotine suitable for receptor binding was investigated, including in vivo biodistribution studies.

Methods.—Using 5-DL-bromonicotine as the precursor, radioiodination was done with a copper (I)-assisted nucleophilic exchange reaction in the presence of a reducing agent. The pH, SN(II) salt concentration, ascorbic acid, Cu(I)chloride, and reaction temperature all were varied to optimize the reaction conditions. The radioiodinated product was purified by high-performance liquid chromatography, and its specific binding was assessed in rat brains by autoradiography. The in vivo biodistribution of 5-[^{131}I]-iodonicotine was determined in rats by well counting and autoradiography.

Results.—The iodinated nicotine product had a radiochemical purity of greater than 98%, with a radiochemical yield of 55% and a specific activity of 5 GBq/μmol or greater. On specific binding studies, an excess of nonradioactive nicotine displaced radioactivity from the specific structures (Fig 2). The equilibrium dissociation constant and maximum receptor number were 13 nmol/L and 22 fmol/mg protein, and unspecific binding was approximately 40%. In vivo distribution studies showed peak brain activity within 0.5 minute after injection, followed by a biexponential washout. Activity in the cerebral cortex was at first 1.5 to 2.0 times greater than in the cerebellum, although homogeneous distribution was achieved by about 15 minutes after injection.

Conclusions.—The technique described in this study permits synthesis of ^{131}I-, ^{125}I-, or ^{123}I-labeled 5-iodo-DL-nicotine with sufficient specific activity for receptor studies. Although these products show specific binding to nicotine receptors in the rat brain, nonspecific binding occurs to a substantial degree after IV injection. This phenomenon results from flow-dependent tissue retention, suggesting that blood flow may have a greater effect on distribution than the presence of specific binding sites.

▶ This agent has rapid blood clearance and high uptake in the cortex. Although this will make an interesting agent for investigation of receptor

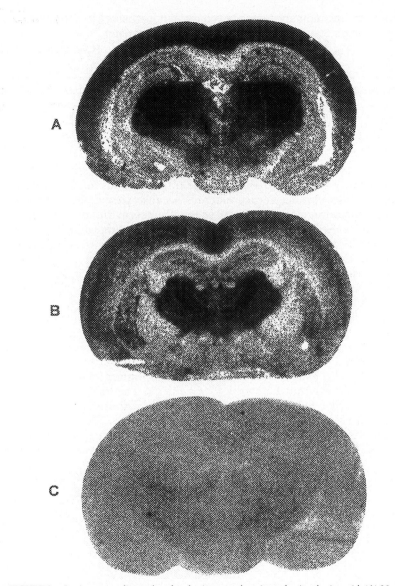

FIGURE 2.—In vivo autoradiography of rat brain coronal sections after incubation with (**A**) 20 nmol/L 5-[^{125}I]iodo-DL-nicotine (specific activity: 5.8 GBq/μmol); (**B**) 10 nmol/L (−)-[N-methyl-H-3]nicotine (specific activity: 2.5 GBq/μmol); (**C**) 20 nmol/L 5-[^{125}I]-iodo-DL-nicotine plus 1 nmol/L nonradioactive nicotine. (Courtesy of Kämpfer I, Sorger D, Schliebs R, et al: Radioiodination of nicotine with specific activity high enough for mapping nicotinic acetylcholine receptors. *Eur J Nucl Med* 23:157–162, 1996. Copyright Springer-Verlag.)

changes, the rapid blood clearance will make it necessary to correct receptor measurements for the regional distribution of perfusion.

H.W. Strauss, M.D.

Reproducibility of Technetium-99m Mercaptoacetyltriglycine Clearance
Piepsz A, Tondeur M, Kinthaert J, et al (Hôpital Saint-Pierre, Brussels, Belgium)
Eur J Nucl Med 23:195–198, 1996   12–12

Introduction.—Technetium-99m mercaptoacetyltriglycine (MAG₃) has become widely accepted as a glomerular tracer and has been suggested for use in overall clearance measurements. Because part of the objective of clearance measurements is to monitor renal function and to assess changes in function over time, it is essential to evaluate the reproducibility of the technique. The precision of ^{99m}Tc MAG₃ clearance was assessed and compared with that of chromium-51 ethylenediamine tetraacetic acid (EDTA).

Methods.—Twelve healthy young adult volunteers were studied on 2 occasions, 8 days apart and under similar physiologic conditions. Both ^{99m}Tc MAG₃ and ^{51}Cr-EDTA were injected intravenously, with 15 blood samples obtained over the subsequent 3–240 minutes. After a biexponential fit was adapted to the plasma disappearance curves, the Sapirstein method was used to calculate the clearances, with correction for body surface area.

Results.—The mean clearance was 226 mL/min/1.73 m² for ^{99m}Tc MAG₃ vs. 110 mL/min/1.73 m² for ^{51}Cr EDTA. The ^{51}Cr EDTA clearance studies showed a mean difference between the first and second measurements of 2.1% of the mean of the 2 successive values. The difference was less than 12% in 10 cases, 15% in one case, and 18% in 1. By comparison, the ^{99m}Tc MAG₃ studies showed a mean difference between the first and

---

TABLE 1.—Overall Results of the Clearance Measurements

Patient no.	Clearance (ml/min/1.73 m²)				Differences (%)	
	EDTA 1	EDTA2	MAG3 1	MAG3 2	EDTA	MAG3
1	101.2	100.3	209.8	223.6	0.92	−6.36
2	91.2	98.7	181.4	249.1	−7.92	−31.44
3	122.6	120.8	192.4	279.2	1.48	−36.82
4	105.6	118.8	271.4	288.8	−11.76	−6.18
5	109.2	105.0	224.1	229.1	3.86	−2.18
6	113.7	118.1	297.7	255.3	−3.84	15.32
7	117.3	122.8	167.3	235.6	−4.12	−33.90
8	111.4	117.5	234.0	233.0	−5.30	0.44
9	113.3	94.6	199.8	224.8	18.02	−11.76
10	127.3	129.7	165.4	318.9	−1.86	−63.40
11	85.0	85.0	109.0	207.0	0.00	−62.02
12	103.0	119.9	200.9	215.3	−14.68	−6.90

second measurements of −20% of the mean of the 2 successive values. The difference was less than 12% in 6 cases, between 15% and 40% in 4 cases, and greater than 60% in 2 cases (Table 1).

Conclusions.—Clearance studies using ^{99m}Tc MAG$_3$ are not precise, i.e., reproducible on a day-to-day basis. This is a serious disadvantage that could stem from methodological or physiologic factors. Clearance studies using ^{51}Cr EDTA show fairly good reproducibility.

▶ This is a troubling and important paper. Several laboratories are using the clearance of MAG$_3$ as an indication of renal function. These data should be viewed with caution in light of the differences of MAG$_3$, which were greater than 30% when the ^{51}Cr EDTA clearances differed by less than 10% in these same patients. One potential explanation for the discrepant results is the difference in count rate between the 2 agents. Early ^{99m}Tc MAG$_3$ samples may have had enough activity to cause substantial dead time in the well counter, resulting in lower values.

H.W. Strauss, M.D.

Ischemic and Reperfused Myocardium Detected With Technetium-99m-Nitroimidazole

Fukuchi K, Kusuoka H, Watanabe Y, et al (Osaka Univ, Japan)
J Nucl Med 37:761–766, 1996   12–13

Purpose.—The use of reperfusion to treat acute myocardial infarction requires imaging techniques to determine whether reperfusion is successful and to differentiate reperfused myocardium from nonreperfused or infarcted myocardium. The radiopharmaceutical nitroimidazole can provide information on the status of tissue oxygenation. The new hypoxia tracer propyleneamine oxime-1,2-nitroimidazole (BMS-1811321) was studied in rats for the detection of ischemic or reperfused myocardium.

Methods.—Experiments were done in anesthetized, mechanically ventilated rats that had undergone thoracotomy. Each animal's left coronary artery was ligated for 15–60 minutes to produce ischemia followed by reperfusion, or simply ligated for 60 minutes without reperfusion. All animals underwent dual-tracer autoradiography with BMS and iodine-125 iodoantipyrine. The BMS was injected just before the start of ischemia, 1 minute before reperfusion, or 15 minutes before reperfusion.

Results.—As assessed by [^{125}I]iodoantipyrine, regional myocardial blood flow (rMBF) in the area at risk returned to the level of the non-ischemic septum in all hearts except those subjected to 60 minutes of occlusion without reperfusion. In "stunned" myocardium—that reperfused after 15 minutes of ischemia—a significant increase in normalized BMS uptake (%BMS) in the area at risk was noted only when the BMS was injected before ischemia. Injecting BMS before 60 minutes of ischemia or just before reperfusion led to a significantly higher %BMS at the marginal zone of the infarct than in the infarct itself (Fig 6). Hearts with 60 minutes

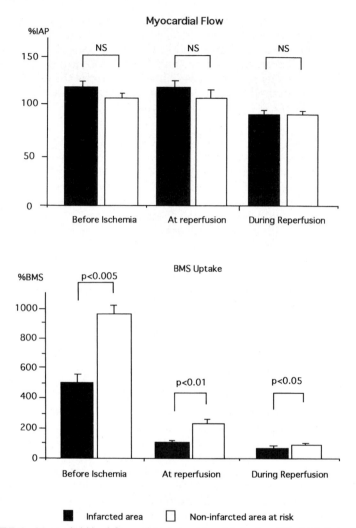

FIGURE 6.—Myocardial blood flow and percent uptake of technetium-99m–labeled nitroimidazole (*BMS*) by the area of 60 minutes of ischemia. Before ischemia, at reperfusion, and during reperfusion indicate the times when BMS was injected. (Reprinted by permission of the Society of Nuclear Medicine, from Fukuchi K, Kusuoka H, Watanabe Y, et al: Ischemic and reperfused myocardium detected with technetium-99m-nitroimidazole. *J Nucl Med* 37:761–766, 1996.)

of occlusion and no reperfusion showed significantly decreased rMBF and %BMS in the area at risk (Fig 7). The peripheral zone of the area at risk showed a significant reduction in rMBF but a significant increase in %BMS.

Conclusions.—The radiotracer BMS may image stunned myocardium only if injected before the onset of ischemia, according to this animal study. In myocardium with prolonged ischemia, the area at risk can be imaged as long as BMS is injected before reperfusion. If BMS is injected

^{125}I-IAP   BMS-181321

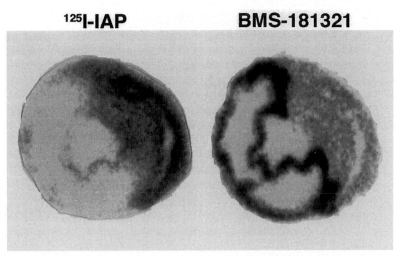

FIGURE 7.—Dual-tracer autoradiograms obtained with iodine-125 iodoantipyrine and technetium-99m–labeled nitroimidazole after 60 minutes of coronary occlusion without reperfusion (permanent occlusion). (Reprinted by permission of the Society of Nuclear Medicine, from Fukuchi K, Kusoka H, Watanabe Y, et al: Ischemic and reperfused myocardium detected with technetium-99m-nitroimidazole. *J Nucl Med* 37:761–766, 1996.)

after reperfusion, negative visualization of the infarcted area can be achieved. The information provided by BMS is different from that provided by other tracers and can help in identifying hypoxic but potentially salvageable myocardium.

▶ The authors present a new radiopharmaceutical that detects an important physiologic phenomenon. It is unfortunate that the agent does not achieve greater contrast in the lesions. However, the data depicted in the figures show the feasibility of this agent to identify ischemic but viable myocardium.

H.W. Strauss, M.D.

Generator-produced Copper-62-PTSM as a Myocardial PET Perfusion Tracer Compared With Nitrogen-13-Ammonia
Tadamura E, Tamaki N, Okazawa H, et al (Kyoto Univ, Japan)
J Nucl Med 37:729–735, 1996   12–14

Background.—Previous research has indicated that copper-62 pyruvaldehyde bis(N^4-methylthiosemicarbazone) (PTSM) appears to be promising in the assessment of myocardial perfusion. The suitability of ^{62}Cu PTSM for evaluating myocardial blood flow (MBF) in patients with coronary artery disease and in healthy individuals was compared with that of nitrogen-13/ammonia.

Methods and Findings.—Thirteen patients with CAD and 9 healthy individuals underwent PET with ^{62}Cu PTSM and ^{13}N ammonia at rest and after pharmacologic vasodilation. The healthy individuals had signifi-

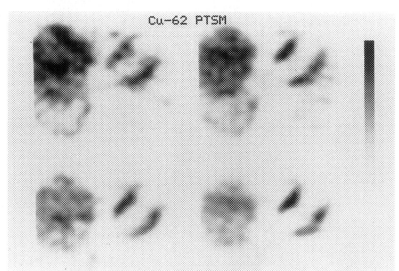

FIGURE 5.—Copper-62 pyruvaldehyde bis(N⁴-methylthiosemicarbazone) (*PTSM*) (**top**) and nitrogen-13 ammonia (**bottom**) contiguous transaxial images obtained at baseline in a patient with anterior myocardial infarction. The tracer distribution in the myocardium correlates closely. Note the high liver activity in the ⁶²Cu PTSM study compared with the ¹³N ammonia study. (Reprinted by permission of the Society of Nuclear Medicine, from Tadamura E, Tamaki N, Okazawa H, et al: Generator-produced copper-62-PTSM as a myocardial PET perfusion tracer compared with nitrogen-13-ammonia. *J Nucl Med* 37:729–735, 1996.)

cantly higher myocardial tracer distribution in the inferior wall in the ⁶²Cu PTSM studies and lower tracer distribution in the lateral wall in the ¹³N ammonia studies. Values for the product of the extraction fraction and MBF showed a linear correlation for both tracers in a low-flow range. However, the extraction fraction and MBF values in a high-flow range for ⁶²Cu PTSM were nonlinearly proportional to the increase of those for ¹³N ammonia. Percent uptake for both tracers at baseline had a good linear correlation. After pharmacologic vasodilation, blood flow with ⁶²Cu PTSM was underestimated compared with that for ¹³N ammonia at high flows (Figs 5 and 6).

Conclusions.—The MBF estimates obtained with ⁶²Cu PTSM in a low-flow range may be as accurate as those obtained with ¹³N ammonia. However, in a high-flow range, the extraction fraction of ⁶²Cu PTSM is considered lower than that of ¹³N ammonia. This may limit the estimation of MBF with ⁶²Cu PTSM after pharmacologic vasodilation.

▶ Another reminder of the importance of characterizing perfusion agents. Most perfusion agents have the characteristic of overestimating tissue flow at low flow and underestimating tissue perfusion at high flow. In the case of thallium, this high-flow "roll-off" may reduce tissue uptake by about 10% to 15%. Sestamibi has a similar decrease in extraction with increased flow, and tetrofosmin appears to have a greater change, perhaps as much as 20%.

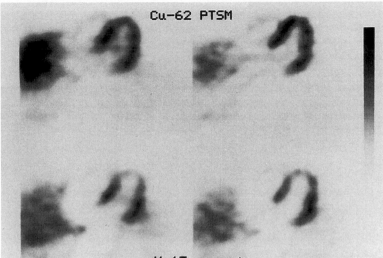

FIGURE 6.—Copper-62 pyruvaldehyde bis(N^4-methylthiosemicarbazone) (*PTSM*) (**top**) and nitrogen-13 ammonia (**bottom**) contiguous transaxial images obtained at baseline in a patient with coronary artery disease after dipyridamole infusion. Coronary angiography showed 75% to 90% stenosis in the right and left anterior descending coronary artery in this patient. Note that the dipyridamole-induced perfusion defect in the anteroseptal region was more prominent with ^{13}N ammonia than with ^{62}Cu PTSM. (Reprinted by permission of the Society of Nuclear Medicine, from Tadamura E, Tamaki N, Okazawa H, et al: Generator-produced copper-62-PTSM as a myocardial PET perfusion tracer compared with nitrogen-13-ammonia. *J Nucl Med* 37:729–735, 1996.)

Tadamura et al. show that ^{62}Cu PTSM also has a marked change compared with ammonia at high flows, suggesting that the contrast between lesion and normal myocardium will be diminished, as shown in Figure 6.

H.W. Strauss, M.D.

Bifunctional NHS-BAT Ester for Antibody Conjugation and Stable Technetium-99m Labeling: Conjugation Chemistry, Immunoreactivity and Kit Formulation
Eisenhut M, Lehmann WD, Becker W, et al (Univ of Heidelberg, Germany; Univ of Erlangen-Nürnberg, Germany; Univ of Frankfurt, Germany; et al)
J Nucl Med 37:362–370, 1996   12–15

Objective.—Several different approaches to improve binding of complexed technetium-99m to antibodies or antibody fragments have been investigated. Coagulation chemistry and kit-binding approaches to binding the NHS ester of 6-(4'-(4"-carboxyphenoxy)butyl)-2,10-dimercapto-2,10-dimethyl-4,8-diazaundecane (NHS-BAT ester) (Fig 1) to monoclonal antibodies (MAbs) were investigated. The study included functional testing of the resulting BAT conjugated and ^{99m}Tc-labeled MAbs BW 431/26, MAb 425, and bispecific MDX210.

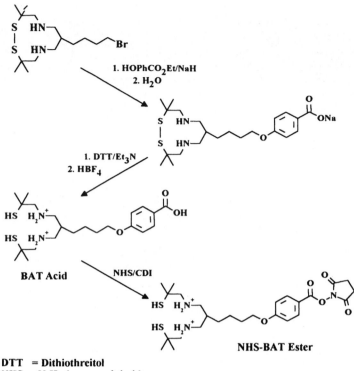

DTT = Dithiothreitol
NHS = N-Hydroxysuccinimide
CDI = N-(3-dimethylaminopropyl)-N'-ethylcarbodiimide

FIGURE 1.—Synthesis of 6-(4'-(4"carboxyphenoxy) butyl)-2,10-dimercapto-2,10-dimethyl-4,8-diaza-undecane (*NHS-BAT*) ester. (Reprinted by permission of the Society of Nuclear Medicine, from Eisenhut M, Lehmann WD, Becker W, et al: Bifunctional NHS-BAT ester for antibody conjugation and stable technetium-99m labeling: Conjugation chemistry, immunoreactivity and kit formulation. *J Nucl Med* 37:362–370, 1996.)

Methods.—High-performance liquid chromatography, size-exclusion chromatography, and positive fast-atom bombardment mass spectra were used for kinetic and chemical assessment of the conjugation reaction. A number of different immunoreactivity assays were used to evaluate the ^{99m}Tc BAT-MAbs. Rat studies were performed to examine the biodistribution of ^{99m}Tc BAT-BW, which was compared with directly labeled BW 431/26.

Results.—The NHS-BAT ester showed high reactivity at a pH of 8.5 and a temperature of 25°C, showing 90% completion after 30 minutes. A 30% conjugation yield was noted with 19 µmol/L MAb and 228 µmol/L NHS-BAT, with higher BAT-to-MAb ratios observed at higher NHS-BAT concentrations. Hydrolysis was completed by conjugation at the NHS ring, the results of positive fast-atom bombardment mass spectra suggested. By 5 minutes, nearly quantitative ^{99m}Tc labeling was obtained. The ^{99m}Tc-BAT antibodies had greater than 90% immunoreactivity and were insensitive to BAT-to-MAb ratios as high as 10.

Whereas organ distribution of ^{99m}Tc BAT-BW 431/26 was comparable with that of directly labeled BW 431/26, urinary excretion was lower. The biological functions of ^{99m}Tc BAT-BW 431/26 and ^{99m}Tc BAT-MAb 425 were shown in vivo by immunoscintigraphy.

Conclusions.—The NHS-BAT ester appears to be a nondestructive and universal bifunctional ligand with which to introduce stable ^{99m}Tc protein-binding sites. This technique can be used to bind not just intact antibodies but also proteins of the molecular size of HSA, F(ab')$_2$ and Fab fragments, and recombinant products. With the use of kit formulations, little time or experience is needed to perform conjugation and labeling.

▶ The difficult chemistry of ^{99m}Tc continues to yield its secrets to the dedicated chemists pursuing new conjugation chemistry. Nuclear medicine needs a variety of approaches to couple ^{99m}Tc to chemical species of interest. The availability of coupling tools that have well-defined characteristics makes it easier for investigators to develop innovative radiopharmaceuticals. This chelate binds well to the antibody and maintains immunoreactivity.

H.W. Strauss, M.D.

Complexes of Technetium-99m With Tetrapeptides Containing One Alanyl and Three Glycyl Moieties

Vanbilloen HP, de Roo MJ, Verbruggen AM (KU Leuven, Belgium; UZ Gasthuisberg, Leuven, Belgium)
Eur J Nucl Med 23:40–48, 1996   12–16

Purpose.—With direct labeling at alkaline pH, previous studies have shown efficient technetium-99m labeling of tetrapeptides. Replacing the mercaptoacetyl moiety of mercaptoacetyltriglycine (MAG$_3$) produces derivative tetrapeptides, and C-methyl–substituted ^{99m}Tc MAG$_3$ derivatives have shown some interesting biological properties. Technetium-99m complexes with tetrapeptides containing 3 glycyl (G) and 1 D- or L-alanyl (A) moiety were studied (Fig 1).

Findings.—The complexes ^{99m}Tc-L-GAGG, ^{99m}Tc-D-GAGG, and ^{99m}Tc-L-GGAG had high and rapid renal excretion in mice, as ^{99m}Tc MAG$_3$ does. The D and L isonomers of ^{99m}Tc-L-AGGG and ^{99m}Tc-D-GAGG showed lower renal handling, whereas ^{99m}Tc-L-GGGA and ^{99m}Tc-D-GGGA had much lower renal handling. Baboon studies showed greater 1-hour plasma clearance with ^{99m}Tc-L-AGGG, ^{99m}Tc-D-AGGG, and ^{99m}Tc-L-GAGG than with ^{99m}Tc-MAG$_3$. Plasma clearance was lower with ^{99m}Tc-D-GAGG, ^{99m}Tc-L-GAGG, and ^{99m}Tc-D-GGGA. Plasma clearance was very low with ^{99m}Tc-L-GGGA and ^{99m}Tc-D-GGGA.

Of the 3 complexes with the greatest plasma clearance in baboons, ^{99m}Tc-L-AGGG and ^{99m}Tc-L-GAGG had plasma clearance comparable to that of ^{99m}Tc-MAG$_3$. Lower plasma clearance was apparent, accompanied by visible liver uptake, with ^{99m}Tc-D-AGGG. On renograms, moderate kidney accumulation was noted with ^{99m}Tc-L-AGGG and ^{99m}Tc-D-AGGG.

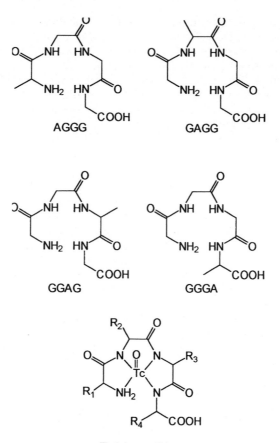

FIGURE 1.—Structure of tetrapeptides containing 1 alanyl L or D and 3 glycyl moieties, alanylglycyl-glycylglycine (*AGGG*), glycylalanylglycylglycine (*GAGG*), glycylglycylalanylglycine (*GGAG*) and glycyl-glycylglycylalanine (*GGGA*), and proposed structure of technetium-99m–Tc-tetrapeptide complexes. (Courtesy of Vanbilloen HP, de Roo MJ, Verbruggen AM: Complexes of technetium-99m with tetrapeptides containing one alanyl and three glycyl moieties. *Eur J Nucl Med* 23:40–48, 1996. Copyright Springer-Verlag.)

In contrast, renography with ^{99m}Tc-L-GAGG showed excellent renal shape, with a somewhat higher maximal kidney concentration than ^{99m}Tc MAG$_3$.

Conclusions.—The methyl substituent of ^{99m}Tc tetrapeptides has a major impact on their biological behavior. The tetrapeptides are an interesting new class of Tc-binding N$_4$-tetraligands. Continued research on derivatives of these tetrapeptides may identify some complexes of value in areas other than renal function studies.

▶ The authors have developed several variations on a theme to define the behavior of a series of potential renal imaging agents. Small differences in configuration resulted in substantial changes in clearance, confirming the remarkable specificity of biological systems. An additional point is the authors' simple and direct method of labeling at a very alkaline pH. These studies suggest that we have not seen the end of the potential parade of interesting renal agents.

H.W. Strauss, M.D.

A Miniaturized Rapid Paper Chromatographic Procedure for Quality Control of Technetium-99m Sestamibi
Patel M, Sadek S, Jahan S, et al (Kuwait Cancer Control Ctr; Kuwait Univ)
Eur J Nucl Med 22:1416–1419, 1995   12–17

Objective.—Technetium-99m–labeled sestamibi is widely used for various indications in clinical nuclear medicine. The manufacturer's recommended technique to assess for impurities calls for the use of thin-layer chromatography with Baker Flex aluminum oxide–coated plates developed in ethanol. This procedure is complicated and time consuming. A simple, miniaturized rapid paper chromatographic (MRPC) technique for quality control of ^{99m}Tc-labeled sestamibi was evaluated.

Methods.—The new MRPC technique was performed using 6.0 x 0.5-cm Whatman 3MM paper strips developed in ethyl acetate. This procedure was compared with the manufacturer's recommended thin-layer chromatographic system and with the mini-paper chromatographic technique described by Hung et al., the solvent system of which has some toxic effects.

Results.—The MRPC technique took only 3 minutes to perform, compared with 4 minutes for the Hung et al. technique and 30–35 minutes for the manufacturer's technique. The new technique had an R_f range of 0.5 to 0.75, compared with 0.9 to 1.0 for the other 2 techniques. All 3 techniques had percent labeling efficiencies of 96% to 98%.

Conclusions.—The new MRPC technique offers a quick and effective method to test for contaminants in ^{99m}Tc-labeled sestamibi preparations. It will be very useful for routine quality control purposes.

▶ Fast and simple.

H.W. Strauss, M.D.

Interaction of Metaiodobenzylguanidine With Cardioactive Drugs: An In Vitro Study
Huguet F, Fagret D, Caillet M, et al (Tours Univ, France; Grenoble Univ, France; Poitiers Univ, France)
Eur J Nucl Med 23:546–549, 1996   12–18

Introduction.—The noradrenaline analogue metaiodobenzylguanidine (MIBG) is used to study the function and integrity of the sympathetic nerve endings of the human heart. Although [iodine-123]MIBG appears to be well suited for use in routine clinical evaluations of myocardial noradrenaline levels, drugs that inhibit the noradrenaline transport system also may block the uptake of MIBG. The effects of various cardiologic drugs on MIBG uptake were studied using an in vitro human blood platelet model.

Methods and Results.—The study model consisted of a platelet preparation from healthy humans incubated with [iodine-125]MIBG alone or with varying concentrations of different cardiologic drugs. The drugs with a significant inhibitory effect on [^{125}I]MIBG uptake were labetalol and propranolol. In contrast, even at doses of over 50 µmol/L, [^{125}I]MIBG uptake was unaffected by other β-blockers, calcium inhibitors, digoxin, and amiodarone. For labetalol, the dose that inhibited 50% of [^{125}I]MIBG uptake was less than the concentrations used clinically. For propranolol, the inhibitory dose exceeded clinical concentrations.

Conclusions.—Labetalol and propranolol may affect myocardial [^{125}I]MIBG uptake in humans. The in vitro model used in this study can predict these inhibitory effects, if the plasma concentration and perhaps the pretreatment period are taken into account.

▶ An interesting piece of research, providing useful data for a complex test. The MIBG images are difficult to interpret, particularly when there is a question about the potential confounding role of other drugs taken by the patient. These investigators used an in vitro incubation of platelets taken from healthy volunteers with the addition of cardiac drugs to define the relative inhibition of MIBG uptake. Only 2 agents, labetalol and propranolol, inhibited platelet uptake, suggesting that other common drugs, such as calcium-channel blockers, amiodarone, and digoxin, will not effect uptake. These data will help ease the concerns of investigators using MIBG imaging to evaluate patients with heart failure.

H.W. Strauss, M.D.

13 Physics and Dosimetry

Introduction

The lead article by Rosenthal et al. (Abstract 13–1) serves as an excellent overview of all of the components of SPECT imaging and reconstruction algorithms. This is followed by 3 articles describing new collimation geometries being developed for tomographic imaging in nuclear medicine. These new developments continue to illustrate that nuclear medicine is a very dynamic and constantly evolving modality. Applying concepts based on slant hole, parallel hole, half-cone beam, and pinhole collimation shows the incredible variety of methods that can be used to acquire projection data in nuclear medicine. Fan beam geometry is already well established in today's imaging routine; by understanding these newer, evolving geometries, we can anticipate new directions for camera designs in the near future.

Coupled with new hardware developments, we continue to see interesting new developments in software reconstruction algorithms. Iterative reconstruction schemes have already established themselves in routine clinical use. We can appreciate improvements in the emission image and the attenuation correction in the 2 articles by Lee et al. and Knešaurek et al. (Abstracts 13–5 and 13–6). Dealing with improved reconstruction methods and attenuation corrections has been one of the central developments during the past few years. More recently, we have seen improved methods for correcting the scatter component that degrades clinical images. The following 3 articles deal with this correction and our attention to improved quantitative images. One of the most interesting new concepts being developed here uses the transmission image (typically used for attenuation correction) as a map for dealing with the scatter component more exactly. My belief is that the use of the transmission image for improved scatter correction will prove to be the next important step we take toward improved quantitative reconstructions.

Improved reconstructions, of course, lead to improved interpretations of the diagnostic images. The next 2 articles demonstrate 2 important characteristics that we read from the clinical image: tracer concentration and object size. The apparent concentration of radiopharmaceutical in a volume unfortunately is influenced by its size. The interplay of these 2 confounding concepts can be appreciated in the 2 articles by Zito et al. and Wang et al. (Abstracts 13–10 and 13–11).

Over the years, we have followed algorithms for registering patient images; this year, we see further development in automating this important image processing step presented by Eberl (Abstract 13–12). Also, being able to image 511-keV photons using conventional nuclear medicine cameras is one of the most exciting recent developments in our field. We are certainly looking forward to many articles next year describing high-energy collimation and coincidence counting using 2-headed Anger cameras. Our quality control can only be as good as the tools we use. One of the most important quality control tools is the uniform flood source, and the next article in this chapter teaches us more about its characteristics.

This year, we have included 5 articles covering dosimetry topics in nuclear medicine. As was true for the imaging section, this section also has an excellent overview article that covers general principles (commandments) for radiation protection. This article by Strom (Abstract 13–15) is a good one to distribute to your staff. The next 3 articles give detailed dosimetry estimates for important radiopharmaceuticals used in our field. And finally, we would like to report on the availability of the Medical Internal Radiation Dose estimation method, which is now available and has a very convenient, user-friendly computer program.

And speaking of computers, who can ignore the Internet? Our concluding article reminds us that nuclear medicine is just as prominent and just as important as all of the other services and information centers available on the World Wide Web. If you don't know about nuclear medicine's place on the Web, then you need to go out and start surfing.

I. George Zubal, Ph.D.

Quantitative SPECT Imaging: A Review and Recommendations by the Focus Committee of the Society of Nuclear Medicine Computer and Instrumentation Council

Rosenthal MS, Cullom J, Hawkins W, et al (Univ of Pittsburgh, Pa; Emory Univ, Atlanta, Ga; Univ of Nebraska Med Ctr, Omaha; et al)
J Nucl Med 36:1489–1513, 1995   13–1

Purpose.—There is growing interest in the use of quantitative SPECT imaging and in improving the quality of SPECT images. This interest has prompted the Computer and Instrumentation Council of the Society of Nuclear Medicine to report on the various factors affecting quantitative SPECT imaging and to make recommendations for SPECT practitioners.

Recommendations.—The report provides a detailed review of the physics of quantitative imaging, its advantages and disadvantages, and instrumentation and reconstruction techniques involved. Special attention is paid to the mechanisms that can affect the accuracy of SPECT images and to techniques of improving image quality and quantitation. It is important to correct SPECT images, but the extent to which attenuation correction and scatter compensation are used will depend on the availability of personnel who can develop these corrective procedures. Recommendations vary for different nuclear medicine groups, but improving image quality will usually be the first step.

All departments should examine their quality assurance and control programs with the goal of improving image quality. They should check out the available software and decide which reconstruction algorithms and filters will provide the best diagnostic images for a specific study. Small departments may be advised not to perform any improvements unless the manufacturer provides some simple software procedure. For departments with a physicist available inhouse, decay and attenuation should be corrected—simple techniques of scatter correction can improve image quality, and perhaps quantitative accuracy, by about 10%. Implementation of full attenuation correction and scatter compensation for quantitative imaging should be considered by research-oriented departments. The goal, in addition to improved image quality, should be true tissue-specific activity for research purposes. Recommendations on the actual techniques to be used at each type of department are presented as well.

Clinical Considerations.—The review focuses on what effects must be managed to obtain quantitative images and assumes that volumes or counts per unit volume are the measures of interest. However, these measures may be inadequate for clinical purposes. In addition to compensating for physical effects, the sensitivity of the entire image acquisition and reconstruction process must be calibrated. Still, even with appropriate phantom studies, the information obtained may not be clinically useful. Quantitative images can be useful if all required data and good statistics are available. In any case, diagnostic value should be enhanced by improved image quality.

Discussion.—The physics, instrumentation, and reconstruction methods used in quantitative SPECT imaging are reviewed, and recommendations are offered. The most important outcome of applying corrections is improved image quality. Although accurate quantitative data are desirable, they cannot always be obtained. With continuing progress in the correction of SPECT data and the development of faster computer systems, data correction and quantitative SPECT will become a clinical reality.

▶ This article should be required reading for anyone involved in SPECT imaging. The authors have done an excellent job of discussing the basic principles involved in nuclear medicine tomographic imaging. These 24 pages should be studied in depth to better understand how a SPECT image is formed and what it represents.

I.G. Zubal, Ph.D.

Transmission Imaging of Large Attenuators Using a Slant Hole Collimator on a Three-headed SPECT System

King MA, Luo D, Dahlberg ST, et al (Univ of Massachusetts, Worcester; Univ of Chicago; Picker Internatl, Bedford Heights, Ohio)

Med Phys 23:263–272, 1996

13–2

Introduction.—Attenuation correction relies on the determination of an accurate, patient-specific attenuation map. With 3-headed SPECT systems with slant hole collimators, conjugate views can be combined to create truncation-free attenuation profiles. The reconstruction algorithms used with slant hole collimators were discussed, along with the potential for image artifacts.

Methods and Findings.—Considering the size of objects that can be imaged without truncation and the size of the overlap region in conjugate views, a 15-degree slant angle was identified as optimal. Subsequent experiments were performed with a 30-degree slant hole collimator and phantom with a lateral width of 56 cm (Fig 1). These studies confirmed that slant-hole transmission could provide an accurate, truncation-free attenuation map. The slant angle and the radius of rotation of the slant collimator were major determinants of the center of rotation. Also, spatial resolution in the transaxial plane of the attenuation map depended on the radius of rotation not of the uncollimated transmission source but of the slant hole collimator.

Transmission Imaging On A 3-Headed SPECTsystem

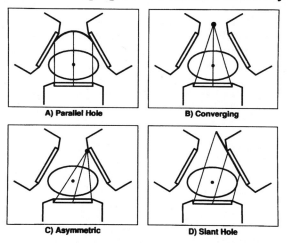

A) Parallel Hole

B) Converging

C) Asymmetric

D) Slant Hole

FIGURE 1.—Drawings illustrating the transmission imaging of a 50-cm-diameter patient on a three-headed SPECT system with 40-cm field of view camera heads using (A) parallel, (B) symmetric fan beam, (C) asymmetric fan beam, and (D) slant hole collimators. In this drawing, head 1 is at 6 o'clock, head 2 is at 2 o'clock, and head 3 is at 10 o'clock, as they would be at the start of a SPECT acquisition. The starting position of head 1 is taken as of 0° for counterclockwise gantry rotation. (Courtesy of King MA, Luo D, Dahlberg ST, et al: Transmission imaging of large attenuators using a slant hole collimator on a three-headed SPECT system. *Med Phys* 23:263–272, 1996.)

Conclusions.—The use of slant hole collimators on 3-headed SPECT systems permits the creation of truncation-free attenuation maps of large patients. The findings suggest that accurate attenuation maps can be created in a short time. A 15-degree collimator appears to offer the best balance between the combination of size of the combined field of view and overlaps of conjugate views. The study also includes an evaluation of a multiline transmission source for use in estimating the attenuation map in technetium-99m–labeled sestamibi perfusion studies.

▶ The dual modality of transmission and emission imaging in nuclear medicine is slowly emerging into clinical applications. Transmission imaging has been attempted using various geometries. A drawback of some of these geometries is that the transmission data are truncated, resulting in a transmission image that is full of artifacts. This article uses a geometric and reconstruction algorithm producing artifact-free transmission images in a large-volume object like the thorax. This takes transmission imaging one step further for acceptance in applying attenuation corrections.

I.G. Zubal, Ph.D.

Half-cone Beam Collimation for Triple-camera SPECT Systems
Li J, Jaszczak RJ, van Mullekom A, et al (Duke Univ, Durham, NC; North Carolina State Univ, Raleigh; Nuclear Fields, St Mary's, Australia)
J Nucl Med 37:498–502, 1996   13–3

Introduction.—The use of cone-beam collimation for triple-camera SPECT systems enhances the detectability of brain lesions, compared with parallel- and fan-beam collimation techniques. With a full-cone beam, however, it is difficult to position the collimator close to the patient's head.

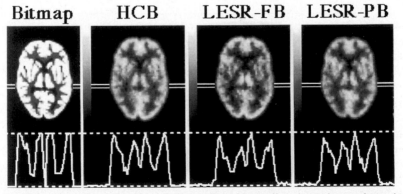

FIGURE 5.—Transverse sectional images and profiles of the Hoffman brain phantom from a high-count density scan. Also shown is the corresponding slice of the bitmap of this phantom. This slice was about 6 cm from the central plane of the half-cone beam collimator. (Reprinted by permission of the Society of Nuclear Medicine, from Li J, Jaszczak RJ, Van Mullekom A, et al: Half-cone beam collimation for triple-camera SPECT systems. *J Nucl Med* 37:498–502, 1996.)

An approach designed to clear the patient's shoulders uses a half-cone beam (HCB) collimator.

Methods.—The performance characteristics of HCB for SPECT imaging of the brain were compared with parallel-beam and fan-beam collimators with similar resolution characteristics. Simultaneous projections were acquired with all 3 collimators, using the 3-dimensional Hoffman brain phantom and 3 patients. A filtered backprojection reconstruction algorithm was used to reconstruct SPECT data.

Results.—Compared with the parallel-beam and fan-beam collimators, the HCB collimator provided much higher sensitivities. When 10 cm from the collimator surface, the planar spatial resolutions for the 3 collimators were 39.7 (parallel-beam), 55.6 (fan-beam), and 85.6 cts/(sec-MBq) (HCB). Results of Hoffman brain phantom and patient imaging showed that the deeper gray matter was more clearly visualized in the half-cone beam scans. In the phantom, the HCB reconstructed image closely resembled the corresponding slice of the bitmap (Fig 5). In patients, the HCB showed better noise characteristics compared with the other collimators.

Conclusion.—The specially designed high-resolution HCB collimator allows the patient's shoulders to be cleared, thereby improving spatial resolution and increasing the useful field of view. Images obtained with the triple-camera SPECT system showed enhanced image quality and noise characteristics.

▶ It seems that a new collimator geometry is developed each year. In going back through past YEAR BOOKS OF NUCLEAR MEDICINE, you will see at least one new geometry that has been presented each year. Converging collimation is the preferred design for brain imaging; the novel new collimator presented here has the advantages of better positioning with respect to the patient and improved image quality.

I.G. Zubal, Ph.D.

Ultra-high Resolution SPECT System Using Four Pinhole Collimators for Small Animal Studies

Ishizu K, Mukai T, Yonekura Y, et al (Kyoto Univ, Japan)
J Nucl Med 36:2282–2287, 1995   13–4

Background.—Small animal studies are needed to assess newly developed radiopharmaceuticals. Although high-resolution imaging of small animals can be performed using parallel-hole collimators, sensitivity is very low. Because of geometric magnification, easily made pinhole collimators can permit high-resolution imaging. A new ultrahigh-resolution SPECT system using 4 pinhole collimators for small animal imaging was developed.

Methods.—Imaging was performed with a clinical 4-head SPECT scanner and specially designed pinhole collimators. Pinholes of different configurations were designed with effective aperture sizes of 1, 2, and 4 mm

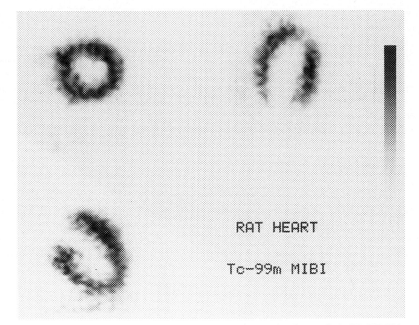

RAT HEART

Tc-99m MIBI

FIGURE 7.—Myocardial perfusion technetium-99m–methoxyisobutyl isonitrile (MIBI) SPECT images in the rat. Left ventricular wall and cardiac activity are clearly visualized. (Reprinted by permission of the Society of Nuclear Medicine, from Ishizu K, Mukai T, Yonekura Y, et al: Ultra-high resolution SPECT system using four pinhole collimators for small animal studies. *J Nucl Med* 36:2282–2287, 1995.)

and rotating radii of 40 and 50 mm. The fixed distance from the axis of rotation to the scintillator was 180 mm. After fan-beam-to-parallel-beam data conversion, the SPECT images were reconstructed using a filtered backprojection algorithm.

Results.—With the optimal types of pinholes, the system achieved a reconstructed spatial resolution of 1.65 mm (FWHM) and a sensitivity of 4.3 kcps/μCi/mL. Rat studies using technetium-99m–hexamethyl-propyleneamine oxime (HMPAO) showed small brain structures clearly, and ^{99m}Tc–methoxyisobutyl isonitrile (MIBI) studies showed clear separation of the myocardium and cardiac cavity (Fig 7). Iodine-123–iomazenil dynamic SPECT imaging of the brain proved feasible as well.

Conclusions.—An ultrahigh-resolution SPECT system for imaging small animals can provide in vivo data on the regional distribution of radiolabeled tracers and may prove useful in the development of new radiopharmaceuticals and in the study of various disease models in animals.

▶ This article once again demonstrates that the physical resolution limit of SPECT is much smaller than that of PET. Single-photon emission CT is not blurred by the path lengths of the positron nor by the variation away from 180 degrees of the 2 photons. For that reason, SPECT resolution can surpass the approximately 3-mm limit of PET and could conceivably approach sub-millimeter resolution. We continue to dream that such resolutions can be achieved for clinical patient studies.

I.G. Zubal, Ph.D.

Bayesian Image Reconstruction in SPECT Using Higher Order Mechanical Models as Priors
Lee S-J, Rangarajan A, Gindi G (State Univ of New York, Stony Brook; Yale Univ, New Haven, Conn)
IEEE Trans Med Imaging 14:669–680, 1995   13–5

Purpose.—Emission tomography is widely performed by the maximum-likelihood (ML) approach using the expectation-maximization (EM) algorithm. However, the ill-posed nature of the reconstruction problem makes the ML-EM method unstable and divergent at higher iteration numbers. Bayesian reconstruction methods have the potential to overcome the instability problem while maintaining a principled means of incorporating the imaging model. Prior information is induced using a spatial smoothness regularizer, and more elaborate smoothness constraints may be used to capture actual spatial information about the object being studied. Previously described prior distributions have assumed a piecewise constant source distribution. A more accurate model, using higher order mechanical models as priors—the weak plate model—is proposed as a more expressive alternative to a piecewise linear model.

The Weak Plate Model.—The key feature of the weak plate prior model is that it favors piecewise linear ramplike regions; it is actually an extension of the weak membrane to higher order. In addition to preserving edges, this model permits piecewise ramplike regions in the reconstruction. For SPECT, these regions appear in ground-truth source distributions as primate autoradiographs of regional cerebral blood flow radionuclides.

The investigators incorporated the weak plate prior in a maximum a posteriori approach, modeling it as a Gibbs distribution and using a Generalized Expectation-Maximization (GEM) formulation for optimization. This GEM model was compared quantitatively with another GEM algorithm with a prior favoring piecewise constant regions and with the ML-EM algorithm, using pointwise regional bias and variance of ensemble image reconstructions as measures of image quality. Compared with the ML-EM technique, the weak plate and membrane priors showed better bias and variance in most regions incorporating edge structure and in smooth regions.

Conclusion.—The weak point prior described in this study compares favorably in terms of bias and variance with other reconstruction models. Variance is reduced in all types of regions, piecewise constant as well as linear ramplike regions. The results are encouraging, although the behavior of weak point priors with regard to hyperparameters and annealing schedule remains to be completely quantified.

▶ Iterative reconstruction algorithms that use additional information (other than just the camera data) to reconstruct the clinical image are referred to as "Bayesian." Knowing the characteristic (typical) distribution properties of the radiopharmaceutical at edges and within structures (texture) can be used as a very powerful tool to reconstruct an image that more closely represents the real distribution within the patient. We need to be sure that we do not impose too high an expectation of what we think is typical (otherwise we will find exactly what we expect), but some prior knowledge of how tracers distribute in tissue can certainly drastically improve the clinical image, as shown here.

I.G. Zubal, Ph.D.

A New Iterative Reconstruction Technique for Attenuation Correction in High-resolution Positron Emission Tomography
Knešaurek K, Machac J, Vallabhajosula S, et al (Mount Sinai Med Ctr, New York)
Eur J Nucl Med 23:656–661, 1996   13–6

Background.—Transmission scans often have a high amount of noise, which propagates to resulting emission scans during the attenuation correction. The filtered backprojection (FBP) method, which permits a trade-off between resolution and noise in reconstructed images, is the most common PET reconstruction method. A new method decreases the amount of noise in the reconstructed images without sacrificing resolution.

Methods and Findings.—The new iterative reconstruction technique (NIRT) uses transmission data for nonuniform attenuation correction. A cost functional including a noise term was derived using the general inverse problem theory. A weighted-least-square maximum a posteriori conjugate gradient (CG) technique was used to minimize the cost functional. In the procedure, the Hessian of the cost function was changed by adding an additional term. Two phantoms were studied. The first phantom was a cylinder uniformly filled with distributed activity of 74 MBq of fluorine-18 and in which 2 inserts were placed. In addition, a Hoffman brain phantom filled with uniformly distributed activity of 7.4 MBq of ^{18}F was studied. The NIRT was compared with a standard FBP method in the resulting reconstructed images. The new technique converged rapidly and provided good image reconstructions. The NIRT images showed better noise properties than the images obtained by the FBP method. The noise (measured as rms% noise) was less by a factor of 1.75 in images reconstructed by NIRT compared with those reconstructed by FBP. The distances between the Hoffman brain slice reconstructed by FBP and by NIRT and the perfect PET Hoffman brain slice created from the MR image were 0.526 and 0.328, respectively (Fig 7).

Conclusions.—The amount of noise in PET images can be significantly reduced by NIRT with no reduction in resolution, resulting in better PET image quality. The disadvantage of NIRT is that computing time per slice

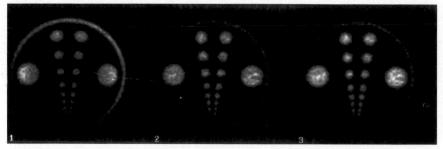

FIGURE 7.—Reconstructed emission scan through the resolution area of the phantom: *(1)* without attenuation correction, *(2)* with attenuation correction and reconstructed by the standard method based on filtered backprojection, and *(3)* with attenuation correction and reconstructed by the new iterative reconstruction technique. (Courtesy of Knešurek K, Machac J, Vallabhajosula S, et al: A new iterative reconstruction technique for attenuation correction in high-resolution positron emission tomography. *Eur J Nucl Med* 23:656–661, 1996. Copyright Springer-Verlag.)

is approximately 15 times longer than with the standard method. However, computing time may be decreased by optimizing the software code.

▶ One of the advantages of iterative reconstruction techniques is the noise suppression in low-count areas. This can be seen by comparing image 3 with image 2 in Figure 7. The intensity values calculated by iterative reconstruction also more closely correspond to the real activities found in the structures. This can be appreciated by reviewing the quantitative presentations contained in the full article.

I.G. Zubal, Ph.D.

Comparative Assessment of Nine Scatter Correction Methods Based on Spectral Analysis Using Monte Carlo Simulations
Buvat I, Rodriguez-Villafuerte M, Todd-Pokropek A, et al (Institut Gustave-Roussy, Villejuif, France; Univ College London)
J Nucl Med 36:1476–1488, 1995   13–7

Introduction.—Blurring caused by photon scatter is a major problem in SPECT. A number of different scatter correction methods have been proposed, all different in their underlying hypotheses and complexity. Monte Carlo simulations were performed to compare 9 different scatter correction methods.

Methods.—Histories of photons emitted from a realistic technetium-99m phantom were generated by means of a Monte Carlo simulation. Information on history, location, and energy of photons detected in a particular projection was gathered and evaluated to test the underlying assumptions of each of the 9 scatter correction methods, including dual- and triple-window techniques, spectral analysis techniques, and factor analysis techniques (Table 1). For each corrected image, the relative and absolute quantification and signal-to-noise ratio were analyzed.

TABLE 1.—Summary of the Performance of 9 Scatter Correction Methods

Method	Requires parameter(s)	Relative quantification	Absolute quantification for high U	Absolute quantification for low U (30 < U < 130)	SNR	Number of spectral windows
M1 Photopeak window acquisition	no +	poor –	poor – ϵ > 30%	poor – ϵ > 65%	good + 19.2	1 +
M2 Dual photopeak window	yes –	poor –	good + ϵ < 10% for U > 130	approx. 10% < ϵ < 80%	good + 19.6; 18.9	2
M3 Channel ratio	yes –	poor –	good + ϵ ~ 10% for U > 130	approx. 10% < ϵ < 45%	poor – 9.6	2
M4 Photopeak energy distribution analysis	yes –	poor –	poor – ϵ ~ 40%	poor – ϵ > 40%	poor – 10.5	2
M5 Dual-energy window	yes or no	poor –	good + ϵ ~ 5% for U > 230	approx. 15% < ϵ < 45%	inter. 14.9; 15.9	2
M6 Trapezoidal approximation	no +	approx.	good + ϵ ~ 10% for U > 330	approx. 10% < ϵ < 45%	poor – 9.0	3
M7 Triangular approximation	no +	approx.	good + ϵ < 10% for U > 130	approx. 5% < ϵ < 35%	inter. 14.1	3
M8 Constrained factor analysis	no +	good +	approx. ϵ < 15% for U > 130	approx. 20% < ϵ < 50%	good + 18.8	6 (list-mode) –
M9 FAMIS-TAS	no +	good +	good + ϵ ~ 10% for U > 130	approx. 10% < ϵ < 25%	good + 17.8	30 (list-mode) –

Abbreviations: +, merit; –, inconvenience; ϵ, relative error; U, number of unscattered photons per pixel U(i); *approx,* approximate; *inter,* intermediate. (Reprinted by permission of the Society of Nuclear Medicine, from Buvat I, Rodriguez-Villafuerte M, Todd-Pokropek A, et al: Comparative assessment of nine scatter correction methods based on spectral analysis using Monte Carlo simulations. *J Nucl Med* 36:1476–1488, 1995.)

Results.—Two of the techniques studied did not permit activity quantification for the simulated data. For methods in which some parameters had to be calibrated, the dual-energy window method offered the best balance between accuracy and ease of implementation. However, it introduced some bias in relative quantification, in which regard a triple-energy window technique was more accurate. Stable quantitative accuracy, with an error of about 10%, was achieved with a factor analysis approach across a wide range of activity. However, this technique necessitated a more sophisticated acquisition mode of 20 energy windows. From both a theoretical and practical viewpoint, the factor analysis of medical image sequences using targeted-apex seeking technique was superior to constrained factor analysis.

Conclusions.—Nine different scatter correction techniques for SPECT were compared, and the findings suggest that applying a spectral analysis technique for scatter correction can significantly improve quantification. Of the spectral analysis techniques tested, the triangular approximation performs better than the trapezoidal approximation, and offers a valuable alternative to the dual-energy window method. The factor analysis of medical image sequences using targeted-apex seeking technique appears to be useful for scatter correction not only for ^{99m}Tc but also for imaging isotopes with more complex spectra.

▶ Correction for scattered radiation remains a major obstacle for improved quantitation in SPECT. Several methods for correcting scattered photons have been reviewed in this YEAR BOOK during the past few years. Being able to compare 9 of these proposed scatter correction methods in one investigation is truly a great help. We get not only an introduction and description of how each correction method works, but also a quantitative measure of the relative error each method contains. If you need a good overview of scatter correction techniques, this is a great manuscript with which to start.

I.G. Zubal, Ph.D.

Effects of Scatter Correction on the Measurement of Infarct Size From SPECT Cardiac Phantom Studies
O'Connor MK, Caiati C, Christian TF, et al (Mayo Clinic, Rochester, Minn; Fondazione Clinica del Lavoro, Cassano Murge, Bari, Italy)
J Nucl Med 36:2080–2086, 1995   13–8

Objective.—Scatter has important negative effects on the quality of thallium-201–labeled and technetium-99m–labeled sestamibi images of the heart. Recently developed gamma cameras have enhanced resolution characteristics as well as hardware and software to perform scatter correction. A series of phantom studies was performed to determine how these advances have affected the quantitation of defect size in tomographic images of the heart.

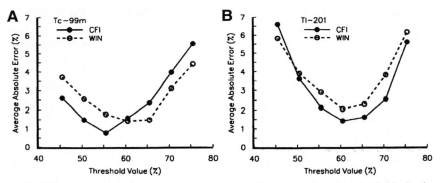

FIGURE 5.—Average absolute error in estimating defect size as a function of the threshold value for scatter corrected (*CFI*) and conventional (*WIN*) image data acquired with (**A**) technetium-99m and (**B**) thallium-201. (Reprinted by permission of the Society of Nuclear Medicine, from O'Connor MK, Caiati C, Christian TF, et al: Effects of scatter correction on the measurement of infarct size from SPECT cardiac phantom studies. *J Nucl Med* 36:2080–2086, 1995.)

Methods.—Both [201]Tl- and ^{99m}Tc-sestamibi images, with and without scatter correction, were obtained from cardiac phantoms with no defects and with defects ranging from 5% to 70% of total myocardial mass. Data acquisition was performed using a newer generation gamma camera with an energy resolution of 8.7% at 140 keV. Circumferential count profiles were generated from 5 representative conventional short-axis slices of the heart. The fraction of radians below a certain threshold value in each of the 5 count profiles was used to compute the defect size. Image contrast was assessed as the nadir value of count profiles in each study.

Results.—Correlation coefficients of greater than 0.99 were obtained with threshold values of 55% to 60% for both ^{201}Tl and [99m]Tc. These values yielded the lowest average absolute error in estimating defect size, i.e., less than 2.1%. With scatter correction, the average absolute error was 1.4% for ^{201}Tl and 0.8% for [99m]Tc (Fig 5). At the same time, nadir values decreased and image quality improved significantly for both isotopes.

Conclusions.—Cardiac phantom studies suggest that scatter correction with newer generation gamma cameras significantly reduces error in measurement of infarct size with both ^{201}Tl and ^{99m}Tc-sestamibi SPECT imaging. Image contrast and image quality are improved as well. The improvements in image quality should reduce differences in quantitative analysis of ^{201}Tl and ^{99m}Tc studies and encourage the use of dual isotope studies and comparison of clinical studies performed at different times.

▶ This article shows the reason that investigators are developing new scatter correction methods like those outlined by Buvat and associates in Abstract 13–7. As shown in Figure 5, the various correction techniques can make up to a few percent difference in evaluating defect size. This can be important for clinical evaluation.

I.G. Zubal, Ph.D.

A Transmission-map-based Scatter Correction Technique for SPECT in Inhomogeneous Media

Welch A, Gullberg GT, Christian PE, et al (Univ of Utah, Salt Lake City; Ohio Imaging of Picker Internatl, Bedford Heights)

Med Phys 22:1627–1635, 1995   13–9

Background.—A significant number of the measured photons undergoing one or more Compton interactions before detection degrade the qualitative and quantitative accuracy of SPECT images. Recent advances in computer hardware technology have made it possible to use iterative methods for reconstructing SPECT data. The compensation for the effects of scattered events may significantly improve reconstructed SPECT images if an accurate model for scatter can be developed and incorporated in the model of the imaging system. A method of modeling the distribution of scattered events in emission projection data for objects with nonuniform attenuation was described.

Transmission-map–based Scatter Correction Technique for SPECT in Inhomogeneous Media.—A transmission map is used to define the inhomogeneous scattering object. Line integrals calculated as part of the attenuation correction method form the basis of the scatter model. The probability of a photon being scattered through a given angle and being detected in the emission energy window was approximated using a Gaussian function. The only free model parameters are the Gaussian parameters, determined by Monte Carlo simulated parallel-beam scatter line spread functions from a nonuniformity attenuating phantom. The broad shape of the scatter line spread functions for a parallel-beam and fan-beam acquisition geometry is reproduced, suggesting that the accuracy of the technique is mainly independent of the acquisition geometry used.

This model was incorporated into a projector-backprojector and used with the expectation-maximization–maximum-likelihood algorithm to reconstruct phantom data. The scatter correction performed well for a phantom that varied slowly in the axial direction. The correction significantly improved the blood pool contrast in a more clinically realistic torso phantom. However, this improvement was not sufficient to restore the contrast to that shown in a reconstruction from scatter-free data.

Conclusions.—Although the scatter correction made possible by the current model may yield some benefits clinically, a 3-dimensional version of the algorithm is needed to realize full benefit. Future research will focus on optimizing the backprojection operation, which may permit extension to 3 dimensions, thus expanding the clinical usefulness of this technique.

▶ Transmission maps are of course obtained to apply improved attenuation corrections. These transmission maps can, however, be used for improved scatter correction methods. Only a small number of investigators are looking into this advanced scatter correction method. However, as computers get faster and memory size gets larger, I believe these methods will make their way into clinical application.

I.G. Zubal, Ph.D.

Single-photon Emission Tomographic Quantification in Spherical Objects: Effects of Object Size and Background
Zito F, Gilardi MC, Magnani P, et al (Univ of Milan, Italy)
Eur J Nucl Med 23:263–271, 1996   13–10

Background.—Because of its anatomical localization abilities and contrast characteristics, single-photon emission tomography (SPET) may be well suited for measurement of volume and radioactivity concentration in organs and lesions. The accuracy of SPET is limited by the attenuation of primary photons; its limited spatial resolution contributes to underestimation of radioactivity in small structures. Kessler et al. have proposed a theoretical model of the effects of spatial resolution on the measurement of radioactivity in small spherical objects. This model, developed for PET, is validated in SPET.

Methods.—The model of Kessler et al. used a gaussian system point-spread function to describe system spatial resolution and considered image counts distribution as a linear system. The model was developed to deal with the partial volume effect, which causes underestimation of the radioactivity concentration in small sources; and spillover from the background, which increases the concentration estimate. A brain-dedicated SPET system with a high-resolution parallel hole collimator was used to acquire tomographic data for the study. Using measurements in experimental phantoms, the model was validated in terms of object size and source/background contrast.

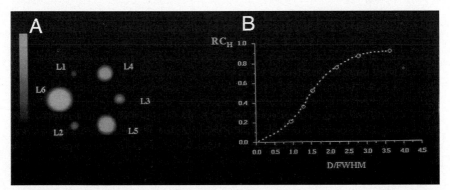

FIGURE 1.—Hot spots in a cold background experiment. **A,** representative single-photon emission tomographic cross-section image showing the apparent decrease in radioactivity concentration as a function of the sphere size, as a result of the partial volume effect. **B,** hot spot recovery coefficient (RC_H) values as a function of sphere diameter (D), normalized to system full width at half maximum. The curve is extrapolated to 0 using a cubic function. (Courtesy of Zito F, Gilardi MC, Magnani P, et al: Single-photon emission tomographic quantification in spherical objects: Effects of object size and background. *Eur J Nucl Med* 23:263–271, 1996. Copyright Springer Verlag.)

Results.—In experiments assessing hot spots on a hot background, the radioactivity concentrations measured by SPET corresponded well to those predicted by the model (Fig 1). On comparison of model-corrected and true radioactivity concentration ratios, the model was accurate within 8.5% across the range of objects assessed, i.e., 9.4 to 36.5 mm. The model appeared to be suitable for clinical use in correcting for partial volume effect in spillover in situations where the anatomical structure of interest is approximately spherical and of known size.

Conclusions.—The accuracy of SPET in measuring radioactivity in anatomical structures depends on the size of the object and the contrast between the lesion and background. This study validates a model to improve the quantitative accuracy of SPET in clinical studies, such as tumor or neuroreceptor studies.

▶ The authors tackle 2 of the most difficult corrections that need to be made for quantitative SPET imaging. As the size of the object changes, the apparent concentration of radiopharmaceutical and level of contamination from the background level vary considerably. Although this is easy to model and to correct using spherical objects, applying this to biological shapes such as the striatum or a tumor still may leave large quantitation errors. Although the authors have done an excellent job in characterizing errors of simple geometry, we should not be complacent that these errors are representative of clinical geometries.

I.G. Zubal, Ph.D.

A 3-D Method for Delineation of Activity Distributions and Assessment of Functional Organ Volumes With SPECT

Wang Y, Jacobsson H, Jacobson SH, et al (Karolinska Inst, Stockholm)
Acta Radiol 36:536–544, 1995   13–11

Background.—Information on an organ's distribution volume is clinically relevant in many situations. Several different techniques have been proposed for use in making volume assessments. A new 3-dimensional technique for delineation of the distribution outline and volume determination was developed.

Methods.—The new technique used SPECT image sets with 3-dimensional operators. Activity distributions were delineated and functional organ volumes evaluated by means of smoothing, differentiation, image relaxation, and voxel counting. The inherent thickness of the voxel-based outline was corrected for by means of a special routine. Phantom experiments were performed using a SPECT system with an LEGP-collimator and a 64 × 64 acquisition matrix with a 6.3- × 6.3-mm² pixel size.

Results.—The phantom studies showed good correlation between the measured volumes and the true volumes. At volumes greater than 120 cc, the experiments showed a correlation coefficient of 0.9999, with a standard error of 1.0 cc and an average relative deviation of 0.49%. Low

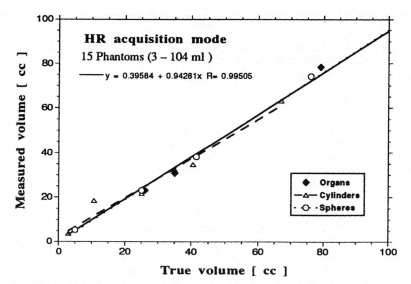

FIGURE 6.—Linear fitting between the measured and the true volumes of 15 phantoms between 3 and 104 cc obtained with high-resolution mode SPECT. Also indicated are the linear fits for the cylinders and the spheres, respectively. (Courtesy of Wang Y, Jacobsson H, Jacobson SH, et al: A 3-D method for delineation of activity distributions and assessment of functional organ volumes with SPECT. *Acta Radiol* 36:536–544, 1995.)

resolution power led to less accuracy at smaller volumes. This problem was addressed by using an LEHR-collimator and a 4.1- × 4.1-mm^2 pixel size. A correlation coefficient of 0.9921, with a standard error of 0.74 cc, was obtained in measurements of 15 phantoms of various shapes and volumes ranging between 3 and 104 cc (Fig 6). At the lowest end of the volume range, the difference between the true and assessed volumes was only 0.6 cc. Reproducibility was within 3% for volumes of greater than 120 cc and within 7% for lesser volumes.

Conclusions.—An accurate 3-dimensional method for delineation of the distribution outline and volume determination in SPECT images is recommended for use in various clinical and research SPECT applications. Volume assessments, especially of small-volume targets, are likely to become increasingly accurate in the near future.

▶ This article follows up on the work described by Zito and colleagues (Abstract 13–10). Here we attempt to determine the volume of a structure. If we rely on SPECT to deliver the total number of counts out of a structure, then, determining the size of the structure, we can solve for the concentration.

I.G. Zubal, Ph.D.

Automated Interstudy Image Registration Technique for SPECT and PET

Eberl S, Kanno I, Fulton RR, et al (Royal Prince Alfred Hosp, Camperdown, Australia; Univ of New South Wales, Sydney, Australia; Research Inst for Brain and Blood Vessels, Akita City, Japan)
J Nucl Med 37:137–145, 1996   13–12

Background.—Precise 3-dimensional registration of data sets is essential when tomographic studies obtained at different times are compared. Previous reports have proposed a number of manual, semiautomated, and fully automated techniques to register reconstructed studies. A fully automated technique for 3-dimensional spatial registration of SPECT and PET studies was developed.

Methods.—The technique was designed to register SPECT-to-SPECT, PET-to-PET, and SPECT-to-PET studies of various organ systems on the basis of functional-anatomical information contained in voxel data. When dealing with a misaligned data set, the algorithm iteratively reslices it until the sum of the absolute differences (SAD) from the reference data set is minimized. Brain and thorax phantom studies were performed to examine registration accuracy. Three different cost functions were compared with the SAD: the stochastic sign change criterion, the sum of products, and the standard deviation of ratios. The technique was also evaluated in clinical neurologic and myocardial perfusion studies, in which accuracy was estimated by the relative locations of landmarks in the reference and registered data sets.

Results.—The brain phantom studies showed registration accuracy of −0.07 for translation, with a maximum error of 1.2 mm, and rotation accuracy of −0.01 degree, with a maximum error of 0.8 degree. Of the cost functions evaluated, the SAD proved the most accurate and reliable. The thoracic phantom studies showed registration errors of 3.1 mm. In the clinical neurologic studies, mean accuracy for 2.0 mm for SPECT-to-SPECT registrations and 1.8 mm for PET-to-SPECT registrations. In the clinical myocardial perfusion studies, registration accuracy averaged 2.1 mm. The algorithm was also useful in other clinical SPECT and PET studies, even studies using tracers with different activity distributions (Fig 8).

Conclusions.—A fully automated technique for 3-dimensional spatial registration of SPECT and PET studies is described. The technique provides accurate registration of both phantom and clinical studies. It permits direct comparison of data sets obtained at different times and by different imaging modalities and can be applied retrospectively. The new algorithm requires minimal operator time and almost completely eliminates the need for data reanalysis.

▶ A currently hot topic is the automated registration of 2 modality images of the same patient. These methods work quite well for rigid structures like the human head, but problems always arise when these registration tech-

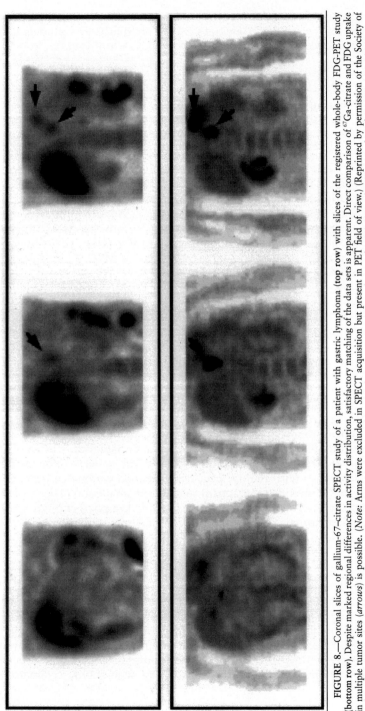

FIGURE 8.—Coronal slices of gallium-67–citrate SPECT study of a patient with gastric lymphoma (top row) with slices of the registered whole-body FDG-PET study (bottom row). Despite marked regional differences in activity distribution, satisfactory matching of the data sets is apparent. Direct comparison of ^{67}Ga-citrate and FDG uptake in multiple tumor sites (*arrows*) is possible. (*Note:* Arms were excluded in SPECT acquisition but present in PET field of view.) (Reprinted by permission of the Society of Nuclear Medicine, from Eberl S, Kanno I, Fulton RR, et al: Automated interstudy image registration technique for SPECT and PET. *J Nucl Med* 37:137–145, 1996.)

niques are applied to the rest of the body. The fact that this method does quite well for registering ^{67}Ga-citrate SPECT with FDG-PET studies is a real tribute to this algorithm.

I.G. Zubal, Ph.D.

SPECT Imaging of Fluorine-18

Leichner PK, Morgan HT, Holdeman KP, et al (Univ of Nebraska, Omaha; Picker Internatl Inc, Bedford Heights, Ohio)
J Nucl Med 36:1472–1475, 1995   13–13

Objective.—There are several uses for metabolic imaging of positron-emitting radiopharmaceuticals. Although SPECT systems are less sensitive and specific than PET scanners in imaging 511-keV photons, SPECT imaging of high-energy photons would have several practical advantages, including increased access to diagnostic studies using positron-emitting radiopharmaceuticals. The clinical potential of SPECT imaging of 511 ke-V annihilation photons was evaluated.

Methods.—The study used the Pricker Prism 3,000, a triple-headed SPECT system for brain and body tomography. Ultrahigh-energy parallel collimators for 511-keV photons were used to image fluorine-18. Measurements of FWHM and FWTM were made in air and for a unit-density scattering medium, and sensitivity measurements were obtained. Image quality was assessed in tomographic phantom studies.

Results.—The 3 cameras were equivalent in their sensitivity. The FWHM was 13 mm and the FWTM 29 mm at a source-to-collimator distance of 100 mm. These figures were similar to those reported for other collimators rated for 511-keV photons. Fluorine-18–filled spheres measuring 20 mm in diameter inside a water-filled phantom were imaged with good resolution. Because of finite resolution capabilities, the sizes of hot lesions were overestimated and those of cold lesions were underestimated.

Conclusions.—With the use of a triple-headed gamma camera, SPECT imaging of ^{18}F provides a practical method of imaging 511-keV photons. The reconstructed slices obtained in this study are good enough for use in some clinical studies. There is only minimal septation of the ultrahigh-energy collimator.

▶ Imaging 511-keV photons with typical nuclear medicine cameras has seen some very exciting developments during the past few years. Building a collimator that stops radiation and that is not perpendicular to the face of the detector requires very thick septa. It is virtually impossible to build a collimator for clinical use that does not leave its structure shadowed onto the image. Filters, as shown here, can remove these artifacts. Admittedly this works well. However, using 2-headed cameras operating in coincidence mode is a strong competitor for heavy, bulky, high-energy collimators. My belief is that operating opposing detectors in coincidence mode is the superior way to image annihilation radiation.

I.G. Zubal, Ph.D.

Influence of High-energy Photons From Cobalt-57 Flood Sources on Scintillation Camera Uniformity Images
Sokole EB, Heckenberg A, Bergmann H (Univ of Amsterdam; Vienna Univ Hosp; Ludwig Boltzmann Inst of Nuclear Medicine, Vienna)
Eur J Nucl Med 23:437–442, 1996   13–14

Background.—System flood-field uniformity checks of scintillation camera performance often involve cobalt-57 flood sources, which are currently available in large sizes and with high activities. However, artifacts occur on uniformity images using new ^{57}Co sources that do not occur on uniformity images from technetium-99m flood sources of the same activity. The images obtained seem to be influenced by the high-energy photons emitted by ^{57}Co and cobalt isotope impurities. How and to what extent the high-energy photons in a ^{57}Co flood source affect uniformity measures were investigated.

Methods and Findings.—Energy spectra and uniformity images of 3 ^{57}Co flood sources of different age were measured on 3 different scintillation cameras. On the flood-field images acquired with the ^{57}Co sources, nonuniformity patterns dependent on the age of the cobalt source, the distance of the course to the collimator, and the specific camera type were observed. These findings were confirmed by quantification of the uniformity images. Energy spectra of a new ^{57}Co source were acquired with an external 1,024-channel analyzer connected to the camera. A broad tail of high-energy photons above the 122-keV photopeak resulted from Compton scatter and collimator penetration. With older sources and increased source to collimator distance, this tail declined, demonstrating that fewer high-energy photons were being measured by the camera system in both situations (Table 3).

Discussion.—Cobalt-57 flood sources, especially the new ones, will produce nonuniformity effects. To minimize problems, the amount of ^{57}Co flood source activity used for quality control should be no greater than 370 MBq, preferably only 180 MBq, although data acquisition time will be prolonged. Also, to establish that there are no artifacts, the uniformity measured using a new cobalt source should be compared with a reference measure, such as that from an old cobalt source, a ^{99m}Tc flood source, or an intrinsic ^{99m}Tc flood image. Placing the cobalt source at about 50 cm from the collimator will reduce the count rate contribution from high-energy photons. The source may need to be stored for some time to permit cobalt isotope impurity decay. Manufacturers should produce ^{57}Co flood sources with no detectable radioactive contaminants.

TABLE 3.—Decay Characteristics and Main Gamma Emissions of Cobalt Isotopes

Nuclide	Half-life (days)	Main gamma emission approximate energy (keV)	Approximate intensities (% of total decay events)
^{57}Co	271	122	87
		136	11
		692	0.16
^{56}C	78.8	511	38
		847	100
		1038	14
		1238	67
		1771	16
		2035	8
		2600	17
		3254	7
^{58}Co	70.8	511	30
		811	100
^{60}Co	1923	1332	100
		1173	100

(Courtesy of Sokole ED, Heckenberg A, Bergmann H: Influence of high-energy photons from cobalt-57 flood sources on scintillation camera uniformity images. *Eur J Nucl Med* 23:437–442, 1996. Copyright Springer-Verlag.)

► So, you thought that a cobalt flood field only contained ^{57}Co? As you can see from Table 3, several isotopes of cobalt are found in most flood sources. This article does a very nice job of describing the artifacts you would expect from these "contaminants."

I.G. Zubal, Ph.D.

Ten Principles and Ten Commandments of Radiation Protection
Strom DJ (Pacific Northwest Natl Lab, Richland, Wash)
Health Phys 70:388–393, 1996   13–15

Background.—For decades the basics of radiation protection have been summarized as "time, distance, and shielding." These 3 principles are probably the most important ones for protection from external radiation sources. However, workers must also protect themselves from intakes of radioactive materials and skin contamination.

Ten Principles of Radiation Protection.—The first principle is *time*: individuals in a radiation field or radioactive atmosphere must hurry, without being hasty, to minimize the exposure or intake time. The second principle is *distance*: individuals must maximize the distance between the source and themselves. The third is *dispersal*: radioactive materials are to be dispersed or diluted, miminizing their concentration. The fourth principle is *source reduction*: the production and use of radiation and radioactive material need to be minimized. The fifth is *source barrier*: sources are shielded to minimize the release of such material. The sixth principle is *personal barrier*: individuals must protect themselves from external radiation fields through the use of personal protective equipment, such as lead aprons, gloves, thyroid shields, and thick glasses. The seventh principle is *decorporation*: after intake or ontake (skin contamination), the uptake of materials must be minimized by maximizing their removal. The eighth is *effect mitigation*, or decreasing the effect of a given individual or collective dose of radioactive materials. The principle of *optimal technology* is that of choosing the best technology to maximize the risk-benefit-cost figure of merit. The final principle is *limitation of others exposures*: individuals should not compound risks by engaging in behaviors such as smoking.

Conclusions.—The basic, time-tested principles of time, distance, and shielding in protection from radiation exposure were expanded to 10. The effective application of these principles relies on knowledge of the radiologic conditions to be managed.

▶ The title of this article is very apt. It very clearly covers the basics. It is an ideal article to photocopy and distribute to junior personnel and staff training within a nuclear medicine department.

I.G. Zubal, Ph.D.

Biodistribution and Dosimetry of Technetium-99m-Hydrazino Nicotinamide IgG: Comparison With Indium-111-DTPA-IgG
Callahan RJ, Barrow SA, Abrams MJ, et al (Massachusetts Gen Hosp, Boston; Harvard Med School, Boston; Johnson Matthey Pharmaceutical Research, West Chester, Pa)
J Nucl Med 37:843–846, 1996   13–16

Background.—Indium-111–labeled human polyclonal IgG is a useful radiopharmaceutical for imaging focal sites of inflammation. The acquisition of high-count density images should enable early lesion detection. Unfortunately, the photon flux of the usual administered ^{111}In-IgG is limited, and the acquisition times needed to record a sufficient count density are long, making it difficult to image the early stage of the inflammatory process. This problem may be solved by the use of a technetium-99m–labeled IgG preparation.

Methods.—The biological behavior of human polyclonal IgG radiolabeled with ^{99m}Tc by a nicotinyl hydrazine derivative (^{99m}Tc-HYNIC-IgG) was assessed in healthy volunteers. Initial biodistribution and dosimetry assessments were done in 6 men. In addition, ^{99m}Tc-IgG and ^{111}In-DTPA-IgG were co-injected into 6 volunteers for scintillation camera images obtained 6 and 18 hours later. Serial blood and urine samples were also collected. Region-of-interest analysis was performed to measure biodistribution of both radiopharmaceuticals. Images were crossover corrected in the dual-injection group.

Findings.—Radiolabeled IgG injections were tolerated with no evident ill effects. The biodistribution of the 2 antibody preparations were very similar. The liver and abdominal activity associated with the ^{111}In preparation was increased. The tissue-to-blood ratios of ^{99m}Tc and ^{111}In-labeled IgG were correlated linearly at both times. The regression line slopes were

TABLE 3.—Radiation Dosimetry of Technetium-HYNIC-IgG and Indium-111-DTPA-IgG in Human Subjects

Organ	rads/mCi	
	^{99m}Tc-HYNIC-IgG	^{111}In-DTPA-IgG*
Lung	0.029	0.649
Liver	0.042	1.42
Spleen	0.045	0.753
GI tract	0.022	0.45
Kidney	0.037	0.727
Muscle	0.018	0.48
Total body	0.019	0.467

* From Macroscint Clinical Imaging Guide, McNeil Pharmaceutical, Springhouse, Pa.
Abbreviation: GI, gastrointestinal.
(Reprinted by permission of the Society of Nuclear Medicine, from Callahan RJ, Barrow SA, Abrams MJ, et al: Biodistribution and dosimetry of technetium-99m-hydrazino nicotinamide IgG: Comparison with indium-111-DTPA-IgG. *J Nucl Med* 37:843–846, 1996.)

0.97 at 6 hours and 0.76 at 18 hours. Compared with ^{111}In-IgG, the beta phase of the blood clearance of ^{99m}Tc-HYNIC-IgG was delayed significantly. The volumes of distribution and urinary excretions did not differ significantly (Table 3).

Conclusions.—The biodistribution properties of ^{99m}Tc-HYNIC-IgG and ^{111}In-DTPA-IgG are almost identical in healthy humans. If these findings are generalizable to patients with focal sites of infection or inflammation, the greater general availability and superior imaging properties of ^{99m}Tc may make it an important agent in clinical imaging.

▶ Table 3 is a good quick reference for estimating the doses received from IgG. An earlier article by Datz et al.[1] contains a similar table, including several additional internal organs.

I.G. Zubal, Ph.D.

Reference

1. Datz FL, Castronovo FP, Christian PE, et al: Biodistribution and dosimetry of indium-111-polyclonal IgG in normal subjects. *J Nucl Med* 36:2372–2379, 1995.

Radiation Dosimetry for Bolus Administration of Oxygen-15-Water
Brihaye C, Depresseux J-C, Comar D (Université de Liège, Belgium)
J Nucl Med 36:651–656, 1995   13–17

Background.—Oxygen-15–labeled water is commonly used to assess regional cerebral blood flow using PET. It has also been proposed for other purposes. Kearfott estimated the absorbed ^{15}O-water doses based on a tracer distribution proportional to the water content of different organs and of the whole body. Kinetic methods are based on a model in which ^{15}O-water distributes as a function of blood flow instead of the volume of

TABLE 4.—Absorbed Dose Estimates for the Adult in μGy/MBq (mRad/mCi)

Organ	Radiation Absorbed Dose	
	Present Study	Kearfott (21)
Brain	0.71 (2.63)	0.16 (0.58)
Breast	1.16 (4.28)	—
GB Wall	1.20 (4.45)	—
Lower large intestine	1.54 (5.68)	0.59 (2.2)
Small intestine	1.05 (3.90)	0.57 (2.1)
Stomach	1.21 (4.46)	0.57 (2.1)
Upper large intestine	1.26 (4.66)	0.57 (2.1)
Heart Wall	0.67 (2.49)	0.57 (2.1)
Kidneys	0.95 (3.52)	0.57 (2.1)
Liver	0.75 (2.76)	0.54 (2.0)
Lungs	0.57 (2.10)	0.54 (2.0)
Muscle	0.15 (0.57)	0.54 (2.0)
Ovaries	1.79 (4.39)	0.57 (2.1)
Pancreas	1.21 (4.48)	0.54 (2.0)
Red marrow	1.49 (5.51)	0.32 (1.2)
Bone surface	1.12 (4.14)	0.21 (0.78)
Skin	1.07 (3.94)	0.57 (2.1)
Spleen	1.19 (4.41)	0.57 (2.1)
Testes	1.11 (4.11)	0.59 (2.2)
Thyroid	1.11 (4.09)	0.51 (1.9)
UB Wall	1.16 (4.31)	0.35 (1.3)
Uterus	1.20 (4.44)	0.51 (1.9)
Total Body	0.42 (1.55)	0.43 (1.6)

(Reprinted by permission of the Society of Nuclear Medicine, from Brihaye C, Depresseux J-C, Comar D: Radiation dosimetry for bolus administration of oxygen-15-water. *J Nucl Med* 36:651–656, 1995.)

water distribution. The Kearfott dose estimates were reevaluated in dynamic conditions, and a new method for more accurately estimating the organ dose values was proposed.

Methods and Findings.—The model included the right heart chambers, lungs, left heart chambers, brain, liver, kidneys, muscles, gastrointestinal tract, and the remainder of the body. Radiation absorbed dose values were estimated. An effective dose equivalent H_E of 1.16 μSv/MBq and an effective dose E of 1.15 μSv/MBq were determined. The cumulated activities in selected organs measured on PET images were similar to the calculated values. Accepting an effective dose of 10 mSv, 8,700 MBq of ^{15}O-water can be administered (Table 4).

Conclusions.—This biokinetic model of the distribution of a bolus of ^{15}O-water is based on its distribution as a blood flow tracer rather than as a volume tracer. The values of effective dose equivalent and effective dose for bolus administration calculated in this model are nearly 3 times more than those published previously.

▶ This table reminds us that we should always be conservative when administering radioactive therapy. The earlier dose estimates presented in this table are much less than those more recently calculated. Using the earlier estimates and allowing patients to receive the maximum permissible dose could have resulted in patients receiving unreasonably high exposures. Perhaps the same diagnostic information could have been achieved with lower activities. The point we are trying to make is that despite the most dedicated efforts, the dose to the patient may be higher than our dosimetrists tell us. Keeping doses "as low as reasonably achievable" is always the best policy.

I.G. Zubal, Ph.D.

Estimated Radiation Dose to the Newborn in FDG-PET Studies
Ruotsalainen U, Suhonen-Polvi H, Eronen E, et al (Turku Univ, Finland; Åbo Akademi Univ, Finland)
J Nucl Med 37:387–393, 1996   13–18

Background.—Few researchers have studied FDG in PET examinations in newborn infants. Thus, the distribution of this tracer in the whole body and the absorbed dose caused by the tracer are unknown. The radiation dose from IV injection of FDG in infants undergoing PET was estimated.

Methods.—Twenty-one infants were studied. Radioactivity concentrations were measured in the brain and bladder. Individual organ masses were estimated according to whole-body and brain masses, and the absorbed dose per unit cumulated activity was calculated.

Findings.—Whole-body distribution of FDG in infants differed from that in adults. A higher proportion of the injected activity accumulated in the brain and less was excreted to urine. The measured cumulated activity was 0.25 MBq • hr/MBq in the brain and 0.04 MBq • hr/MBq in the bladder, the latter showing great individual variation. The calculated absorbed doses were 0.24 mGy/MBq and 1.03 mGy/MBq in the brain and bladder wall, respectively. The effective dose was estimated to be 0.43 mSv/MBq (Table 2).

Conclusions.—The dose to the bladder wall in infants was lower than that in adults. The higher activity remaining in the body may raise doses to other organs. Compared with adults and conventional nuclear medicine studies of infants, the effective dose in the current series was lower.

TABLE 2.—Estimated Absorbed Dose (mGy/MBq) to Selected Organs

Organ	Patient no.																						Avg.	s.d.
	1	2	3	4	5	6	7	8	9	10	11	12	13	14	15	16	17	18	19	20	21	Avg.	s.d.
Adrenals	0.32	0.28	0.26	0.25	0.26	0.23	0.23	0.21	0.21	0.20	0.19	0.20	0.20	0.20	0.19	0.19	0.10	0.17	0.13	0.16	0.13	0.21	0.05
Bladder wall*	0.35	4.30	0.69	0.89	0.29	0.24	0.55	0.77	0.34	0.41	0.26	0.22	0.20	0.50	0.25	0.35	0.29	0.33	9.90	0.30	0.13	1.03	2.10
Brain*	0.27	0.34	0.28	0.30	0.28	0.37	0.24	0.26	0.23	0.28	0.28	0.23	0.21	0.19	0.20	0.20	0.21	0.17	0.17	0.17	0.23	0.24	0.05
Stomach wall	0.32	0.28	0.26	0.25	0.25	0.23	0.23	0.21	0.21	0.20	0.19	0.20	0.19	0.19	0.19	0.19	0.17	0.17	0.13	0.16	0.12	0.21	0.05
Small intestine wall	0.32	0.29	0.26	0.25	0.26	0.23	0.23	0.21	0.21	0.20	0.19	0.20	0.19	0.20	0.19	0.19	0.18	0.17	0.16	0.16	0.12	0.21	0.05
ULI wall	0.32	0.28	0.26	0.25	0.26	0.23	0.23	0.21	0.21	0.20	0.19	0.20	0.19	0.20	0.19	0.19	0.18	0.17	0.15	0.16	0.12	0.21	0.05
LLI wall	0.32	0.28	0.25	0.24	0.25	0.23	0.22	0.21	0.20	0.19	0.19	0.19	0.19	0.19	0.19	0.18	0.17	0.16	0.18	0.15	0.12	0.20	0.04
Heart wall	1.50	1.40	1.20	1.10	1.10	1.10	0.98	0.92	0.88	0.86	0.83	0.81	0.78	0.78	0.76	0.74	0.68	0.63	0.56	0.58	0.43	0.89	0.26
Kidneys	0.83	0.76	0.65	0.64	0.65	0.62	0.56	0.52	0.50	0.49	0.47	0.47	0.45	0.45	0.44	0.43	0.40	0.37	0.32	0.34	0.26	0.51	0.14
Liver	0.66	0.60	0.52	0.51	0.52	0.49	0.45	0.42	0.41	0.40	0.38	0.38	0.37	0.37	0.36	0.35	0.33	0.30	0.27	0.28	0.22	0.41	0.11
Lungs	0.31	0.27	0.25	0.24	0.25	0.22	0.22	0.20	0.20	0.19	0.18	0.19	0.18	0.18	0.18	0.18	0.16	0.16	0.12	0.15	0.11	0.20	0.05
Pancreas	1.30	1.20	1.00	1.00	1.00	0.98	0.87	0.81	0.78	0.76	0.73	0.72	0.69	0.69	0.67	0.65	0.60	0.55	0.50	0.51	0.37	0.78	0.20
Red marrow	0.49	0.44	0.38	0.37	0.38	0.36	0.32	0.30	0.29	0.28	0.27	0.27	0.26	0.26	0.26	0.25	0.23	0.21	0.18	0.20	0.15	0.29	0.08
Spleen	0.35	0.31	0.27	0.27	0.27	0.25	0.24	0.23	0.22	0.21	0.20	0.21	0.20	0.21	0.20	0.20	0.18	0.18	0.14	0.17	0.13	0.22	0.05
Testes	0.50	—	0.39	—	—	0.36	0.33	—	0.30	—	—	—	0.27	0.27	—	—	0.23	0.22	0.26	0.20	0.14	0.29	0.09
Thyroid	0.31	0.27	0.24	0.24	0.24	0.22	0.22	0.20	0.20	0.19	0.18	0.19	0.18	0.18	0.18	0.18	0.17	0.16	0.11	0.15	0.12	0.20	0.05
Remainder of the body	0.30	0.26	0.23	0.23	0.23	0.21	0.20	0.19	0.19	0.18	0.17	0.17	0.17	0.17	0.17	0.16	0.15	0.15	0.12	0.14	0.11	0.19	0.04

* Calculated from measured cumulative activities.
(Reprinted by permission of the Society of Nuclear Medicine, from Ruotsalainen U, Suhonen-Polvi H, Eronen E, et al: Estimated radiation dose to the newborn in FDG-PET studies. *J Nucl Med* 37:387–393, 1996.)

MIRDOSE: Personal Computer Software for Internal Dose Assessment in Nuclear Medicine

Stabin MG (Oak Ridge Inst, Tenn)
J Nucl Med 37:538–546, 1996   13–19

Introduction.—Internal dose estimates are calculated by adding the radiation absorbed in various target tissues from source organs containing radioactive material. This is usually done by the Medical Internal Radiation Dose (MIRD) committee method, which is somewhat tedious and repetitive for routine use. The MIRDOSE computer program was developed to perform these calculations, freeing the analyst to perform other tasks.

Structure.—The program estimates radiation dose per unit of administered activity, based on user-entered source organ residence times for a given radionuclide and one or more phantoms. It includes libraries of radionuclide decay data and specific absorbed fractions for use in developing S values for the specified source and target organs. Estimates of radiation dose are provided in SI and traditional units, with the 2 organs accounting for the first and second highest percentages of total dose. The program output includes all model output and assumptions, and tables of S values for all source and target organs can be provided if desired. The program data libraries, calculational framework, and creation of S-value tables are discussed in detail. The program includes the standard and most up-to-date models used in internal dosimetry, including a gastrointestinal tract model, a dynamic bladder model, a region-specific bone and marrow model, and a module to calculate absorbed dose to small, unit density spheres.

Conclusions.—An overview of the MIRDOSE software program focuses on the differences between program versions 2 and 3. This program greatly simplifies the calculation of internal radiation dose estimates by the MIRD technique. Once the user has entered organ residence time, the program creates radiation dose estimates for all organs, including the effective dose equivalent and effective dose. The standardized radiation dose estimates provided should facilitate the interpretation of dose estimates by users, manufacturers, and regulators.

▶ Gone are the days when you had to look up the S factors in the MIRD pamphlet No. 11 to calculate internal doses for patients. Given a personal computer and a copy of this software, you can easily and accurately carry out these internal dose calculations. The original article gives Michael Stabin's address for more information; you can also e-mail him at: StabinM@orau.gov.

I.G. Zubal, Ph.D.

An Internet-based Nuclear Medicine Teaching File

Wallis JW, Miller MM, Miller TR, et al (Washington Univ, St Louis)
J Nucl Med 36:1520–1527, 1995   13–20

Background.—A network-accessible electronic teaching file has several advantages over a traditional film-based file. Cases are more easily indexed and accessed, are readily available over any distance, cannot be lost from files, and can display dynamic studies. An Internet-based nuclear medicine teaching file, using a Mosaic application for image display and searching, was studied for its suitability.

Description.—A World-Wide-Web server, configured to run on a UNIX work station, is connected to the hospital network and, using a microwave relay, to an Internet gateway on a nearby campus. Access to the teaching file is possible from Apple Macintosh and IBM-PC compatible computers, and from UNIX work stations. Data can be displayed with diagnoses or as unknown cases. Hypertext Markup Language links text to appropriate images and other text pages. Case entry uses a specific form, displayed on the screen, and requires the use of a password. Cases are reviewed by faculty before release onto the network. Direct image transfer to the teaching file from clinical interpretation work stations is possible.

Results.—Access time is generally less than 10 seconds, using Ethernet or Internet. Access using a 14.4K modem requires about 50 seconds. Initial entry of a simple nuclear medicine case requires around 10 minutes. Pre-entry research and text writing can, of course, take much longer. Using image compression, a 300- $\times$ 400-pixel whole-body bone scintigraph can be stored in 56K bytes. A relatively complex case with multiple images fills around 1.25 megabytes.

Conclusion.—This Teaching File-Web application allows ease of access, ease of new case entry, and widespread availability of a collection of nuclear medicine teaching cases.

▶ Where else but in the physics section could we make mention of the role that the Internet is playing in nuclear medicine? Although it's neither "physics" nor "dosimetry," the effect of this "tool" on teaching and information exchange is extremely far reaching. With proper attention paid to confidentiality, the Internet literally connects all computers in all nuclear medicine laboratories to compare and exchange technical and clinical information. The advantage of this is so enormous that mention must be made somewhere.

I.G. Zubal, Ph.D.

Subject Index*

A

Abscess
  brain, discordance between fluorine-18
    fluorodeoxyglucose uptake and
    contrast enhancement in, 95: 74
  intraabdominal, leukocyte vs.
    granulocyte imaging of, and
    ultrasound, 97: 188
  technetium-99m small molecular weight
    complexes in, accumulation of (in
    mice), 96: 105
Absorptiometry
  dual photon, for bone mineral
    measurements with gamma camera,
    95: 158
  x-ray, dual energy
    of body composition, 97: 73
    for bone measurements of lumbar
      spine and femur in women, 97: 74
Acalculous
  cholecystitis, acute, indium-111
    leukocyte positive, normal
    cholescintigraphy in, converse
    photopenic "rim" sign in, 96: 211
Acetate
  carbon-11, in ventricular efficiency
    approach, 96: 350
Acetazolamide
  enhanced technetium-99m HMPAO
    SPECT, of watershed ischemia,
    96: 262
Acetylcholine
  receptors, nicotinic, radioiodination of
    nicotine for mapping of, 97: 354
ACTH
  producing tumor, ectopic,
    technetium-99m sestamibi
    localizing, 96: 176
  secreting bronchial carcinoid,
    somatostatin analogs in, 95: 160
Adenocarcinoma
  advanced, CC49 murine monoclonal
    antibody lutetium-177, 97: 64
  intestine, localization with vasoactive
    intestinal peptide receptor imaging,
    96: 399
  papillary, with thyroid nodule in
    Graves' hyperthyroidism, 97: 127
Adenoma
  hepatocellular, technetium-99m sulfur
    colloid uptake and radiography of,
    97: 201

parathyroid, large, rapid washout of
  technetium-99m MIBI from,
  97: 133
Adenomyosis
  bone scintigraphy of, blood flow and
    blood pool, 95: 249
Adenosine
  SPECT, thallium-201 imaging in
    angiographic evidence of coronary
    artery disease, 96: 329
  technetium-99m sestamibi
    myocardial perfusion SPECT, for
      coronary artery disease detection in
      women, 97: 294
    myocardial tomography in coronary
      artery disease, vs. exercise, 96: 310
    SPECT, of jeopardized myocardium
      after acute myocardial infarction,
      97: 278
    vs. exercise stress thallium-201
      scintigraphy, 96: 309
Adhesion molecule E selectin (see E
  selectin)
Adolescence
  chondroblastoma of patella presenting
    as knee pain during, 97: 333
  spinal disorders during, scintigraphy of,
    95: 136
Adrenal
  masses
    clinically silent, scintigraphic
      evaluation, 96: 174
    incidentally discovered bilateral,
      scintigraphy of, 97: 199
    indeterminate, with cancer, PET
      2-[F-18]-fluoro-2-deoxy-D-glucose,
      96: 175
    solid, differential diagnosis with
      adrenocortical scintigraphy,
      96: 173
Adrenergic
  myocardial derangement, anthracycline
    related, assessment by iodine-123
    metaiodobenzylguanidine
    scintigraphy, 96: 361
  tumors, iodine-131
    metaiodobenzylguanidine for,
    95: xxiv
Adrenocorticotropin (see ACTH)
Adriamycin
  cardiomyopathy, myocardial substrate
    utilization and left ventricular
    function in, 95: 337

---

* All entries refer to the year and page number(s) for data appearing in this and previous
editions of the YEAR BOOK.

Author Index